Advances in Esophageal and Gastric Cancer

Editor

DAVID H. ILSON

SURGICAL ONCOLOGY
CLINICS OF NORTH AMERICA

www.surgonc.theclinics.com

Consulting Editor
NICHOLAS J. PETRELLI

April 2017 • Volume 26 • Number 2

ELSEVIER

1600 John F. Kennedy Boulevard • Suite 1800 • Philadelphia, Pennsylvania, 19103-2899

http://www.theclinics.com

SURGICAL ONCOLOGY CLINICS OF NORTH AMERICA Volume 26, Number 2
April 2017 ISSN 1055-3207, ISBN-13: 978-0-323-52435-3

Editor: John Vassallo (j.vassallo@elsevier.com)
Developmental Editor: Meredith Madeira

Surgical Oncology Clinics of North America (ISSN 1055-3207) is published quarterly by Elsevier Inc., 360 Park Avenue South, New York, NY 10010-1710. Months of publication are January, April, July, and October. Business and Editorial Offices: 1600 John F. Kennedy Blvd., Ste. 1800, Philadelphia, PA 19103-2899. Customer Service Office: 3251 Riverport Lane, Maryland Heights, MO 63043. Periodicals postage paid at New York, NY and additional mailing offices. Subscription prices are $296.00 per year (US individuals), $490.00 (US institutions) $100.00 (US student/resident), $337.00 (Canadian individuals), $620.00 (Canadian institutions), $205.00 (Canadian student/resident), $418.00 (foreign individuals), $620.00 (foreign institutions), and $205.00 (foreign student/resident). Foreign air speed delivery is included in all *Clinics* subscription prices. All prices are subject to change without notice. **POSTMASTER:** Send address changes to *Surgical Oncology Clinics of North America,* Elsevier Health Science Division, Subscription Customer Service, 3251 Riverport Lane, Maryland Heights, MO 63043. **Customer Service: 1-800-654-2452 (US and Canada). 314-447-8871 (outside US and Canada). Fax: 314-447-8029. E-mail:** journalscustomerservice-usa@elsevier.com **(for print support);** journalsonline support-usa@elsevier.com **(for online support).**

Reprints. For copies of 100 or more, of articles in this publication, please contact the Commercial Reprints Department, Elsevier Inc., 360 Park Avenue South, New York, New York 10010-1710. Tel. 212-633-3874; Fax: 212-633-3820; E-mail: reprints@elsevier.com.

Surgical Oncology Clinics of North America is covered in *MEDLINE/PubMed (Index Medicus)* and *EMBASE/ Excerpta Medica, Current Contents/Clinical Medicine, and ISI/BIOMED.*

Contributors

CONSULTING EDITOR

NICHOLAS J. PETRELLI, MD, FACS
Bank of America Endowed Medical Director, Helen F. Graham Cancer Center & Research Institute, Christiana Care Health Systems, Newark, Delaware

EDITOR

DAVID H. ILSON, MD, PhD
Attending Physician, Memorial Sloan Kettering Cancer Center; Professor of Medicine, Weill Cornell Medical College, New York, New York

AUTHORS

ARRHCHANAH BALACHANDRAN, MBBS (Hons)
Department of Gastroenterology and Hepatology, Lyell McEwin Hospital, Elizabeth Vale, South Australia, Australia

ELLIOTT BIRNSTEIN, MD
Division of Gastroenterology and Nutrition Service, Department of Medicine, Memorial Sloan Kettering Cancer Center, New York, New York

MARIA IGNEZ BRAGHIROLI, MD
Advanced Oncology Fellow, Gastrointestinal Oncology Service, Memorial Sloan Kettering Cancer Center, New York, New York

MICHAEL R. CASSIDY, MD
Fellow, Department of Surgery, Memorial Sloan Kettering Cancer Center, New York, New York

DANIEL V.T. CATENACCI, MD
Associate Director, Gastrointestinal Oncology Program, Section of Hematology/Oncology; Assistant Professor of Medicine, University of Chicago Comprehensive Cancer Center, Chicago, Illinois

STEPHEN G. CHUN, MD
Assistant Professor, Department of Radiation Oncology, The University of Texas MD Anderson Cancer Center, Houston, Texas

SEPIDEH GHOLAMI, MD
Fellow, Department of Surgery, Memorial Sloan Kettering Cancer Center, New York, New York

DAVID H. ILSON, MD, PhD
Attending Physician, Memorial Sloan Kettering Cancer Center; Professor of Medicine, Weill Cornell Medical College, New York, New York

YELENA Y. JANJIGIAN, MD
Assistant Attending Physician, Gastrointestinal Oncology Service, Memorial Sloan Kettering Cancer Center; Assistant Professor of Medicine, Weill Cornell Medical College, New York, New York

DOREEN KOAY, MB BCh BAO, MRCP
Department of Gastroenterology and Hepatology, Lyell McEwin Hospital, Elizabeth Vale, South Australia, Australia

GEOFFREY Y. KU, MD
Gastrointestinal Oncology Service, Department of Medicine, Memorial Sloan Kettering Cancer Center, New York, New York

YUKINORI KUROKAWA, MD, PhD
Associate Professor, Department of Gastrointestinal Surgery, Osaka University Graduate School of Medicine, Suita, Osaka Prefecture, Japan

LORI LUTZKE, LPN
Senior Research Coordinator, Barrett's Esophagus Unit, Division of Gastroenterology and Hepatology, Mayo Clinic, Rochester, Minnesota

STEVEN B. MARON, MD
Section of Hematology/Oncology, Fellow, University of Chicago Comprehensive Cancer Center, Chicago, Illinois

BRUCE D. MINSKY, MD
Professor, Department of Radiation Oncology, The University of Texas MD Anderson Cancer Center, Houston, Texas

QURAT-UL-AIN RIZVI, MBBS, FRACP
Gastroenterology Advanced Trainee, Department of Gastroenterology and Hepatology, Lyell McEwin Hospital, Elizabeth Vale, South Australia, Australia

MITSURU SASAKO, MD, PhD
Specially Appointed Professor, Department of Multidisciplinary Surgical Oncology, Hyogo College of Medicine, Nishinomiya, Hyogo Prefecture, Japan

MARK SCHATTNER, MD
Division of Gastroenterology and Nutrition Service, Department of Medicine, Attending Physician, Memorial Sloan Kettering Cancer Center; Professor of Clinical Medicine, Weill Cornell College of Medicine, New York, New York

PRATEEK SHARMA, MD
Division of Gastroenterology and Hepatology, University of Kansas School of Medicine, VA Medical Center, Kansas City, Missouri

RAJVINDER SINGH, MBBS, MPhil, FRACP, AM, FRCP
Department of Gastroenterology and Hepatology, Lyell McEwin Hospital, Elizabeth Vale, South Australia, Australia

HEATH D. SKINNER, MD, PhD
Assistant Professor, Department of Radiation Oncology, The University of Texas MD Anderson Cancer Center, Houston, Texas

VIVIAN E. STRONG, MD
Associate Attending, Gastric and Mixed Tumor Service, Department of Surgery, Memorial Sloan Kettering Cancer Center, New York, New York

KENNETH K. WANG, MD
Russ and Kathy Van Cleve Professor of Gastroenterology Research, Division of Gastroenterology and Hepatology, Mayo Clinic, Rochester, Minnesota

ELIZABETH WON, MD
Assistant Attending, Gastrointestinal Medical Oncology, Memorial Sloan Kettering Cancer Center, West Harrison, New York

LIAM ZAKKO, MD
Fellow in Gastroenterology and Hepatology, Division of Gastroenterology and Hepatology, Mayo Clinic, Rochester, Minnesota

Contents

> Gastric adenocarcinoma, esophageal adenocarcinoma, and esophageal squamous cell carcinoma are among the most prevalent and deadly of malignancies worldwide. Screening and prevention programs will be critical to finally improving outcomes in these diseases. For gastric adenocarcinoma, screening in high-risk populations has significantly reduced mortality. More research is needed on screening high-risk individuals in low-risk populations. For esophageal adenocarcinoma, work is needed to develop efficient and effective techniques in mass screening programs. For most Western populations, current screening is not cost effective. Avoiding environmental risk factors is critical to reducing the incidence of this deadly illness.

> Esophagogastric cancer accounts for the second most common cause of cancer-related mortality worldwide. Significant efforts have been made to detect these malignancies at an earlier stage through the implementation of screening programs in high-risk individuals using advanced diagnostic techniques. Endoscopic management techniques, such as endoscopic mucosal resection and endoscopic submucosal dissection, have consistently demonstrated excellent outcomes in the management of these lesions. These techniques are associated with a lower risk of morbidity and mortality when compared with traditional surgical management.

> Minimally invasive surgical techniques are an emerging option in the staging and management of gastric cancer in the United States and elsewhere. Although much of the current knowledge about these approaches and their outcomes has been generated in Eastern countries, experience in the United States is growing. This article discusses both laparoscopic and robotic approaches to gastric cancer management. Important aspects of patient selection are emphasized. Surgical and oncologic outcomes are presented and compared with traditional open gastrectomy.

Technical considerations are discussed along with comments on the learning curve to achieve proficiency in each approach.

In East Asia, D2 dissection has been routine surgical procedure for curable advanced gastric cancer. More extended surgery than D2 is reserved for borderline resectable disease with extended nodal metastasis. The addition of radiation therapy to adjuvant chemotherapy failed to improve the outcome after D2 dissection. Because many patients are diagnosed in East Asia with early-stage disease, postoperative adjuvant chemotherapy is preferred, and S-1 monotherapy or capecitabine-oxaliplatin is standard care. Neoadjuvant chemotherapy may be preferred for stage III tumors; for borderline resectable tumors, preoperative chemotherapy is under study given the limitations of postoperative adjuvant chemotherapy in high-risk patients.

Staging of locally advanced gastric cancer includes imaging with computed tomography scan and laparoscopic assessment to rule out peritoneal disease or positive peritoneal washings. Preoperative and postoperative chemotherapy improves survival compared with surgery alone. After primary D2 resection, adjuvant chemotherapy with a fluorinated pyrimidine with or without a platinum agent improves survival. Inclusion of postoperative radiation therapy appears required in combination with chemotherapy in patients with less than a D1-D2 resection. Potential lower rates of R0 resection with preoperative chemotherapy alone in tumors of the gastroesophageal junction argue that combined preoperative chemotherapy and radiotherapy is required.

This review summarizes established adjuvant approaches for locally advanced esophageal cancer (including preoperative, perioperative, or postoperative approaches, which include chemotherapy alone or chemoradiation). It also discusses areas of uncertainty and therapeutic equipoise.

The treatment of locally advanced esophageal cancer is controversial. For patients who are candidates for surgical resection, multiple prospective clinical trials have demonstrated the advantages of neoadjuvant chemoradiation. For patients who are medically inoperable, definitive chemoradiation is an alternative approach with survival rates comparable to trimodality therapy. Although trials of dose escalation are ongoing, the standard radiation dose remains 50.4 Gy. Modern radiotherapy techniques such as image-guided radiation therapy with motion management and intensity-modulated radiation therapy are strongly encouraged with a planning objective to maximize conformity to the intended target volume while reducing dose delivered to uninvolved normal tissues.

This review summarizes completed and ongoing studies evaluating the activity of immune checkpoint inhibitors in esophagogastric cancer.

Gastroesophageal cancer (GEC) remains a major cause of cancer-related mortality worldwide. Although the incidence of distal gastric adenocarcinoma (GC) is declining in the United States, proximal esophagogastric junction adenocarcinoma (EGJ) is increasing in incidence. GEC, including GC and EGJ, is treated uniformly in the metastatic setting. Overall survival in the metastatic setting remains poor. Molecular characterization of GEC has identified mutations and copy number variations, along with other oncogenes, biomarkers, and immuno-oncologic checkpoints that may serve as actionable therapeutic targets. This article reviews these key aberrations, their impact on protein expression, therapeutic implications, and clinical directions within each pathway.

Esophagogastric cancer is a worldwide health problem. The addition of the epidermal growth factor receptor 2 (HER2)-directed antibody trastuzumab to chemotherapy increased the overall survival of patients with metastatic HER2-positive esophagogastric cancer. This article discusses the available data to support HER2 as validated biomarker and recently completed and ongoing clinical trials of HER2-directed agents in metastatic and localized disease. Also reviewed is the mechanisms of resistance for HER2-directed therapy and ongoing research strategies including new imaging techniques and studies with patient-derived xenografts.

Esophageal and gastric cancers are common malignancies, both in the United States and worldwide, that carry significant morbidity and mortality. Malnutrition is a common complication in patients with esophageal and gastric cancers and it portends a poor prognosis. For patients who undergo surgical therapy for these types of cancers, preoperative and postoperative nutritional optimization have been shown to improve outcomes. The support can be accomplished in different manners, including orally, enterally, or parentally. In patients who do not undergo surgery but receive chemotherapy and/or radiation, nutritional support is also an important aspect of the multidisciplinary care approach.

Esophagogastric cancers predominantly affect older adults; however, older patients are less likely to be recommended for both curative and palliative treatment. Older patients have unique challenges that need to be addressed during their oncologic care. Tools such as complete geriatric assessments may help to better identify fit older adults and stratify patients for aggressive treatment strategies. This review evaluates the current knowledge and the remaining challenges in optimally managing elderly patients with esophagogastric cancers.

SURGICAL ONCOLOGY
CLINICS OF NORTH AMERICA

THE CLINICS ARE AVAILABLE ONLINE!
Access your subscription at:
www.theclinics.com

Foreword

Gastric and Esophageal Cancer 2017

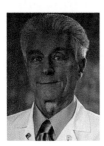

Nicholas J. Petrelli, MD, FACS
Consulting Editor

This issue of the *Surgical Oncology Clinics of North America* discusses esophageal and gastric cancer. The guest editor is David H. Ilson, MD, PhD. Dr Ilson is an attending physician and member of Memorial Sloan Kettering Cancer Center and Professor of Medicine at Weill Cornell Medical College. Dr Ilson is recognized nationally for his special interest and expertise in treating patients who have upper gastrointestinal cancers, particularly those with esophageal and gastric cancer. His research focus is in esophageal and gastric cancer, studying new agents to treat advanced disease and evaluating novel agents in combined modality therapy to treat locally advanced disease. Dr Ilson is a member of the GI Committees of the National Clinical Research Groups, such as the Cancer and Leukemia Group B and the Radiation Therapy Oncology Group. He is also a member of the Upper GI Cancer Guidelines Committee of the National Comprehensive Cancer Network and Senior Committee Member of the Intergroup Esophageal and Gastric Cancer Task Force Committee.

Dr Ilson has invited an outstanding group of experts in the diagnosis and treatment of esophageal and gastric cancer. This group has included an article on novel targeted therapies for esophagogastric cancer by Drs Maron and Catenacci from the Section of Hematology/Oncology at the University of Chicago Comprehensive Cancer Center. Contributions by international colleagues include the article entitled, "The Asian Perspective on the Surgical and Adjuvant Management of Esophagogastric Cancer," by Drs Kurokawa and Sasako from Japan. Last, the emerging role in gastric cancer for minimally invasive surgery is discussed by Drs Cassidy, Gholami, and Strong from the Department of Surgery at Memorial Sloan Kettering Cancer Center.

I would like to thank Dr Ilson for organizing this outstanding group of authors on the subject of esophageal and gastric cancer. This extensive issue of the *Surgical*

Surg Oncol Clin N Am 26 (2017) xiii–xiv
http://dx.doi.org/10.1016/j.soc.2016.11.001
1055-3207/17/© 2016 Published by Elsevier Inc.

surgonc.theclinics.com

Oncology Clinics of North America should be shared with young investigators, and radiation, medical, and surgical residents in training.

Nicholas J. Petrelli, MD, FACS
Helen F. Graham Cancer Center & Research Institute
Christiana Care Health Systems
4701 Ogletown-Stanton Road, Suite 1233
Newark, DE 19713, USA

E-mail address:
npetrelli@christianacare.org

Preface

Updates in Esophagogastric Cancer

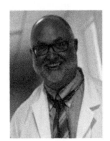

David H. Ilson, MD, PhD
Editor

Taken together, esophageal and gastric cancers are the second leading cause of cancer mortality globally, with a particularly high toll in countries of East Asia. Modest advances have been made in the past decade, with an emerging global consensus about the staging of gastroesophageal (GE) cancer, the optimal surgical approach, the utilization of adjuvant therapy, the management of advanced disease, and the application of endoscopic therapies. This issue of *Surgical Oncology Clinics of North America* is dedicated to an update of the management of esophagogastric cancer from the perspective of the gastroenterologist, surgeon, radiation therapist, and medical oncologist.

The staging and surgical management from both an Eastern and a Western perspective are discussed by Drs Sasako and Strong. An emphasis on adequate surgical staging, including laparoscopy, and the underscoring of the need for consistent and high surgical quality with adoption globally of D2 gastrectomy are made by both authors. The advent of minimally invasive surgery as an acceptable surgical alternative is also reviewed. Drs Sasako, Ilson, and Ku discuss improvement in survival with the use of adjuvant therapy. In Asia, the use of adjuvant chemotherapy after D2 gastrectomy has been proven to be beneficial, with ongoing trials of preoperative therapy in high-risk patients. In the West, perioperative chemotherapy added to surgery has been validated and adopted as standard practice. The need for the addition of adjuvant radiation therapy appears to be dictated by the adequacy of surgical resection performed, with postoperative radiation therapy appearing to benefit patients undergoing less than D1 surgical resection. For cancers of the distal esophageal and GE junction, the combination of preoperative chemotherapy and radiation therapy appears required to achieve negative margin resection and reduce the risk of local tumor recurrence. Drs Chun, Skinner, and Minsky review the role of radiation therapy–based management in cancers of the esophagus and GE junction.

Surg Oncol Clin N Am 26 (2017) xv–xvi
http://dx.doi.org/10.1016/j.soc.2017.01.001
1055-3207/17/© 2017 Published by Elsevier Inc.

surgonc.theclinics.com

Drs Janjigian, Catenacci, and Ku review emerging data for targeted agents and immunotherapy, including therapies targeting HER2 and novel pathways such as the MET and FGF receptors. Drs Wang and Sharma review the role of screening and endoscopic management of precancerous and early esophagogastric cancers. Dr Schattner reviews the importance and contribution of nutritional support as part of multidisciplinary management. Last, given that esophagogastric cancer is largely a disease of the elderly, Dr Won provides perspective on the incorporation of geriatric assessment and age-appropriate variations into treatment paradigms of these diseases.

It is clear from the reviews contained in this issue of *Surgical Oncology Clinics of North America* that the use of a multispecialty team to manage cancers of the esophagus, GE junction, and stomach is required to ensure delivery of state-of-the-art medical care.

David H. Ilson, MD, PhD
Memorial Sloan Kettering Cancer Center
Weill Cornell Medical College
300 East 66th Street, BAIC 1031
New York, NY 10065, USA

E-mail address:
ilsond@mskcc.org

Screening and Preventive Strategies in Esophagogastric Cancer

Liam Zakko, MD[a], Lori Lutzke, LPN[b], Kenneth K. Wang, MD[a],*

KEYWORDS

- Screening • Prevention • Gastric adenocarcinoma • Barrett esophagus
- Esophageal adenocarcinoma • Esophageal squamous cell carcinoma

KEY POINTS

- Gastric adenocarcinoma, esophageal adenocarcinoma, and esophageal squamous cell carcinoma are among the most prevalent and deadly of malignancies.
- Screening in high-risk populations has significantly reduced the mortality of gastric adenocarcinoma; however, screening efficacy for high-risk individuals within low-risk populations is unclear.
- Although esophageal adenocarcinoma has a clear precursor lesion (Barrett esophagus), clearly effective screening techniques and programs are still being developed.
- Screening for esophageal squamous cell carcinoma is not cost-effective; however, avoidance of environmental risk factors (smoking, alcohol abuse) can prevent the disease.

INTRODUCTION

Gastric and esophageal cancers are among the most common tumors that cause significant mortality worldwide, although their incidence is much higher in specific geographic locations. Unfortunately, although new treatment protocols have improved the outcome of most major malignancies, prognosis in gastric and esophageal cancer remains poor. Screening and prevention programs offer the hope of reducing morbidity and mortality from these diseases.

Disclosure Statement: Dr K.K. Wang discloses research support from Nine Point Medical, C2 Therapeutic, CSA Medical, Boston Scientific, and Fujinon. Funding support provided by National Cancer Institute, U01 CA182940 and U54 CA163004. Drs L. Zakko and L. Lutzke have nothing to disclose.
[a] Division of Gastroenterology and Hepatology, Mayo Clinic, 200 2nd St. SW, Rochester, MN 55905, USA; [b] Barrett's Esophagus Unit, Division of Gastroenterology and Hepatology, Mayo Clinic, 200 First Street Northwest, Rochester, MN, USA
* Corresponding author.
E-mail address: wang.kenneth@mayo.edu

GASTRIC CANCER

Gastric cancer is among the most common cancers in the world with more than 900,000 cases in 2012, making it the fifth most common cancer in the world.[1,2] The incidence of gastric cancer, however, is much higher in the developing world, particularly in East Asia where more than 50% of cases occur.[3] Although screening programs have been developed in Asian countries, particularly Japan and Korea, significantly improving outcomes through early detection,[4–6] mortality rates in the West have remained high.[7,8]

Risk Factors

There are numerous risk factors for developing gastric cancer. These risks can be broken down into modifiable and nonmodifiable (Table 1).

Nonmodifiable risk factors

Race and ethnicity are nonmodifiable risk factors for gastric cancer. Although environmental factors likely play a role, they alone cannot explain the high incidence of disease in East Asia; particularly because this increased incidence persists in immigrants and their offspring from East Asia to the West.[9,10] Age is also important, with more than 90% of cases occurring after the age of 45 years.[8] Family history also contributes to risk, with studies from both the West and East showing a first-degree relative with gastric cancer increases a person's risk 2- to 4-fold.[11–13] Gender also plays a role, with men having a 2- to 5-fold increased risk of gastric cancer.[14] Higher estrogen levels seem to protect women from the disease. Increased rates of gastric cancer in women on estrogen-blocking therapies (tamoxifen) and after menopause demonstrate this effect.[15,16] In fact, women seem to develop gastric cancer at a similar rate to men but with a 10 to 15 year lag.[17]

Although gastric cancer is usually sporadic, about 10% of cases seem linked to genetic syndromes.[18] The most common syndrome is hereditary diffuse gastric cancer (HDGC), recently defined by the International Gastric Cancer Linkage Consortium.[19] HDGC is characterized by autosomal dominant inheritance, with about a 60% to 80% increase in the risk of gastric cancer and a 40% to 50% increase in breast cancer. About 40% of HDGC is due to mutations in E-cadherin (CDH1). Mutations in CTNNA1 have also recently been found in a subset of patients with the condition.[18] Other cancer syndromes have been associated with increased risk of gastric cancer, including Lynch syndrome (DNA mismatch repair gene mutation), familial adenomatous polyposis (APC gene mutation), Peutz-Jeghers syndrome (STK11 gene mutation), juvenile-polyposis syndrome (SMAD4 or BMPR1A mutation), hereditary breast and ovarian cancer syndrome (BRCA 1 or BRCA 2 mutation), and Li-Fraumeni syndrome (p53 mutation). However, gastric cancer still remains very uncommon in these syndromes, with rates of occurrence less than 5%.[20]

Table 1
Risk factors for developing gastric cancer

Nonmodifiable Risk Factors	Modifiable Risk Factors
Race or ethnicity (East Asian or Pacific Islander)	H pylori infection
Age (>45 y)	Tobacco smoking
Family history	Obesity (body mass index >30)
Sex (Male) Genetics	High salt diet
	Low fruit or vegetable diet

Modifiable risk factors

The most clear modifiable risk factor for gastric cancer is *Helicobacter pylori* infection. Although gastric cancer develops in only about 1% of infected humans, more than 90% of those with gastric cancer have been infected with *H pylori*.[8] Other modifiable risk factors are less influential. Cigarette use seems to increase the risk of both cardia and noncardia cancer.[21] Obesity (body mass index [BMI] >30) seems to increase the risk of noncardia cancer.[22] A high salt diet also seems to increase the risk, whereas diets high in fruit and vegetables seem to be protective.[23,24]

Precursor Lesions

Chronic gastritis seems to lead to atrophic gastritis, which leads to intestinal metaplasia, which can develop into dysplasia and, ultimately, cancer.[25] Within 5 years of diagnosis, the annual incidence of gastric cancer was 0.1% for patients with atrophic gastritis, 0.25% for intestinal metaplasia, 0.6% for mild-to-moderate dysplasia, and 6% for severe dysplasia.[26] The progression from intestinal metaplasia to gastric cancer also greatly depends on the histologic subtype of intestinal metaplasia. Complete intestinal metaplasia (characterized by normal-appearing goblet cells and crypts) is much less likely to progress to gastric cancer than incomplete intestinal metaplasia (characterized by tortuous crypts and elongated columnar cells).[8]

Screening Techniques for Gastric Cancer

Serology screening

H pylori serology is the least invasive test for gastric cancer but is limited by a very low sensitivity and an inability to detect premalignant lesions.[27] Furthermore, the test may become negative as gastric atrophy progresses, causing false-negative results in those most at risk for the condition.[8]

Alternatively, pepsinogen testing has been studied as part of mass screening protocols. A precursor to pepsin, pepsinogen comes in subtypes I and II. Subtype I is secreted from the chief stomach cells. Subtype II is secreted from all gastric cells. Reductions in levels of subtype I and in the ratio of subtype I and II suggest increasing gastric atrophy. A subtype I cutoff of less than 70 ng/L and pepsinogen I to II ratio less than 3.0 were 77% sensitive and 73% specific for gastric cancer.[28] A case control study also demonstrated a reduction in odds ratio (OR) of death from gastric cancer at 1 and 2 years in subjects screened with pepsinogen levels.[29] However, the test was not found to be effective enough for it to be adopted into currently implemented mass screening programs.[8]

Gastric imaging

Although a barium upper gastrointestinal series only has a sensitivity of 60% to 80%,[30] 2 case control studies from Japan showed a 40% to 60% decline in gastric cancer mortality.[31,32] As such, barium imaging remains part of the mass screening programs of both Korea and Japan.

Endoscopy is the gold standard for gastric cancer screening because it has the highest detection rate (sensitivity of 78%–84%) and allows for biopsies to confirm the diagnosis.[33,34] In areas of high incidence, endoscopy is the mainstay of screening. In countries such as the United States, where gastric cancer is less prevalent and the cost of endoscopy is higher, endoscopic screening is unlikely to be cost-effective.[8]

Studies suggest that narrow-band imaging and digital-based image enhancement technologies, such as computed virtual chromoendoscopy, increase the diagnostic yield and accuracy of gastric neoplasia detection.[8] However, imaging criteria are inconsistent and validation studies have yet to be performed.[8] These techniques cannot be recommended currently.

Current Screening Guidelines

Countries with a high incidence of disease (eg, Japan and Korea) have implemented mass screening programs. Screening starts at age 40 to 50 years with upper gastro-intestinal series or endoscopy every 2 to 3 years.[8] Under these protocols, two-thirds of gastric cancers cases detected are in an early stage, leading to an increased 5-year survival rate.[35,36]

Mass screening programs are thought to be cost-ineffective in low-prevalence populations. However, a cost analysis of performing esophagogastroduodenoscopy at the time of screening colonoscopy in the United States found a cost-effectiveness ratio of $95,559 per quality-adjusted life year saved, less than the $100,000 cutoff for cost-effective screening.[37] Others have noted that a targeted approach to high-risk individuals would be even more cost-effective.[8] Yeh and colleagues[38] recently suggested that serum pepsinogen screening in smokers had a cost-effectiveness ratio of $76,000 per quality-adjusted life year saved.

The American Society of Gastrointestinal Endoscopy (ASGE) 2015 guideline suggests screening for those with known gastric intestinal metaplasia and an increased risk due to ethnic background or family history. With minimal data on screening in the West, the ASGE guidelines offer no guidance on follow-up interval.[39] European guidelines suggest surveillance at 1 to 2 year intervals for all patients with intestinal metaplasia who have greater than 20% metaplasia, incomplete intestinal metaplasia, a first-degree relative with gastric cancer, or are actively smoking. Otherwise, a 3-year interval follow-up is recommended.[40] However, it is noteworthy that Eastern Europe, the Iberian Peninsula, and Italy have higher incidences of gastric cancer.[41]

Prevention

Currently, prevention requires adjusting modifiable risk factors. For instance, H pylori elimination in those with gastric atrophy can lead to normalization of stomach mucosa, significantly reducing risk.[42] Improving lifestyle by reducing obesity, promoting smoking cessation, and increasing fruit and vegetable consumption may also decrease the incidence of gastric cancer, though the evidence for such prevention is less clear.

A recent large cohort study by Cao and colleagues[43] that looked at aspirin as a chemopreventive agent did show a preventative association between gastrointestinal cancer and aspirin use, with a relative risk of 0.85 after multivariate analysis. Although most of this reduction was due to colorectal cancer, in women a relative risk of 0.71 (CI 0.52–0.98) was noted between aspirin use and gastroesophageal cancer on multivariate analysis. Men, however, had a relative risk of 0.94 (CI 0.74–1.21). Whether this represents a true association between aspirin use and reduced gastroesophageal cancer in women requires further study. Furthermore, given the low rates of gastroesophageal cancer, it is unclear whether the benefit of using aspirin solely for cancer prevention would outweigh the risk of adverse events.

ESOPHAGEAL ADENOCARCINOMA

Esophageal adenocarcinoma is the dominant form of esophageal cancer in the developed world. Its incidence has increased 6-fold in the last 40 years but it continues to have a dismal prognosis with mortality rates that almost equal its incidence rates.[44] In fact, nearly half of patients diagnosed are unable to undergo treatment beyond palliative care.[45] However, outcomes with early-stage cancers are much better, particularly with new endoscopic treatment techniques.[46] As such, screening to allow early detection and preventative treatment is recommended.

Risk Factors

Chronic inflammation of the esophagus develops due to gastroesophageal reflux disease (GERD) or other irritants. From this inflammation, intestinal metaplasia can occur in the distal esophagus, termed Barrett esophagus (BE). Continued irritation will lead to low-grade dysplasia, which will progress to high-grade dysplasia and then to adenocarcinoma. Furthermore, a recent study has begun to show genetic lineage between patients with GERD, BE, and esophageal adenocarcinoma (EAC).[47]

Clinical risk factors for Barrett esophagus progression

Although GERD is the strongest risk factor, 15% to 45% of BE develops in patients with no symptoms of GERD. Furthermore, although GERD occurs in 15% to 20% of the Western population, only 10% to 15% of those patients have BE.[48] Although BE is clearly a precursor, it only progresses to EAC at a rate of 0.12% to 0.60% per year.[49] As such, other risk factors are looked for to determine who should be screened for BE (Box 1).

Men with BE develop EAC at more than twice the yearly rate of women, 0.28% to 0.13%, respectively.[50] Other clinical factors include increasing age, central obesity, and active smoking; essentially the same as risk factors for developing BE.[51]

Endoscopic risk factors for Barrett esophagus progression

Evidence of esophagitis or anatomic risk factors for worse reflux (ie, hiatal hernia) has been associated with increased progression from BE to EAC. Furthermore, most investigations into BE segment length suggest the increasing area of disease increases the risk for EAC. Finally, mucosal nodularity, ulcers, and strictures noted on endoscopy have been associated with increased risk of EAC. However, these probably indicate present high-grade dysplasia or EAC instead of risk of future development.

Histologic risk factors for Barrett esophagus progression

Rates of progression increase to about 1% per year for patients with BE that includes low-grade dysplasia and about 7% per year for patients with BE that includes high-grade dysplasia.[52] The use of histology, however, is limited. First, biopsies of BE may miss dysplastic areas, leading to sampling error. Second, interpathologist and intrapathologist agreement in rating dysplasia is poor, leading to interpretative error.[50]

Biomarkers are being developed to improve the accuracy of histologic assessment of BE. P53, a tumor suppression gene, is the most promising and immunostaining is

---

Box 1
Risk factors for developing Barrett esophagus

GERD[50]

Male sex[51]

Increasing age[89]

Central adiposity (visceral adipose tissue area, increased waist-to-hip ratio, or waist or abdominal circumference)[90]

Family history of dysplastic BE or EAC[91]

Smoking[92]

currently recommended by the British Society of Gastroenterology guidelines.[53] Reid and colleagues[54] have promoted the use of aneuploidy and tetraploidy, evidence of genetic instability, as a marker of potential tumor progression. Kastelein and colleagues[55] demonstrated that both p53 overexpression (adjusted relative risk 5.6, 95% CI 3.1–10.3) and p53 loss of expression (adjusted relative risk 14.0, 95% CI 5.3–37.2) were associated with an increased risk of developing high-grade dysplasia or EAC. Other complex combinations of tumor markers are in development but require significant testing before they can be clinically used.

Screening Techniques

Screening can be broken down into (1) techniques to identify those in the population with BE and (2) techniques to identify those in the population with BE most likely to develop EAC, so they can undergo intensive surveillance and treatment.

Identifying Barrett Esophagus

Direct visualization

There are obvious benefits to endoscopic screening, such as direct visualization and the ability to take biopsies for histologic analysis. However, there are also significant limitations, such as that the physical process of the technique is unappealing to patients, it requires an endoscopy suite, and the side effects of sedation. Cost is another limitation, directly because of the need for staffing, equipment, and so forth; and indirectly due to the patients' time off work and decreased productivity.[50]

Capsule endoscopy is a noninvasive way to detect BE. However, the technique has low sensitivity, requires endoscopy to confirm diagnosis and obtain biopsies, and is not cost-effective compared with standard endoscopy.[56] Recently, a tethered capsule endomicroscope, which uses optical frequency domain imaging to provide cross-sectional architectural images of esophageal mucosa, allows identification of BE and dysplasia. Although this is reusable (overcoming some cost-effectiveness issues of capsule endoscopy), its accuracy is unproven and it is unclear patients would find swallowing a tethered pill more appetizing than a sedated endoscopic procedure.[57]

Instead of standard endoscopy, ultrathin transnasal endoscopy (TNE) offers an endoscopy approach that avoids issues with sedation and can be performed outside an endoscopic suite. The procedure does seem to be effective. A meta-analysis of 5 studies (439 subjects) comparing TNE with standard endoscopy in the same subjects showed the pooled sensitivity and specificity of TNE in detecting BE was 91% and 96%, respectively.[58] However, even when a mobile unit brought TNE to patients' neighborhoods, only 48% were willing to undergo the procedure.[59] Furthermore, the technique has not gained widespread acceptance among physicians.[60]

Tissue sampling

Cytosponge is an abrasive sponge encapsulated in gelatin to form a pill attached to a tether. The patient swallows it, the gelatin capsule dissolves, and the sponge is pulled back up through the esophagus, capturing mucosa for analysis. The cytosponge does have good sensitivity and specificity at 73.3% and 93.8%, respectively, with a BE segment with circumferential length greater than or equal to 1 cm; and 90.0% and 93.5%, respectively, with a BE segment with circumferential length greater than 2 cm.[61] Furthermore, cost-effectiveness analysis demonstrated benefit in men older than 50 years with GERD, with a potential reduction of EAC by 19%.[62] However, patient tolerability still seems to be an issue; only 18% of subjects offered the test were willing to proceed in the initial studies.[58]

Unfortunately, tests with blood, urine, or stool to detect those at risk for EAC have not been developed. A promising noninvasive test, however, involves electronic nose technology, in which a device uses reactable compounds to detect different volatile organic compounds in breath samples. In a study of 85 subjects undergoing surveillance for dysplastic BE (43 with biopsy proven active BE and 42 without), the test had 86% specificity and 90% sensitivity. More encouraging, the test had 98% acceptance rate in recruitment.[63] This technology could represent an acceptable, easily used, cost-effective mechanism to screen large populations for BE or EAC.

Identifying Dysplastic Barrett Esophagus

Customarily, random biopsies (taken in 4 quadrants around the circumference of the esophagus) along the BE segment are obtained to try and identify dysplasia. As previously noted, however, this is limited by sampling and interpretative errors. To improve the efficiency of sampling, electronic high-resolution chromoendoscopy (usually narrow band imaging) has been used to obtain better, more detailed, imaging of the vasculature and mucosa. Although randomized controlled trails did not show an increased diagnostic yield for high-grade dysplasia or adenocarcinoma, a meta-analysis of 843 subjects in 14 studies demonstrated an increased diagnostic yield of 34% (95% CI 20%–56%, $P<.0001$) compared with standard endoscopy.[64]

In-procedure histology-level imaging through probe-based confocal endomicroscopy (pCLE) has been shown to enhance detection of BE-associated dysplasia compared with standard endoscopy.[65] pCLE is limited, however, because it has a very limited field of view, requires administration of intravenous fluorescent agents, and needs endoscopists to make a histologic diagnosis. Research in topical fluorescent agents to allow for simplified pCLE is ongoing.

Another optical technique is volumetric laser endomicroscopy (VLE), which uses a frequency domain optical coherence tomography device that can generate wide-field cross-sectional views of the entire distal portion (6 cm) of the human esophagus. The benefits of VLE are that it allows for comprehensive assessment of a significant length of esophageal mucosa and submucosa. However, VLE can effectively distinguish normal squamous epithelium from BE only when highly trained pathologists use specific scoring systems.[66,67] This has prevented widespread application of the technology.

Current Screening Guidelines

No major society recommends general population screening for BE or EAC. Screening is recommended by the American Gastroenterology Association, the British Society of Gastroenterology, the ASGE, and the American College of Gastroenterology for certain high-risk groups (Box 2). If BE is found, then 4 biopsies every 2 cm (for at least 8 biopsies) should be obtained to assess for dysplasia. If Los Angeles grade B, C, or D esophagitis is found, then repeat screening in 8 to 12 weeks after twice a day proton pump inhibitor treatment is recommended to ensure there is no underlying BE. Otherwise, if no BE is found, then repeat screening endoscopy is not recommended.[68]

If no dysplastic BE is found, guidelines still suggest endoscopic screening every 3 to 5 years with 4-quadrant biopsies every 2 cm is reasonable.[68] For patients with indeterminate dysplasia, 2 expert pathologists should confirm the diagnosis. Repeat endoscopy with biopsy samples should be obtained in 3 to 6 months. If dysplasia persists, then endoscopic surveillance yearly with 4-quadrant biopsies every 1 cm is recommended.[68]

Once low-grade dysplasia is found, endoscopic treatment can be considered. Otherwise, yearly endoscopic surveillance with 4-quadrant biopsies every 1 cm

---

Box 2
High-risk groups recommended to undergo Barrett esophagus screening

1 of:
1. Men with >5 y GERD
2. Men with > weekly GERD symptoms (heartburn or acid regurgitation)

And

2 of:
1. Age >50
2. Central obesity (waist circumference >102 cm or waist-to-hip ratio >0.9)
3. White race
4. Active or history of smoking
5. First-degree relative with BE or EAC

Data from Qumseya BJ, Wang H, Badie N, et al. Advanced imaging technologies increase detection of dysplasia and neoplasia in patients with Barrett's esophagus: a meta-analysis and systematic review. Clin Gastroenterol Hepatol 2013;11(12):1562–70.e1-2.

---

should be pursued. If high-grade dysplasia is found and confirmed by 2 expert pathologists, then endoscopic or surgical treatment should be pursued.[68]

Even with these complex screening guidelines, 90% of individuals diagnosed with BE will die from an unrelated condition. Worse, 93% of EA cases are not detected by current screening algorithms, presenting at an advanced stage.[54] To try and further improve efficiency of BE screening, risk predication models have been developed (Table 2).

Prevention

Control of clinical risk factors is the first step in prevention of EAC. Therefore, smoking cessation and prevention or treatment of obesity are important interventions. Treatment of GERD is also important because reduction of the irritating effects of stomach

Table 2
Risk predictor models for presence of Barrett esophagus

Model	Variables	Area Under the Receiver Operating Characteristic Curve (AUROC)
Thrift Clinical Model[93]	Age, sex, smoking status, BMI, highest level of education, and frequency of use of acid-suppressant medications	0.61
Michigan Barrett Esophagus pREdiction Tool[94] (http://mberet.umms.med.umich.edu/)	Weekly GERD, age, waist-to-hip ratio, and pack-years of cigarette smoking	0.72
Thrift Combined Biomarker Model[95]	Biomarkers: IL12p70, IL6, IL8, IL10, and leptin Clinical: GERD frequency and duration, age, sex, race, waist-to-hip ratio, and *H pylori* status	0.85

acid may prevent the development of dysplasia or EAC.[69] Proton pump inhibitors may prevent the development of EAC in patients with BE who do not have heartburn symptoms.[70–72] However, the use of antireflux surgery is only recommended to prevent GERD symptoms, not to improve BE outcomes.[68]

Population studies have shown aspirin users have lower incidence of EAC.[73,74] Preliminary data indicate that nonsteroidal antiinflammatory drugs inhibit inflammatory pathways in the esophagus. Due to its side-effect profile, further data are needed before aspirin can be recommended as a preventive agent.[68]

Being at much higher risk of progression to BE, treatment to eliminate dysplastic BE is thought to be justified. Historically, this meant esophagectomy. Fortunately, endoscopic treatments can now be provided that significantly reduce treatment morbidity. Nodular lesions in dysplastic BE can be resected through either endoscopic mucosal resection or endoscopic submucosal dissection.[75] Pech and colleagues[76] compared endoscopic resection to esophagectomy in a multicenter retrospective cohort study and found complete remission in 98.7% of subjects treated with endoscopic resection. Few subjects undergoing endoscopic resection had complications, whereas 32% had major complications after esophagectomy.

Flat dysplastic BE is treated with radiofrequency ablation (RFA), which uses a high-frequency electromagnetic field from regularly spaced electrodes in an endoscopically attached ablation catheter to produce superficial thermal injury. In a multicenter, sham-controlled, randomized trial, complete eradication of dysplasia was achieved in 91% of cases with low-grade dysplasia and in 81% of cases with high-grade dysplasia.[77] Recent data have shown decreased progression to high-grade dysplasia and to EAC in patients with low-grade dysplasia who received RFA.[78] RFA is a relatively safe procedure, particularly compared with esophagectomy.[75]

ESOPHAGEAL SQUAMOUS CELL CARCINOMA

Although no longer the dominant form in the West, esophageal squamous cell carcinoma (ESCC) remains the most prevalent form of esophageal cancer worldwide. Rates of 100 cases per 100,000 person-years are found in Southeastern Africa and the so-called Asian esophageal cancer belt (Turkey, Iran, Kazakhstan, and Northern and Central China).[79]

Risk Factors

The most important risk factors for ESCC are environmental. Smoking seems to increase the risk of developing the disease.[80] A study from Taiwan showed smokers have an OR of 4.2 and former smokers an OR of 3.4 compared with never smokers for developing ESCC.[81] It does seem that in higher risk regions, smoking is less of a risk factor.[79]

Alcohol is another important risk factor, with increasing relative risk from 2 to 8, depending on the volume of alcohol consumed.[80] Certain areas of increased alcohol consumption do seem to be hotspots for the disease, though alcohol consumption is low in several high-incidence regions of the world.[79]

Eating dietary products high in nitrogenous components was shown to have an OR of 2 for individuals who eat foods rich in such compounds compared with those who do not.[80] The areca nut, commonly chewed like tobacco in India and Southeast Asia, has an OR of 2.3 for developing ESCC in chewers versus nonchewers.[80] Wood burning for heating and cooking has been associated with ESCC in Africa, Iran, and Brazil.[82] This may be related to increased exposure to polycyclic aromatic hydrocarbons.[83]

A genetic basis for ESCC was suggested by family predominance in high-incidence areas and is associated with autosomal dominant diseases such as tylosis.[79] A Chinese population dataset that included 453,852 single nucleotide polymorphisms (SNPs) from 1898 squamous carcinoma subjects and 2100 control subjects was used to identify candidate causal SNPs revealed 3 strong possible genetic pathways to developing ESCC.[84] Genome-wide association studies have shown SNPs for alcohol dehydrogenase 1B (rs1229984), aldehyde dehydrogenase 2 family (rs671), and a region of chromosome 20 (C20orf54).[79,85]

Screening Techniques

It is thought that esophageal squamous dysplasia is the precursor lesion to ESCC, though there are no prospective studies that assess the relationship between dysplasia and ESCC.[86] Chromoendoscopy with Lugol staining is the gold standard for the diagnosis of precancerous squamous lesions.[76] The sensitivity and specificity of white-light endoscopy for the detection of high-grade dysplasia and cancer is 62% and 79%, respectively, compared with a much higher sensitivity of 96% when using Lugol chromoendoscopy.[87]

Cytology techniques without endoscopy and tissue or serum markers of risk have been suggested as alternative screening techniques.[76] Although several nonendoscopic techniques to obtain esophageal cytology exist, these techniques have a sensitivity of only 24% to 47% for dysplasia-cancer and 18% to 44% for cancer, making them unsuitable for screening.[82] Very few studies looked at serum biomarkers but those that exist suggest these could be used in the future.[82]

Screening Guidelines

Due to low incidence in Western countries, screening is clearly not effective. However, guidelines do exist in high-incidence regions (30 cases per 100,000 persons per year), such as in Northern China.[76] Based on economic parameters and management, a comparison study between 12 different existing screening methods in high-risk or high-incidence areas of squamous cell carcinoma in China demonstrated 2 endoscopic screening strategies that were cost-effective.[88] In areas with low income levels and limited health care access, the investigators recommended 1 screening endoscopy at age 50 years, with 5-year follow-up for low-grade dysplasia and 3-year follow-up for high-grade dysplasia. In areas with higher incomes and better health care access, they recommended 3 screening endoscopies at 5-year intervals starting at the age of 40 years, with the equivalent monitoring of low-grade and high-grade dysplasia.

Prevention

Prevention of ESCC requires avoiding the environmental factors that increase the risk of developing the disease. Avoidance of smoking, alcohol, and high-risk food products is important.[77] Good screening programs may help with prevention in high-incidence areas but is not cost-effective in most of the world.

SUMMARY

Gastric adenocarcinoma, EAC, and ESCC are among the most prevalent and deadly of malignancies worldwide. Screening and prevention programs will be critical to finally improving outcomes in these diseases. For gastric adenocarcinoma, screening in high-risk populations has significantly reduced disease mortality. More research is needed to determine how to screen high-risk individuals in low-risk populations. For

EAC, though BE is a clear precursor lesion, more work is needed to develop truly effi-cient and effective techniques to improve mass screening programs. Meanwhile, for most populations, screening for ESCC is not effective. However, avoidance of toxic environmental risk factors is critical to reducing the incidence of this deadly illness.

REFERENCES

1. Ferlay J, Soerjomataram I, Dikshit R, et al. Cancer incidence and mortality world-wide: sources, methods and major patterns in GLOBOCAN 2012. Int J Cancer 2015;136:E359–86.
2. Ferlay J, Soerjomataram I, Ervik M, et al. GLOBOCAN 2012 v1.0, Cancer inci-dence and mortality worldwide: IARC CancerBase No. 11. Lyon (France): Interna-tional Agency for Research on Cancer; 2013. Available at: http://globocan.iarc.fr. Accessed June 1, 2016.
3. Ferlay J, Shin HR, Bray F, et al. Estimates of worldwide burden of cancer in 2008: GLOBOCAN 2008. Int J Cancer 2010;127:2893–917.
4. Isobe Y, Nashimoto A, Akazawa K, et al. Gastric cancer treatment in Japan: 2008 annual report of the JGCA nationwide registry. Gastric Cancer 2011;14:301–16.
5. Jang JS, Shin DG, Cho HM, et al. Differences in the survival of gastric cancer pa-tients after gastrectomy according to the medical insurance status. J Gastric Cancer 2013;13:247–54.
6. Bollschweiler E, Boettcher K, Hoelscher AH, et al. Is the prognosis for Japanese and German patients with gastric cancer really different? Cancer 1993;71: 2918–25.
7. Siegel RL, Miller KD, Jemal A. Cancer statistics, 2015. CA Cancer J Clin 2015;65: 5–29.
8. Kim GH, Liang PS, Bang SJ, et al. Screening and surveillance for gastric cancer in the United States: is it needed? Gastrointest Endosc 2016;84:18–28.
9. Maskarinec G, Noh JJ. The effect of migration on cancer incidence among Jap-anese in Hawaii. Ethn Dis 2004;14:431–9.
10. Lui FH, Tuan B, Swenson SL, et al. Ethnic disparities in gastric cancer incidence and survival in the USA: an updated analysis of 1992-2009 SEER data. Dig Dis Sci 2014;59:3027–34.
11. Palli D, Galli M, Caporaso NE, et al. Family history and risk of stomach cancer in Italy. Cancer Epidemiol Biomarkers Prev 1994;3:15–8.
12. La Vecchia C, Negri E, Franceschi S, et al. Family history and the risk of stomach and colorectal cancer. Cancer 1992;70:50–5.
13. Shin CM, Kim N, Yang HJ, et al. Stomach cancer risk in gastric cancer relatives: interaction between *Helicobacter pylori* infection and family history of gastric can-cer for the risk of stomach cancer. J Clin Gastroenterol 2010;44:e34–9.
14. Brown LM, Devesa SS. Epidemiologic trends in esophageal and gastric cancer in the United States. Surg Oncol Clin N Am 2002;11:235–56.
15. Derakhshan MH, Liptrot S, Paul J, et al. Oesophageal and gastric intestinal-type adenocarcinomas show the same male predominance due to a 17 year delayed development in females. Gut 2009;58:16–23.
16. Sheh A, Ge Z, Parry NM, et al. 17β-estradiol and tamoxifen prevent gastric cancer by modulating leukocyte recruitment and oncogenic pathways in *Helicobacter py-lori*-infected INS-GAS male mice. Cancer Prev Res (Phila) 2011;4:1426–35.
17. Camargo MC, Goto Y, Zabaleta J, et al. Sex hormones, hormonal interventions, and gastric cancer risk: a meta-analysis. Cancer Epidemiol Biomarkers Prev 2012;21:20–38.

18. Hansford S, Kaurah P, Li-Chang H, et al. Hereditary Diffuse Gastric Cancer Syndrome: CDH1 Mutations and Beyond. JAMA Oncol 2015;1(1):23–32.

19. Fitzgerald RC, Hardwick R, Huntsman D, et al, International Gastric Cancer Linkage Consortium. Hereditary diffuse gastric cancer: updated consensus guidelines for clinical management and directions for future research. J Med Genet 2010;47(7):436–44 [Erratum appears in J Med Genet 2011;48(3):216].

20. Colvin H, Yamamoto K, Wada N, et al. Hereditary Gastric Cancer Syndromes. Surg Oncol Clin N Am 2015;24(4):765–77.

21. Ladeiras-Lopes R, Pereira AK, Nogueira A, et al. Smoking and gastric cancer: systematic review and meta-analysis of cohort studies. Cancer Causes Control 2008;19:689–701.

22. Yang P, Zhou Y, Chen B, et al. Overweight, obesity and gastric cancer risk: results from a meta-analysis of cohort studies. Eur J Cancer 2009;45:2867–73.

23. Lunet N, Valbuena C, Vieira AL, et al. Fruit and vegetable consumption and gastric cancer by location and histological type: case-control and meta-analysis. Eur J Cancer Prev 2007;16:312–27.

24. Ge S, Feng X, Shen L, et al. Association between habitual dietary salt intake and risk of gastric cancer: a systematic review of observational studies. Gastroenterol Res Pract 2012;2012:808120.

25. Correa P. Human gastric carcinogenesis: a multistep and multifactorial process - First American Cancer Society Award Lecture on Cancer Epidemiology and Prevention. Cancer Res 1992;52:6735–40.

26. de Vries AC, van Grieken NC, Looman CW, et al. Gastric cancer risk in patients with premalignant gastric lesions: a nationwide cohort study in the Netherlands. Gastroenterology 2008;134:945–52.

27. Ley C, Mohar A, Guarner J, et al. Screening markers for chronic atrophic gastritis in Chiapas, Mexico. Cancer Epidemiol Biomarkers Prev 2001;10:107–12.

28. Dinis-Ribeiro M, da Costa-Pereira A, Lopes C, et al. Validity of serum pepsinogen I/II ratio for the diagnosis of gastric epithelial dysplasia and intestinal metaplasia during the follow-up of patients at risk for intestinal-type gastric adenocarcinoma. Neoplasia 2004;6:449–56.

29. Yoshihara M, Hiyama T, Yoshida S, et al. Reduction in gastric cancer mortality by screening based on serum pepsinogen concentration: a case-control study. Scand J Gastroenterol 2007;42:760–4.

30. Kato M, Asaka M. Recent development of gastric cancer prevention. Jpn J Clin Oncol 2012;42:987–94.

31. Fukao A, Tsubono Y, Tsuji I, et al. The evaluation of screening for gastric cancer in Miyagi Prefecture, Japan: a population-based case-control study. Int J Cancer 1995;60:45–8.

32. Inaba S, Hirayama H, Nagata C, et al. Evaluation of a screening program on reduction of gastric cancer mortality in Japan: preliminary results from a cohort study. Prev Med 1999;29:102–6.

33. Hosokawa O, Hattori M, Takeda T, et al. Accuracy of endoscopy in detecting gastric cancer. J Gastroenterol Mass Surv 2004;42:33–9.

34. Otsuji M, Kouno Y, Otsuji A, et al. Assessment of small diameter panendoscopy for diagnosis of gastric cancer: comparative study with follow-up survey date. Stomach Intest 1989;24:1291–7.

35. Choi KS, Kwak MS, Lee HY, et al. Screening for gastric cancer in Korea: population-based preferences for endoscopy versus upper gastrointestinal series. Cancer Epidemiol Biomarkers Prev 2009;18:1390–8.

36. Korean Statistical Information Service. Cancer registration statistics in 2012. Available at: http://kosis.kr/. Accessed July 15, 2015.
37. Gupta N, Bansal A, Wani SB, et al. Endoscopy for upper GI cancer screening in the general population: a cost-utility analysis. Gastrointest Endosc 2011;74: 610–24.e2.
38. Yeh JM, Hur C, Ward Z, et al. Gastric adenocarcinoma screening and prevention in the era of new biomarker and endoscopic technologies: a cost-effectiveness analysis. Gut 2016;65:563–74.
39. ASGE Standards of Practice Committee, Evans JA, Chandrasekhara V, et al. The role of endoscopy in the management of premalignant and malignant conditions of the stomach. Gastrointest Endosc 2015;82:1–8.
40. Dinis-Ribeiro M, Areia M, de Vries AC, et al. Management of precancerous conditions and lesions in the stomach (MAPS): guideline from the European Society of Gastrointestinal Endoscopy (ESGE), European Helicobacter Study Group (EHSG), European Society of Pathology (ESP), and the Sociedade Portuguesa de Endoscopia Digestiva (SPED). Endoscopy 2012;44:74–94.
41. Bosetti C, Bertuccio P, Malvezzi M, et al. Cancer mortality in Europe, 2005–2009, and an overview of trends since 1980. Ann Oncol 2013;24:2657–71.
42. Liu KS, Wong IO, Leung WK. *Helicobacter pylori* associated gastric intestinal metaplasia: Treatment and surveillance. World J Gastroenterol 2016;22:1311–20.
43. Cao Y, Nishihara R, Wu K, et al. Population-wide Impact of Long-term Use of Aspirin and the Risk for Cancer. JAMA Oncol 2016;2(6):762–9.
44. Pohl H, Sirovich B, Welch HG. Esophageal adenocarcinoma incidence: are we reaching the peak? Cancer Epidemiol Biomarkers Prev 2010;19:1468–70.
45. Auvinen MI, Sihvo EI, Ruohtula T, et al. Incipient angiogenesis in Barrett's epithelium and lymphangiogenesis in Barrett's adenocarcinoma. J Clin Oncol 2002;20: 2971–9.
46. Prasad GA, Wu TT, Wigle DA, et al. Endoscopic and surgical treatment of mucosal (T1a) esophageal adenocarcinoma in Barrett's esophagus. Gastroenterology 2009;137:815–23.
47. Gharahkhani P, Tung J, Hinds D, et al. Chronic gastroesophageal reflux disease shares genetic background with esophageal adenocarcinoma and Barrett's esophagus. Hum Mol Genet 2016;25(4):828–35.
48. Koop H. Reflux disease and Barrett's esophagus. Endoscopy 2000;32:101–7.
49. Rubenstein JH, Shaheen NJ. Epidemiology, diagnosis, and management of esophageal adenocarcinoma. Gastroenterology 2015;142:302–17.
50. Bhat S, Coleman HG, Yousef F, et al. Risk of malignant progression in Barrett's esophagus patients: results from a large population-based study. J Natl Cancer Inst 2011;103:1049–57.
51. Sami SS, Ragunath K, Iyer PG. Screening for Barrett's esophagus and esophageal adenocarcinoma: rationale, recent progress, challenges, and future directions. Clin Gastroenterol Hepatol 2015;13:623–34.
52. Desai TK, Krishnan K, Samala N, et al. Th e incidence of oesophageal adenocarcinoma in non-dysplastic Barrett's oesophagus: a meta-analysis. Gut 2012;61: 970–6.
53. Fitzgerald RC, di Pietro M, Ragunath K, et al. British Society of Gastroenterology guidelines on the diagnosis and management of Barrett's oesophagus. Gut 2014; 63:7–42.
54. Reid BJ, Paulson TG, Li X. Genetic insights in Barrett's esophagus and esophageal adenocarcinoma. Gastroenterology 2015;149:1142–52.

55. Kastelein F, Biermann K, Steyerberg EW, et al. Aberrant p53 protein expression is associated with an increased risk of neoplastic progression in patients with Barrett's oesophagus. Gut 2013;62:1676–83.

56. Rubenstein JH, Inadomi JM, Brill JV, et al. Cost utility of screening for Barrett's esophagus with esophageal capsule endoscopy versus conventional upper endoscopy. Clin Gastroenterol Hepatol 2007;5:312–8.

57. Gora MJ, Sauk JS, Carruth RW, et al. Tethered capsule endomicroscopy enables less invasive imaging of gastrointestinal tract microstructure. Nat Med 2013;19: 238–40.

58. Sami SS, Subramanian V, Ortiz-Fernández-Sordó J, et al. The utility of ultrathin endoscopy as a diagnostic tool for Barrett's oesophagus (BO). Systematic review and meta-analysis United European Gastroenterology Week. Volume UEG13-ABS-2547. Berlin, 2013.

59. Sami SS, Dunagan KT, Johnson ML, et al. A randomized comparative effectiveness trial of novel endoscopic techniques and approaches for Barrett's esophagus screening in the community. Am J Gastroenterol 2015;110:148–58.

60. Atkinson M, Das A, Faulx A, et al. Ultrathin esophagoscopy in screening for Barrett's esophagus at a Veterans Administration Hospital: easy access does not lead to referrals. Am J Gastroenterol 2008;103:92–7.

61. Kadri SR, Lao-Sirieix P, O'Donovan M, et al. Acceptability and accuracy of a non-endoscopic screening test for Barrett's oesophagus in primary care: cohort study. BMJ 2010;341:c4372.

62. Benaglia T, Sharples LD, Fitzgerald RC, et al. Health benefits and cost effectiveness of endoscopic and nonendoscopic cytosponge screening for Barrett's esophagus. Gastroenterology 2013;144:62–73.

63. Chan DK, Lutzke LS, Clemens MA, et al. Detection of Barrett's esophagus by noninvasive breath screening of exhaled volatile organic compounds using an electronic-nose device. Gastroenterolog 2016;150:S67.

64. Qumseya BJ, Wang H, Badie N, et al. Advanced imaging technologies increase detection of dysplasia and neoplasia in patients with Barrett's esophagus: a meta-analysis and systematic review. Clin Gastroenterol Hepatol 2013;11(12): 1562–70.e1-2.

65. Sharma P, Meining AR, Coron E, et al. Real-time increased detection of neoplastic tissue in Barrett's esophagus with probe-based confocal laser endomicroscopy: final results of an international multicenter, prospective, randomized, controlled trial. Gastrointest Endosc 2011;74:465–72.

66. Sauk J, Coron E, Kava L, et al. Interobserver agreement for the detection of Barrett's esophagus with optical frequency domain imaging. Dig Dis Sci 2013;58: 2261–5.

67. Evans JA, Poneros JM, Bouma BE, et al. Optical coherence tomography to identify intramucosal carcinoma and high-grade dysplasia in Barrett's esophagus. Clin Gastroenterol Hepatol 2006;4:38–43.

68. Shaheen NJ, Falk GW, Iyer PG, et al. ACG clinical guideline: diagnosis and management of Barrett's esophagus. Am J Gastroenterol 2016;111:30–50.

69. Singh S, Garg SK, Singh PP, et al. Acid-suppressive medications and risk of oesophageal adenocarcinoma in patients with Barrett's oesophagus: a systematic review and meta-analysis. Gut 2014;63:1229–37.

70. Kastelein F, Spaander MC, Steyerberg EW, et al. Proton pump inhibitors reduce the risk of neoplastic progression in patients with Barrett's esophagus. Clin Gastroenterol Hepatol 2013;11:382–8.

71. Hillman LC, Chiragakis L, Shadbolt B, et al. Proton-pump inhibitor therapy and the development of dysplasia in patients with Barrett's oesophagus. Med J Aust 2004;180:387–91.

72. Nguyen DM, El-Serag HB, Henderson L, et al. Medication usage and the risk of neoplasia in patients with Barrett's esophagus. Clin Gastroenterol Hepatol 2009; 7:1299–304.

73. Gammon MD, Terry MB, Arber N, et al. Nonsteroidal anti-inflammatory drug use associated with reduced incidence of adenocarcinomas of the esophagus and gastric cardia that overexpress cyclin D1: a population based study. Cancer Epidemiol Biomarkers Prev 2004;13:34–9.

74. Corley DA, Kerlikowske K, Verma R, et al. Protective association of aspirin/NSAIDs and esophageal cancer: a systematic review and metaanalysis. Gastroenterology 2003;124:47–56.

75. Chandra S, Gorospe EC, Leggett CL, et al. Barrett's esophagus in 2012: updates in pathogenesis, treatment, and surveillance. Curr Gastroenterol Rep 2013;15:32.

76. Pech O, Bollschweiler E, Manner H, et al. Comparison between endoscopic and surgical resection of mucosal esophageal adenocarcinoma in Barrett's esophagus at two high volume centers. Ann Surg 2011;254:67–72.

77. Shaheen NJ, Sharma P, Overholt BF, et al. Radiofrequency ablation in Barrett's esophagus with dysplasia. N Engl J Med 2009;360:2277–88.

78. Phoa KN, van Vilsteren FG, Weusten BL, et al. Radiofrequency ablation vs endoscopic surveillance for patients with Barrett esophagus and low-grade dysplasia: a randomized clinical trial. JAMA 2014;311:1209–17.

79. Domper Arnal MJ, Ferrández Arenas Á, Lanas Arbeloa Á. Esophageal cancer: risk factors, screening and endoscopic treatment in Western and Eastern countries. World J Gastroenterol 2015;21:7933–43.

80. Wheeler JB, Reed CE. Epidemiology of esophageal cancer. Surg Clin North Am 2012;92:1077–87.

81. Lee CH, Lee JM, Wu DC, et al. Independent and combined effects of alcohol intake, tobacco smoking and betel quid chewing on the risk of esophageal cancer in Taiwan. Int J Cancer 2005;113:475–82.

82. Mlombe YB, Rosenberg NE, Wolf LL, et al. Environmental risk factors for oesophageal cancer in Malawi: A case-control study. Malawi Med J 2015;27:88–92.

83. Kamangar F, Strickland PT, Pourshams A, et al. High exposure to polycyclic aromatic hydrocarbons may contribute to high risk of esophageal cancer in northeastern Iran. Anticancer Res 2005;25:425–8.

84. Yang X, Zhu H, Qin Q, et al. Genetic variants and risk of esophageal squamous cell carcinoma: a GWAS-based pathway analysis. Gene 2015;556:149–52.

85. Zhang HZ, Jin GF, Shen HB. Epidemiologic differences in esophageal cancer between Asian and Western populations. Chin J Cancer 2012;31:281–6.

86. Lin Y, Totsuka Y, He Y, et al. Epidemiology of esophageal cancer in Japan and China. J Epidemiol 2013;23:233–42.

87. Lao-Sirieix P, Fitzgerald RC. Screening for oesophageal cancer. Nat Rev Clin Oncol 2012;9:278–87.

88. Yang J, Wei WQ, Niu J, et al. Cost-benefit analysis of esophageal cancer endoscopic screening in high-risk areas of China. World J Gastroenterol 2012;18: 2493–501.

89. Eloubeidi MA, Provenzale D. Clinical and demographic predictors of Barrett's esophagus among patients with gastroesophageal reflux disease: a multivariable analysis in veterans. J Clin Gastroenterol 2001;33:306–9.

90. Wong A, Fitzgerald RC. Epidemiologic risk factors for Barrett's esophagus and associated adenocarcinoma. Clin Gastroenterol Hepatol 2005;3:1–10.
91. Juhasz A, Mittal SK, Lee TH, et al. Prevalence of Barrett esophagus in first-degree relatives of patients with esophageal adenocarcinoma. J Clin Gastroenterol 2011; 45:867–71.
92. Cook MB, Shaheen NJ, Anderson LA, et al. Cigarette smoking increases risk of Barrett's esophagus: an analysis of the Barrett's and Esophageal Adenocarcinoma Consortium. Gastroenterology 2012;142:744–53.
93. Thrift AP, Kendall BJ, Pandeya N, et al. A clinical risk prediction model for Barrett esophagus. Cancer Prev Res (Phila) 2012;5:1115–23.
94. Rubenstein JH, Morgenstern H, Appelman H, et al. Prediction of Barrett's esophagus among men. Am J Gastroenterol 2013;108:353–62.
95. Thrift AP, Garcia JM, El-Serag HB. A multibiomarker risk score helps predict risk for Barrett's esophagus. Clin Gastroenterol Hepatol 2014;12(8):1267–71.

Endoscopic Management of Early Esophagogastric Cancer

Qurat-ul-ain Rizvi, MBBS, FRACP[a], Arrhchanah Balachandran, MBBS (Hons)[a],
Doreen Koay, MB BCh BAO, MRCP[a], Prateek Sharma, MD[b],
Rajvinder Singh, MBBS, MPhil, FRACP, AM, FRCP[a],*

KEYWORDS

- Endoscopic mucosal resection (EMR) • Endoscopic submucosal dissection (ESD)
- Ablative therapies • Barrett esophagus • Esophageal cancer
- Early gastric cancer (EGC)

KEY POINTS

- Endoscopic management of early esophagogastric cancer is largely dependent on patient factors, the degree of tumour extent and level of medical expertise available.
- Endoscopic mucosal resection is a well-established therapeutic modality in the treatment of early esophageal cancer, early gastric cancer and Barrett esophagus with high-grade dysplasia.
- Ablative therapies are used independently or in combination with endoscopic mucosal resection in the treatment of Barrett esophagus, with or without dysplasia.
- Endoscopic submucosal dissection is superior to other endoscopic treatment modalities in achieving en-bloc or complete resection in tumours greater than 2 cm.
- Endoscopic submucosal dissection has similar outcomes to surgery with respect to the management of esophageal squamous cell carcinoma and early gastric cancer.

INTRODUCTION

Esophagogastric cancers remain some of the most difficult cancers to treat, accounting for approximately 16% of cancer-related mortality worldwide.[1] The emergence of advanced diagnostic techniques—including high-resolution, high-definition white light endoscopy; chromoendoscopy; and narrow band imaging—in addition to the

Disclosures: The authors have nothing to disclose.
[a] Department of Gastroenterology and Hepatology, Lyell McEwin Hospital, Haydown Road, Elizabeth Vale, South Australia 5112, Australia; [b] Division of Gastroenterology and Hepatology, University of Kansas School of Medicine, VA Medical Center, 4801 Linwood Boulevard, Kansas City, MO 64128, USA
* Corresponding author.
E-mail address: Rajvinder.singh@sa.gov.au

Surg Oncol Clin N Am 26 (2017) 179–191
http://dx.doi.org/10.1016/j.soc.2016.10.007
surgonc.theclinics.com

implementation of screening programs in certain high-risk individuals has been largely responsible for the early detection of premalignant and malignant lesions.[2] Traditionally, the gold standard treatment of esophagogastric cancer has been surgery, even at the earliest stages of malignancy. These procedures, however, are associated with increased rates of treatment-related morbidity and mortality.[3] Over the past decade, minimally invasive endoscopic management has become a viable alternative to surgical treatment.[4] Ultimately, the mode of management is determined by local factors, including a patient's age, comorbidities, and personal preference as well as the level of available medical expertise.[2] This review discusses some of the major modes of endoscopic management pertaining to early esophageal and gastric cancer, including its techniques, indications and surrounding controversies.

EARLY ESOPHAGEAL CANCER

Esophageal cancer typically occurs in 2 histologic forms: squamous cell carcinoma and adenocarcinoma. Squamous cell carcinoma is the predominant form of esophageal cancer in Asia and much of the world. Its major risk factors include alcohol and tobacco abuse. Squamous cell carcinoma can develop anywhere in the esophagus but often occurs proximally. Adenocarcinoma is the leading type of esophageal cancer in most Western countries.[1] This is due to the high incidence of Barrett esophagus, a premalignant condition involving replacement of the squamous epithelium in the distal esophagus of any length with columnar epithelium with identifiable intestinal metaplasia on histopathologic assessment.[5]

Early esophageal cancers are classified as low-grade and high-grade intraepithelial neoplasia (dysplasia) and as adenocarcinoma contained within the mucosa. This definition is sometimes extended to include superficial submucosal involvement.[6] Endoscopic therapy has become an integral part of the multidisciplinary management of early esophageal cancer. These approaches include endoscopic mucosal resection (EMR), endoscopic submucosal dissection (ESD), radiofrequency ablation (RFA), photodynamic therapy (PDT), cryotherapy and argon plasma coagulation (APC).

Initial Assessment

The UK National Institute for Health and Care Excellence guidelines recommend that endoscopic procedures (1) need to be carefully considered in high-volume tertiary referral centers with access to a surgeon, (2) should be performed by appropriately trained staff, and (3) must be managed by a multidisciplinary team to optimize patient care. For the best outcomes, patients suitable for endoscopic therapy must be carefully selected to avoid inadequate treatment of advanced cancers. An important aspect of choosing an appropriate management strategy is the accurate assessment of disease extent. It is important to carefully assess the depth of invasion, tumor grade, and degree of lymphovascular invasion to determine the stage of esophageal cancer. Submucosal involvement is the most important prognostic determinant for early esophageal cancer because the presence of lymphatic vessels within the submucosa facilitates dissemination of malignant cells. Modalities, such as endoscopic ultrasound, and histopathologic examination through biopsy and EMR have been shown to accurately predict lymph node involvement.

Endoscopic Mucosal Resection In Early Esophageal Cancer

EMR was first described in 1973 as a novel treatment of colorectal polyps.[7] It has evolved into an effective diagnostic and treatment option for both early esophageal and gastric cancers. According to recently modified guidelines published by the

Japanese Esophageal Society, lesions confined to the mucosal epithelium or lamina propria of the mucosal layer are rarely associated with lymph node metastasis. As such, EMR is suitable to treat these lesions. Lesions reaching the muscularis mucosae or slightly infiltrating the submucosa (up to 200 μm, T1b-SM1) are amenable to EMR but may carry a risk of lymph node metastasis. Therefore, these cases represent relative indications to performing EMR; 50% of lesions invading deeper (greater than 200 μm) into the submucosa (T1b-SM2) are associated with the presence of nodal metastases and should be treated in the same manner as advanced cancers (ie, cancer exceeding the muscularis propria) with esophagectomy.

The literature describes 3 major EMR techniques, including the inject, lift, and cut method; the cap-assisted EMR method; and EMR with ligation. EMR typically involves the injection of normal saline, which may be mixed with dilute adrenaline to allow for a bloodless endoscopic view, and a dye to better identify the target lesion. This submucosal injection both cushions and isolates the tissue before removal of the lesion with a snare. This also reduces the risk of thermal injury, perforation, and hemorrhage as well as facilitating en bloc resection.[8] The cap-assisted technique is frequently used to excise early esophageal cancers (Fig. 1). After submucosal injection, a cap mounted on the head of the endoscope is placed over the target lesion, which is subsequently suctioned into the cap.[9] The snare, placed in the cap, is then closed around the base

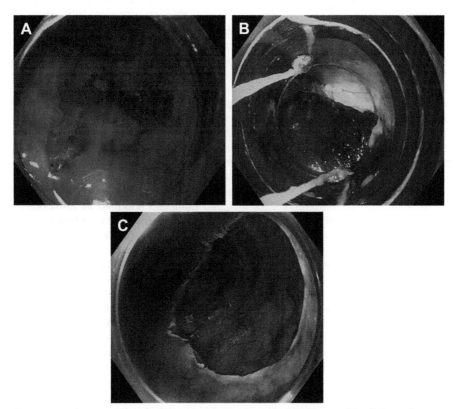

Fig. 1. EMR of an esophageal squamous cell carcinoma. (A) Lesion on white light endoscopy: irregular reddish area measuring approximately 1.5 cm. (B) EMR: resection in progress. (C) Base at the end of the procedure.

and diathermy is used to complete the excision.[10] The banding method, or EMR ligation, is also commonly used. It involves using a band ligation device.[11] The inject, lift and cut method is safe and straightforward but is more frequently used to manage colonic lesions.[12] Larger lesions exceeding 2 cm are not excluded from EMR, although they may require piecemeal resection.[9] Piecemeal resection is associated with tumor recurrence and should be performed with meticulous attention to avoid any residual islands of tissue being left behind.[13]

Endoscopic mucosal resection in barrett esophagus

Endoscopic therapy is not recommended for the treatment of Barrett esophagus without dysplasia. It is the treatment of choice, however, for Barrett esophagus with high-grade dysplasia (HGD) and early mucosal cancer.[14] Visible nodules or lumps in metaplastic Barrett esophagus have a high incidence of invasive cancer. Tissue sampling with biopsies from these lesions tends to underestimate the degree of dysplasia. Multiple studies have shown that EMR leads to better interobserver agreement with respect to the degree of dysplasia and can lead to clarification of the final histologic stage when compared with biopsy specimens.[15] Follow-up of a seminal study conducted by Pech and colleagues[13] found that the rates of recurrence and metachronous neoplasia range from 0% to 30%. Bleeding and stricture formation were the most common complications, which both could be dealt with endoscopically. Bleeding can occur in up to 12% of patients whereas perforation may occur in up to 2.3%.[16,17] Early intervention demonstrated a higher remission rate and faster response time for small and low-grade cancers removed with EMR.[18] A prospective study was conducted in 64 patients with early carcinoma or HGD who were grouped as low-risk or high-risk based on their stage, size and grade of cancer. These results demonstrated a higher complete remission rate for the low-risk group (97%). The mean follow-up period of 12 months revealed a 14% rate of recurrence for metachronous neoplasia.[19] In a case series, recurrences of dysplasia or carcinoma were reported in 12% to 21% of patients after a mean follow-up period of 43 to 63 months. These cases were amenable to repeat endoscopic management. The risk of recurrence was higher in patients with long segment Barrett esophagus, patients with multifocal neoplasia, patients who underwent piecemeal resection and patients who needed a longer period to achieve complete remission.[20] Another study assessed the role of endoscopy in esophageal adenocarcinomas limited to the upper third of the submucosa. The main outcomes included complete endoluminal remission in 87% and long-term remission in 84% of cases. Lymph node metastasis was ultimately found in only 1.9%, and metachronous neoplasia in 19% of cases. With the low rate of lymph node metastasis and an estimated 5-year survival rate of 84%, endoscopic therapy was thought preferable for small, low-risk esophageal cancers with SM1 involvement.[21]

Endoscopic mucosal resection in squamous cell carcinoma

Lymphovascular invasion occurs earlier in squamous cell carcinoma. Lesions confined to the epithelium and lamina propria have up to a 5.6% risk of lymph node metastasis.[22,23] Nodal metastases occur in up to 18% of patients with muscularis mucosae involvement and up to 53% of patients with SM1 involvement.[22,24,25] A Japanese study reported on the outcomes of EMR in superficial esophageal cancer in 396 patients at 80 institutions. En bloc resection rates of 64.3% were achieved in tumors measuring less than 1 cm in diameter and 36.5% in those less than 2 cm in diameter. Patients with submucosal cancers showed significantly worse 5-year survival rates than those with mucosal cancers.[26] In another prospective case series by Pech and colleagues,[27] a total of 179 resections were performed (mean number of resections $\pm$ SD per patient, 2.8 $\pm$ 1.8); 11 of 12 patients (91.7%) with high-grade intraepithelial neoplasia and 51 out of 53 patients (96.2%) with mucosal cancer achieved a complete response during a mean follow-up period of 39.3 $\pm$ 22.8 months. Recurrence of malignancy after achieving a complete response was observed in 16 patients (26%), but these patients all achieved complete response after further endoscopic treatment. Independent risk factors for tumor recurrence included multifocal carcinoma (relative risk 4.1, $P = .018$). The 7-year survival rate calculated for all groups was 77%.[27] Ciocirlan and colleagues[28] performed a retrospective cohort study of 51 patients with early squamous cell carcinoma or HGD. These results demonstrated a complete local remission rate of 91% and a 5-year survival rate of 58%, mandating the need for close endoscopic surveillance after EMR.

Hence, patients with squamous cell carcinoma confined to the superficial mucosa (m1 and m2) may be candidates for EMR. Tumors that have invaded into the deep mucosa or submucosa, however, should be referred for surgical resection.

Ablative therapies

Ablative therapies have become one of the most important endoscopic modalities in the management of Barrett esophagus. They can be used independently or in combination with EMR in the treatment of Barrett-related dysplasia or early adenocarcinoma. A concerning factor for ablative therapies is the risk of recurrence from buried glands where neosquamous epithelium overgrows ablated tissue, potentially masking residual metaplastic or dysplastic tissue.[18]

Radiofrequency ablation

RFA devices deliver alternating currents of electromagnetic waves at high frequency to physically destroy premalignant or malignant tissue. This technique is completed via catheters with inflatable balloons along guidewires or plates, which are attached to the tip or instrumental channel of an endoscope.[9] The American College of Gastroenterology guidelines recommend that in subjects with EMR specimens demonstrating HGD or intramucosal carcinoma, endoscopic ablative therapy for the remaining Barrett esophagus should be performed.[29] Given the costs and side-effect profile associated with PDT, RFA seems the preferred modality of ablative therapy for most patients. This is supported by a large body of data demonstrating its safety and efficacy. RFA is highly effective in the complete eradication of intestinal metaplasia and dysplasia, which has been confirmed by multiple studies, including the landmark Ablation of Intestinal Metaplasia Containing Dysplasia trial.[30–32] In another European multicenter study, focal EMR followed by RFA was found safe and highly effective for the eradication of early Barrett-related adenocarcinoma as well as complete resection of the entire Barrett segment, correlating with success rates of approximately 90%. During a median follow-up of 27 months, the recurrence rate of neoplasia or visible Barrett mucosa remained at less than 10%. Common side effects included dysphagia, stricture formation, bleeding, and, rarely, perforation.[33]

Photodynamic therapy

PDT involves the application of a photosensitizing agent, such as oral 5-aminolevulinic acid or intravenous sodium porfimer. When these photosensitizing agents are exposed to a specific wavelength of light, they produce a form of oxygen that can destroy nearby cells.[34] PDT may be used as an alternative treatment option for Barrett esophagus with dysplasia. In a prospective, double-blind, randomized trial, PDT was compared with a placebo therapy in patients with low-grade dysplasia in Barrett esophagus. In the group exposed to PDT, 89% of patients responded with neosquamous epithelium in the treated area and no further development of dysplasia. Comparatively, no epithelial response was detectable in 67% of patients in the placebo group.[35] Although this technique is effective, it is expensive and has unfavorable side effects, including stricture formation, skin photosensitivity, vomiting and chest pain.[36]

Cryotherapy

Cryotherapy involves snap freezing of the surface epithelium, by using either liquid nitrogen or rapidly expanding carbon dioxide, which is released at high velocity, leading to immediate apoptosis.[2] Cell injury occurs during reperfusion by the generation of free radicals in the frozen tissue as it is reoxygenated. Johnston and colleagues[37] described the use of cryotherapy in 11 patients with Barrett esophagus. Histologic reversal of Barrett esophagus was identified in 78% of patients (n = 9) after a 6-month follow-up period without any major complications. Several other small studies have shown benefit with cryotherapy, particularly with patients excluded from surgery or who have failed other endoscopic treatments.[34] Longitudinal studies are further required to determine the durability of benefits from cryotherapy at any stage of Barrett esophagus.

Argon plasma coagulation

APC causes thermal injury to the mucosa through energy delivery from ionized argon plasma via monopolar electrocautery.[38] It is a recognized technique in the treatment of nondysplastic Barrett esophagus.[2,38] Success rates of 70% to 86% have been reported when used in isolation for the eradication of Barrett esophagus with or without HGD.[39–41] APC can lead to complications, however, such as postprocedural chest pain, ulceration, bleeding and stricture development. Buried glands may also occur in up to 30% of cases, which is considerably more common compared with other ablative therapies.[34,42] Since the development of RFA, it has been used less frequently in the management of nondysplastic Barrett esophagus.[38]

Endoscopic Submucosal Dissection In Early Esophageal Cancer

ESD was pioneered in Japan in the 1990s to overcome the shortfalls of endoscopic management for early gastric cancer (EGC).[43] It is an advanced endoscopic technique, which first involves marking the target lesion with several vertical and lateral markings around its margin. The submucosa is then lifted with an injection solution similar to that used in EMR. The mucosa is then incised using a range of electrocautery knives. This allows for direct dissection of the submucosal layer until complete removal of the target lesion is achieved (Fig. 2).[9] The advantage of ESD is its ability to achieve en bloc margin-negative resection of tumors greater than 2 cm. It also reduces the need for piecemeal resection, which is associated with high rates of local recurrence.[44] Due to the narrow lumen of the esophagus, which is prone to stricture formation, the Japanese Esophageal Society developed absolute and relative indications for performing ESD. Absolute indications include T1a esophageal carcinomas involving the epithelium or lamina propria and less than two-thirds of the circumference of the esophagus. Relative indications include esophageal carcinomas involving the muscularis mucosae or less than 200 μm of the submucosa.[45] Most of the published literature stems from Japanese centers, given the high incidence of squamous cell carcinoma. Results of a recent survey suggested that only 12 of 340 published articles were reported from Western countries.[46] Studies have still shown that the incidence of lymph node metastasis with T1a esophageal adenocarcinoma may be up to

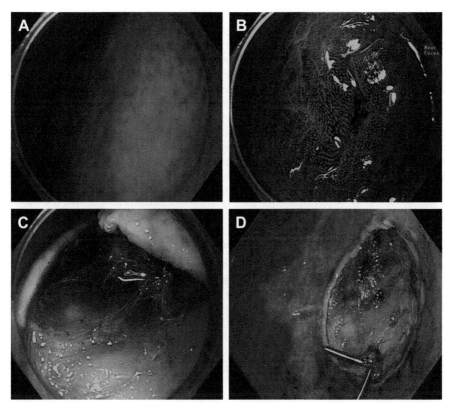

Fig. 2. ESD of an EGC. (*A*) Lesion on white light endoscopy: mildly erythematous area. (*B*) Lesion on narrow band imaging and magnification: irregular pit pattern and friability. (*C*) Dissection of the submucosal plane during ESD. (*D*) Base at the end of the procedure.

2.6%, which is comparatively less than the mortality rate after esophagectomy.[47–49] Therefore, it seems reasonable to consider ESD in the management of early esophageal cancer.

EARLY GASTRIC CANCER

EGC is defined as cancer that does not invade beyond the submucosa regardless of lymph node involvement. EGC carries an excellent prognosis, with reported 5-year survival rates of greater than 99% if confined to the mucosa and greater than 96% if confined to the submucosa.[50] The increasing incidence of EGC may be attributed to the increasing use of screening endoscopies, particularly in Asian countries, as well as advances in endoscopic diagnostic techniques. EGC represents 40% to 60% of all gastric cancers in Japan.[50] In Eastern Asia, up to one-half of resections for gastric adenocarcinoma represent EGC.[51] By contrast, in Western countries, EGC accounts for 15% to 21% of gastric adenocarcinomas.[52]

Recent advancements in endoscopic management techniques have altered the entire management of EGC in Eastern Asia. Standard gastrectomy, however, remains the definitive locoregional treatment of EGC given that endoscopic therapies are not recognized as a first-line standard of care worldwide. This section focuses on the recent developments in the endoscopic management of EGC. The Japanese Gastric

Cancer Association recently modified guidelines regarding the endoscopic management of EGC.[53,54] Their indications are based on tumor size and morphology, which are amenable to endoscopic resection and are at low risk of lymph node metastasis. These guidelines propose 2 separate sets of indications for endoscopic management: (1) an absolute set of criteria for endoscopic therapy (including EMR and ESD) and (2) an expanded set of criteria for ESD as an investigational treatment. With respect to the absolute indications, the tumor must meet all of the following criteria, which are (1) well-differentiated adenocarcinoma, (2) no ulceration, (3) stage T1a, and (4) having a diameter of less than 2 cm. The expanded criteria are modified to account for the improved resection capabilities of ESD, compared with EMR, for tumors that have a very low probability of lymph node metastasis. This includes tumors clinically diagnosed as T1a and are (1) a well-differentiated type without ulceration but greater than 2 cm in diameter, (2) a differentiated type with ulceration and less than 3 cm in diameter, or (3) an undifferentiated type without ulceration and less than 2 cm in diameter.[54]

Endoscopic Mucosal Resection In Early Gastric Cancer

Similar to early esophageal cancer, EMR is a well-established therapeutic modality for the treatment of EGC, including those that are differentiated and no more than 2 cm in size. Manner and colleagues[55] performed a study in which EMR was performed in 39 patients with EGC; 38 of 39 patients achieved complete remission after a mean period of 1.3 ± 0.6 EMR sessions. Recurrent or metachronous lesions were observed in 11 patients (29%) during a follow-up period of 57 months. All lesions were successfully treated by repeat endoscopic resection. No tumor-related deaths occurred during the follow-up period.[55] In another cross-sectional, retrospective cohort study, the local recurrence rate of piecemeal resection in patients with a differentiated adenocarcinoma localized to the mucosa was investigated by annual surveillance endoscopy over a 10-year period. En bloc EMR was performed in 66 cases and piecemeal resection was performed in 83 cases. The local recurrence rate was 30% (95% CI, 20%–40%) at both 5 and 10 years in the piecemeal resection group. No recurrence was observed in the en bloc group.[56] A retrospective analysis of 551 patients who underwent either complete EMR or curative surgical resection revealed there were no significant differences in the risk of mortality or tumor recurrence. Although patients who underwent EMR had a higher risk of metachronous gastric cancers, all recurrent or metachronous gastric cancers after EMR were successfully retreated without affecting the overall survival rate.[57]

Endoscopic Submucosal Dissection In Early Gastric Cancer

ESD increases the success rate of en bloc and complete resection, thus decreasing the chance of recurrence. In a retrospective study, EMR and ESD were compared in terms of en bloc resection rate, histologically complete resection rate, operation time, complications and local recurrence rate. En bloc and histologically complete resection rates were significantly higher with ESD than with EMR, regardless of tumor size. Furthermore, no patient experienced recurrence in the ESD group.[46] Two further retrospective, single-center studies sampling a large number of cases compared EMR and ESD in the treatment of EGC. Both reports confirmed that ESD achieved a higher en bloc resection rate and a lower local recurrence rate.[58,59] ESD was associated with significantly more complications, however, including hemorrhage and perforation.

In another study documenting the tumor recurrence and survival rates of EGC after ESD, en bloc resection was achieved in 94.9% of subjects (n = 559) with larger lesions at higher risk of piecemeal resection. Furthermore, 94.7% of lesions (n = 550) were deemed to have undergone curative resection. En bloc resection was the only significant contributor to curative ESD. Patients with noncurative resection developed local recurrence more frequently. The 5-year overall and disease-specific survival rates were 97.1% and 100%, respectively.[60] In a retrospective, multicenter study sampling 1000 cases of EGC, the rates of en bloc resection, complete en bloc resection, vertical incomplete resection, and piecemeal resection were 95.3%, 87.7%, 1.8%, and 4.1%, respectively. The rates of delayed bleeding, significant bleeding, perforation, and surgery related to complications were 15.6%, 0.6%, 1.2%, and 0.2%, respectively.[61]

There is limited evidence concerning ESD versus gastrectomy. A recent retrospective study conducted in Hong Kong attempted to compare the outcomes of ESD against gastrectomy in an analysis of 114 patients with either severe dysplasia or EGC. All patients underwent endoscopic ultrasound and image-enhanced endoscopy prior to either procedure. Follow-up for ESD consisted of routine endoscopy at 3-month intervals for 2 years, followed by 6-month intervals until 5 years after the procedure. A total of 40 patients underwent radical gastrectomy whereas 74 patients received treatment with ESD. ESD (obtaining en bloc resection) was successful in 68 of 74 cases. The overall complication rate was higher in the gastrectomy group, although the study found no significant difference between the groups with respect to the 3-year survival rates.[62] In a systematic review comparing endoscopic resection (EMR and ESD) to gastrectomy in the treatment of EGC, the 5-year survival rates were similar between endoscopic resection and gastrectomy. Endoscopic resection offers a shorter hospital stay, however, and fewer complications in the treatment of EGC.[63]

SUMMARY

The increasing incidence of esophagogastric cancer, which may be attributed to the increasing use of surveillance programs in high-risk populations, has led to advancements in various endoscopic imaging and management strategies. Hybrid therapy that involves EMR of visible lesions, followed by endoscopic ablation of metaplastic epithelium, has been shown an effective therapy in the management of Barrett esophagus. ESD is an effective treatment modality with comparable results to surgery in the treatment of esophageal squamous cell carcinoma and EGC.

REFERENCES

1. Ferlay J, Shin HR, Bray F, et al. Estimates of worldwide burden of cancer in 2008: GLOBOCAN 2008. Int J Cancer 2010;127(12):2893–917.
2. Singh R, Yeap SP, Cheong KL. Detection and characterization of early malignancy in the esophagus: what is the best management algorithm? Best Pract Res Clin Gastroenterol 2015;29(4):533–44.
3. Enestvedt BK, Ginsberg GG. Advances in endoluminal therapy for esophageal cancer. Gastrointest Endosc Clin N Am 2013;23(1):17–39.
4. Barnes JA, Willingham FF. Endoscopic Management of Early Esophageal Cancer. J Clin Gastroenterol 2015;49(8):638–46.
5. Wang KK, Sampliner RE. Updated guidelines 2008 for the diagnosis, surveillance and therapy of Barrett's esophagus. Am J Gastroenterol 2008;103(3):788–97.
6. Wani S, Drahos J, Cook MB, et al. Comparison of endoscopic therapies and surgical resection in patients with early esophageal cancer: a population-based study. Gastrointest Endosc 2014;79(2):224–32.e1.
7. Deyhle P, Jenny S, Fumagalli I. Endoscopic polypectomy in the proximal colon. A diagnostic, therapeutic (and preventive?) intervention. Dtsch Med Wochenschr 1973;98(5):219–20 [in German].

8. Uraoka T, Saito Y, Yamamoto K, et al. Submucosal injection solution for gastrointestinal tract endoscopic mucosal resection and endoscopic submucosal dissection. Drug Des Devel Ther 2009;2:131–8.

9. Testoni PA, Arcidiacono PG, Mariani A. Endoscopic management of gastrointestinal cancer and precancerous conditions. 1st edition. Turin (Italy): Edizioni Minerva Medica; 2015.

10. Inoue H, Takeshita K, Hori H, et al. Endoscopic mucosal resection with a cap-fitted panendoscope for esophagus, stomach, and colon mucosal lesions. Gastrointest Endosc 1993;39(1):58–62.

11. Tanabe S, Koizumi W, Kokutou M, et al. Usefulness of endoscopic aspiration mucosectomy as compared with strip biopsy for the treatment of gastric mucosal cancer. Gastrointest Endosc 1999;50(6):819–22.

12. Soetikno RM, Gotoda T, Nakanishi Y, et al. Endoscopic mucosal resection. Gastrointest Endosc 2003;57(4):567–79.

13. Pech O, Manner H, Ell C. Endoscopic resection. Gastrointest Endosc Clin N Am 2011;21(1):81–94.

14. Eloubeidi MA, Mason AC, Desmond RA, et al. Temporal trends (1973-1997) in survival of patients with esophageal adenocarcinoma in the United States: a glimmer of hope? Am J Gastroenterol 2003;98(7):1627–33.

15. Cameron GR, Jayasekera CS, Williams R, et al. Detection and staging of esophageal cancers within Barrett's esophagus is improved by assessment in specialized Barrett's units. Gastrointestinal endoscopy 2014;80(6):971–83.e971.

16. Chadwick G, Groene O, Markar SR, et al. Systematic review comparing radiofrequency ablation and complete endoscopic resection in treating dysplastic Barrett's esophagus: a critical assessment of histologic outcomes and adverse events. Gastrointest Endosc 2014;79(5):718–31.e3.

17. Sgourakis G, Gockel I, Lang H. Endoscopic and surgical resection of T1a/T1b esophageal neoplasms: a systematic review. World J Gastroenterol 2013;19(9): 1424–37.

18. Smith I, Kahaleh M. Endoscopic versus surgical therapy for Barrett's esophagus neoplasia. Expert Rev Gastroenterol Hepatol 2015;9(1):31–5.

19. Ell C, May A, Gossner L, et al. Endoscopic mucosal resection of early cancer and high-grade dysplasia in Barrett's esophagus. Gastroenterology 2000;118(4): 670–7.

20. Pech O, Behrens A, May A, et al. Long-term results and risk factor analysis for recurrence after curative endoscopic therapy in 349 patients with high-grade intraepithelial neoplasia and mucosal adenocarcinoma in Barrett's oesophagus. Gut 2008;57(9):1200–6.

21. Manner H, Pech O, Heldmann Y, et al. Efficacy, safety, and long-term results of endoscopic treatment for early stage adenocarcinoma of the esophagus with low-risk sm1 invasion. Clin Gastroenterol Hepatol 2013;11(6):630–5 [quiz: e45].

22. Eguchi T, Nakanishi Y, Shimoda T, et al. Histopathological criteria for additional treatment after endoscopic mucosal resection for esophageal cancer: analysis of 464 surgically resected cases. Mod Pathol 2006;19(3):475–80.

23. Tajima Y, Nakanishi Y, Ochiai A, et al. Histopathologic findings predicting lymph node metastasis and prognosis of patients with superficial esophageal carcinoma: analysis of 240 surgically resected tumors. Cancer 2000;88(6):1285–93.

24. Araki K, Ohno S, Egashira A, et al. Pathologic features of superficial esophageal squamous cell carcinoma with lymph node and distal metastasis. Cancer 2002; 94(2):570–5.

25. Shimada H, Nabeya Y, Matsubara H, et al. Prediction of lymph node status in patients with superficial esophageal carcinoma: analysis of 160 surgically resected cancers. Am J Surg 2006;191(2):250–4.

26. Kodama M, Kakegawa T. Treatment of superficial cancer of the esophagus: a summary of responses to a questionnaire on superficial cancer of the esophagus in Japan. Surgery 1998;123(4):432–9.

27. Pech O, May A, Gossner L, et al. Curative endoscopic therapy in patients with early esophageal squamous-cell carcinoma or high-grade intraepithelial neoplasia. Endoscopy 2007;39(1):30–5.

28. Ciocirlan M, Lapalus MG, Hervieu V, et al. Endoscopic mucosal resection for squamous premalignant and early malignant lesions of the esophagus. Endoscopy 2007;39(1):24–9.

29. Shaheen NJ, Falk GW, Iyer PG, et al. ACG Clinical Guideline: Diagnosis and Management of Barrett's Esophagus. Am J Gastroenterol 2016;111(1):30–50; quiz 51.

30. Haidry RJ, Dunn JM, Butt MA, et al. Radiofrequency ablation and endoscopic mucosal resection for dysplastic barrett's esophagus and early esophageal adenocarcinoma: outcomes of the UK National Halo RFA Registry. Gastroenterology 2013;145(1):87–95.

31. Shaheen NJ, Sharma P, Overholt BF, et al. Radiofrequency ablation in Barrett's esophagus with dysplasia. N Engl J Med 2009;360(22):2277–88.

32. Dunn JM, Banks MR, Oukrif D, et al. Radiofrequency ablation is effective for the treatment of high-grade dysplasia in Barrett's esophagus after failed photodynamic therapy. Endoscopy 2011;43(7):627–30.

33. Phoa KN, Pouw RE, van Vilsteren FG, et al. Remission of Barrett's esophagus with early neoplasia 5 years after radiofrequency ablation with endoscopic resection: a Netherlands cohort study. Gastroenterology 2013;145(1):96–104.

34. Garman KS, Shaheen NJ. Ablative therapies for Barrett's esophagus. Curr Gastroenterol Rep 2011;13(3):226–39.

35. Ackroyd R, Brown NJ, Davis MF, et al. Photodynamic therapy for dysplastic Barrett's oesophagus: a prospective, double blind, randomised, placebo controlled trial. Gut 2000;47(5):612–7.

36. Overholt BF, Lightdale CJ, Wang KK, et al. Photodynamic therapy with porfimer sodium for ablation of high-grade dysplasia in Barrett's esophagus: international, partially blinded, randomized phase III trial. Gastrointest Endosc 2005;62(4):488–98.

37. Johnston MH, Eastone JA, Horwhat JD, et al. Cryoablation of Barrett's esophagus: a pilot study. Gastrointest Endosc 2005;62(6):842–8.

38. Leggett CL, Gorospe EC, Wang KK. Endoscopic therapy for Barrett's esophagus and early esophageal adenocarcinoma. Gastroenterol Clin North Am 2013;42(1):175–85.

39. Dulai GS, Jensen DM, Cortina G, et al. Randomized trial of argon plasma coagulation vs. multipolar electrocoagulation for ablation of Barrett's esophagus. Gastrointest Endosc 2005;61(2):232–40.

40. Sharma P, Wani S, Weston AP, et al. A randomised controlled trial of ablation of Barrett's oesophagus with multipolar electrocoagulation versus argon plasma coagulation in combination with acid suppression: long term results. Gut 2006;55(9):1233–9.

41. Attwood SE, Lewis CJ, Caplin S, et al. Argon beam plasma coagulation as therapy for high-grade dysplasia in Barrett's esophagus. Clin Gastroenterol Hepatol 2003;1(4):258–63.

42. Hornick JL, Mino-Kenudson M, Lauwers GY, et al. Buried Barrett's epithelium following photodynamic therapy shows reduced crypt proliferation and absence of DNA content abnormalities. Am J Gastroenterol 2008;103(1):38–47.

43. Fukami N. Endoscopic submucosal dissection. 1st edition. New York: Springer; 2015.

44. Cao Y, Liao C, Tan A, et al. Meta-analysis of endoscopic submucosal dissection versus endoscopic mucosal resection for tumors of the gastrointestinal tract. Endoscopy 2009;41(9):751–7.

45. Kuwano H, Nishimura Y, Oyama T, et al. Guidelines for Diagnosis and Treatment of Carcinoma of the Esophagus April 2012 edited by the Japan Esophageal Society. Esophagus 2015;12:1–30.

46. Oka S, Tanaka S, Kaneko I, et al. Advantage of endoscopic submucosal dissection compared with EMR for early gastric cancer. Gastrointest Endosc 2006; 64(6):877–83.

47. Dunbar KB, Spechler SJ. The risk of lymph-node metastases in patients with high-grade dysplasia or intramucosal carcinoma in Barrett's esophagus: a systematic review. Am J Gastroenterol 2012;107(6):850–62 [quiz: 863].

48. Li Z, Rice TW, Liu X, et al. Intramucosal esophageal adenocarcinoma: primum non nocere. J Thorac Cardiovasc Surg 2013;145(6):1519–24.e1-3.

49. Markar SR, Karthikesalingam A, Thrumurthy S, et al. Volume-outcome relationship in surgery for esophageal malignancy: systematic review and meta-analysis 2000-2011. J Gastrointest Surg 2012;16(5):1055–63.

50. Baptista V, Singh A, Wassef W. Early gastric cancer: an update on endoscopic management. Curr Opin Gastroenterol 2012;28(6):629–35.

51. Shimizu S, Tada M, Kawai K. Early gastric cancer: its surveillance and natural course. Endoscopy 1995;27(1):27–31.

52. Everett SM, Axon AT. Early gastric cancer in Europe. Gut 1997;41(2):142–50.

53. Hirasawa T, Gotoda T, Miyata S, et al. Incidence of lymph node metastasis and the feasibility of endoscopic resection for undifferentiated-type early gastric cancer. Gastric cancer 2009;12(3):148–52.

54. Japanese gastric cancer treatment guidelines 2014 (ver. 4). Gastric cancer: official journal of the International Gastric Cancer Association and the Japanese Gastric Cancer Association 2016:1–19.

55. Manner H, Rabenstein T, May A, et al. Long-term results of endoscopic resection in early gastric cancer: the Western experience. Am J Gastroenterol 2009;104(3): 566–73.

56. Horiki N, Omata F, Uemura M, et al. Risk for local recurrence of early gastric cancer treated with piecemeal endoscopic mucosal resection during a 10-year follow-up period. Surg Endosc 2012;26(1):72–8.

57. Choi KS, Jung HY, Choi KD, et al. EMR versus gastrectomy for intramucosal gastric cancer: comparison of long-term outcomes. Gastrointest Endosc 2011; 73(5):942–8.

58. Watanabe K, Ogata S, Kawazoe S, et al. Clinical outcomes of EMR for gastric tumors: historical pilot evaluation between endoscopic submucosal dissection and conventional mucosal resection. Gastrointest Endosc 2006;63(6):776–82.

59. Tanabe S, Ishido K, Higuchi K, et al. Long-term outcomes of endoscopic submucosal dissection for early gastric cancer: a retrospective comparison with conventional endoscopic resection in a single center. Gastric cancer 2014;17(1): 130–6.

60. Isomoto H, Shikuwa S, Yamaguchi N, et al. Endoscopic submucosal dissection for early gastric cancer: a large-scale feasibility study. Gut 2009;58(3):331–6.

61. Chung IK, Lee JH, Lee SH, et al. Therapeutic outcomes in 1000 cases of endoscopic submucosal dissection for early gastric neoplasms: Korean ESD Study Group multicenter study. Gastrointest Endosc 2009;69(7):1228–35.
62. Chiu PW, Teoh AY, To KF, et al. Endoscopic submucosal dissection (ESD) compared with gastrectomy for treatment of early gastric neoplasia: a retrospective cohort study. Surg Endosc 2012;26(12):3584–91.
63. Wang S, Zhang Z, Liu M, et al. Endoscopic resection compared with gastrectomy to treat early gastric cancer: a systematic review and meta-analysis. PLoS One 2015;10(12):e0144774.

Minimally Invasive Surgery

The Emerging Role in Gastric Cancer

Michael R. Cassidy, MD[a,1], Sepideh Gholami, MD[a,1], Vivian E. Strong, MD[b,*]

KEYWORDS

- Gastric cancer • Laparoscopic gastrectomy • Robotic gastrectomy
- Minimally invasive gastrectomy

KEY POINTS

- Minimally invasive approaches to the treatment of gastric cancer are emerging as a preferred option for well-selected patients.
- Appropriate patient selection is important.
- Minimally invasive techniques allow for decreased blood loss, less pain, and enhanced recovery.
- Laparoscopic and robotic approaches can provide equivalent oncologic outcomes when compared with open gastrectomy.
- Most data on minimally invasive gastrectomy come from Eastern countries, but the Western experience is growing.

INTRODUCTION

Although gastric cancer is less common in the United States than in other areas of the world, it remains an important contributor to cancer death and is associated with worse survival than in Eastern countries.[1] In 2012, there were an estimated 951,600 new diagnoses of gastric cancer and 723,100 deaths due to gastric cancer worldwide.[2] The overall incidence of gastric cancer in the United States is increasing from 22,000 to 25,000 new cases per year, with a particular increase in incidence of gastroesophageal junction and gastric cardia tumors. Additionally, in the young population of 25 to 39 year olds, the United States has seen a 70% increase in noncardia gastric cancer over the past several years.[3] Moreover, gastric cancer may manifest in a variety of histologic, anatomic, and genetic patterns, which influences the surgical approach and requires a customized and multimodality treatment plan for each

The authors have nothing to disclose.
[a] Department of Surgery, Memorial Sloan Kettering Cancer Center, 1275 York Avenue, C-1272, New York, NY 10065, USA; [b] Gastric and Mixed Tumor Service, Department of Surgery, Memorial Sloan Kettering Cancer Center, 1275 York Avenue, H-1217, New York, NY 10065, USA
[1] Contributed equally to this work.
* Corresponding author.
E-mail address: strongv@mskcc.org

Surg Oncol Clin N Am 26 (2017) 193–212
http://dx.doi.org/10.1016/j.soc.2016.10.001

patient. Gastrectomy with curative intent remains the only treatment that can offer potential for cure in gastric cancer patients. Over the past 20 years, minimally invasive techniques have emerged that enhance the surgical armamentarium of approaches to both complete gastric cancer staging and curative resection. Multiple randomized trials comparing laparoscopic to open gastrectomy have proved oncologic equivalency of the 2 approaches and have demonstrated favorable outcomes in postoperative recovery with minimally invasive approaches.[4-9] As a result, minimally invasive surgery is emerging as a preferred option in the treatment of well-selected gastric cancer patients. As knowledge grows regarding the conduct and outcomes of robotic-assisted approaches, this new technique is being adopted both in the United States and elsewhere, with favorable outcomes in retrospective series. This article discusses the emerging role of both laparoscopic and robot-assisted approaches to gastric cancer management.

THE ROLE OF DIAGNOSTIC LAPAROSCOPY AND PERITONEAL WASHING CYTOLOGY

Laparoscopy has emerged as an important staging modality for locally advanced gastric cancer. Patients who are found to have T3 or greater disease or node-positive disease, by CT scan and/or endoscopic ultrasonography (EUS), benefit from staging laparoscopy because the findings may alter the management strategy and treatment intent in a significant proportion of patients.

In a study of 657 patients at Memorial Sloan Kettering Cancer Center (MSKCC), diagnostic laparoscopy was performed for patients with gastric adenocarcinoma and staging CT scans showing no definitive evidence of metastatic disease. In the entire study population, visible peritoneal metastases were identified in 31% of patients, suggesting a high incidence of radiographically occult metastatic disease.[10] Clinicopathologic predictors of identifying radiographically occult peritoneal metastases were location of the tumor at the gastroesophageal junction or involving the entire stomach, poor differentiation on histology, and age less than or equal to 70 years. Imaging predictors of identifying peritoneal metastases at laparoscopy were lymphadenopathy greater than 1 cm and T3/T4 tumors. EUS may also be used to stratify risk for radiographically occult metastatic disease. EUS findings in 94 patients were correlated with their diagnostic laparoscopy results in a retrospective study that identified patients as high risk when EUS showed T3, T4, and/or N1 disease; all others were considered low risk. The high-risk group had a 25% likelihood of peritoneal metastatic disease compared with 4% in the low-risk group.[11] Because peritoneal metastatic disease changes treatment intent from curative to palliative, diagnostic laparoscopy, therefore, can alter the goals of therapy in a large proportion of patients considered to have locally advanced disease at presentation.

Diagnostic laparoscopy additionally provides the opportunity to collect peritoneal washings for cytology, in the absence of visible peritoneal disease. Several studies have demonstrated that the presence of cancer cells in peritoneal washings of gastric cancer patients is a significant predictor of mortality from the disease. In a study of 1297 patients with gastric cancer who underwent peritoneal lavage, the population with positive cytology had a 5-year survival rate of only 2%.[12] At MSKCC, in a study of 371 patients who underwent R0 resection for gastric cancer, those who had positive peritoneal cytology had a significantly reduced median survival of 14.8 months compared with 98.5 months in those with negative cytology. In multivariate analysis, positive cytology was the strongest predictor of death from gastric cancer.[13] Other studies have also convincingly demonstrated reduced survival in those with positive peritoneal cytology.[14-17] Owing to this evidence, positive peritoneal cytology is considered metastatic (M1) disease according to the American Joint Committee on Cancer staging system. As such, laparoscopy plays a vital role in the staging of gastric cancer patients.

SELECTIVE USE OF LAPAROSCOPIC APPROACHES

Appropriate selection of patients and optimal technical approach are paramount for good outcomes and require deep understanding of gastric cancer and the underlying differences in biological behavior and natural history of diffuse and intestinal types of the disease. Thin patients with few comorbidities and early cancers are the most ideal patients for a laparoscopic approach. As the learning curve progresses and the surgeon's understanding of the biological behavior of the disease matures, indications may be broadened.

As with any novel surgical approach and technique, a relative contraindication includes technical expertise of the surgeon and experience. It is crucial to keep in mind that the primary goal is to provide an oncologically equivalent operation via the minimally invasive approach. For a surgeon who is early in his or her learning curve, relative contraindications include patients with a high body mass index and more advanced tumors that require possible en bloc resection of associated invading organs and structures. Patients with comorbidities, including severe pulmonary or cardiac disease, may benefit from a shorter anesthetic time and thus an open approach. Lastly, patients with multiple previous abdominal operations or extensive adhesions as well as those who have completed neoadjuvant therapy may have more technically complicated cases and should therefore be selected judiciously.

OUTCOMES OF LAPAROSCOPIC GASTRECTOMY

A large volume of research regarding outcomes for the laparoscopic approach compared with the open approach has been published since the first report by Kitano and colleagues[18] in 1994. Given the increased incidence of early gastric cancer in East Asia, the Eastern experience with laparoscopic gastrectomy has been more robust than in the United States, where laparoscopic approaches for gastric cancer have been more slowly accepted. Given different results comparing outcomes of gastric cancer surgery in the East and the West as well as differing epidemiology of cases, Eastern-derived data should be extrapolated cautiously with regard to Western patients.[1] Table 1 lists the major findings of several recent randomized trials of laparoscopic compared with open gastrectomy.

Perioperative Factors

In a recent meta-analysis of 7 randomized controlled trials totaling 390 patients comparing laparoscopic versus open distal gastrectomies, the laparoscopic approach was found to have longer operative time but was also associated with less blood loss, fewer analgesics administered, faster recovery, and shorter postoperative hospital stay.[19] Similar findings have been reported by Viñuela and colleagues[20] looking at various factors comparing the laparoscopic and open approaches. Specifically, operative time was found on average 48 minutes longer via the laparoscopic approach compared with the open procedure. Some studies suggest this difference is related to learning curve issues. This study also found operative blood loss lower for the laparoscopic approach.

Multiple other retrospective series as well as randomized controlled trials have demonstrated less postoperative pain and postoperative ileus, earlier oral intake

Table 1
Recent randomized clinical trials of laparoscopic versus open gastrectomy for the treatment of gastric cancer

Study, Year	Eligibility	Procedure	Lymph Node Dissection Extent	Number of Patients	Operative Time Less	Blood Loss Less	Number of Lymph Nodes Retrieved	Hospital Stay	Morbidity	Mortality
Kitano et al,[5] 2002	cT1	LADG/ODG	NR	14/14	ODG	LADG	Equivalent	Equivalent	Equivalent	Equivalent
Fujii et al,[41] 2003	cT1	LADG/ODG	NR	10/10	ODG	Equivalent	NR	NR	Equivalent	Equivalent
Hayashi et al,[21] 2005	cT1	LADG/ODG	NR	14/14	ODG	Equivalent	Equivalent	LADG	NR	Equivalent
Huscher et al,[7] 2005	cT1-4 N0-2	TLGD/ODG	D1, D2	30/29	Equivalent	TLGD	Equivalent	TLGD	Equivalent	Equivalent
Lee et al,[6] 2005	cT1	LADG/ODG	D2	24/23	ODG	Equivalent	Equivalent	Equivalent	LADG	NR
Kim et al,[8] 2008	cT1 N0-1	LADG/ODG	D1, D2	82/82	ODG	LADG	ODG	LADG	NR	NR
Kim et al,[9] 2010	cT1-2N0-1	LADG/ODG	D1, D2	179/163	ODG	LADG	NR	NR	Equivalent	Equivalent
Cai et al,[36] 2011	cT2-3	LAG/OG	D2	49/47	OG	Equivalent	Equivalent	Equivalent	Equivalent	NR
Sakuramoto et al,[37] 2013	cT1	LADG/ODG	D1	31/32	ODG	LADG	Equivalent	Equivalent	Equivalent	NR
Takiguchi et al,[72] 2013	cTNMI	LADG/ODG	D1, D2	20/20	ODG	LADG	Equivalent	LADG	NR	NR
Aoyama et al,[73] 2014	cTNMI	LADG/ODG	D1, D2	13/13	ODG	LADG	Equivalent	NR	Equivalent	Equivalent

Abbreviations: LADG, laparoscopic-assisted distal gastrectomy; LAG, laparoscopic-assisted gastrectomy; NR, not reported; ODG, open distal gastrectomy; OG, open gastrectomy; TLDG, totally laparoscopic distal gastrectomy.

From Son T, Hyung WJ. Laparoscopic gastric cancer surgery: current evidence and future perspectives. World J Gastroenterol 2016;22(2):731; with permission.

and ambulation, and better postoperative respiratory function in favor of the laparo-scopic group.[5,21–29]

Length of stay has been reported lower in many Western series; however, this finding is more likely correlated to differences in practice patterns comparing Western and Eastern countries. In the recent meta-analysis,[21] discussed previously, the investigators analyzed this outcome and found that hospital stay was significantly reduced by more than 3 days after laparoscopic distal gastrectomy compared with the conventional open procedure.

Postoperative Morbidity and Mortality

The 30-day postoperative complication rates of laparoscopic gastrectomy have been reported to range between 10% and 20% in Eastern country studies[9,30] whereas studies from Western countries have demonstrated a slightly higher morbidity rate (20% to 30%).[7,22] Possible explanations include an older cohort of patients with increased comorbidities in Western countries. In a recent updated meta-analysis of 14 randomized controlled trials, which compared safety and efficacy of laparoscopic gastrectomy with open gastrectomy for resectable gastric cancer totaling 2307 patients (1163 in laparoscopic and 1144 in open), laparoscopic gastrectomy was associated with decreased blood loss, length of hospital stay, and overall postoperative morbidity and improved postsurgical recovery. In addition, the laparoscopic group demonstrated accelerated time to first flatus, first walking, and oral intake as well as reduced frequency of analgesic administration. No significant difference in number of retrieved lymph nodes, mortality, recurrence, or long-term overall survival and disease-free survival was observed.[31]

Perioperative Complications

Unexpected intraoperative events are usually the major reason for conversion from a laparoscopic to an open procedure. Most of these are associated by direct handling of organs with retractors and dissection devices.[32] To prevent a catastrophic outcome, it is crucial that the surgical team is aware of these potential issues and prepared for immediate conversion to an open procedure without any delays if such an incident occurs. Factors, such as higher body mass index and more extensive lymphadenectomies, have been described as associated with a higher risk of intraoperative events.

These complications are in general rare. Most conversions to an open procedure are related to bleeding events. One retrospective study from Korea calculated a 2.6% rate of intraoperative complications; 56% were bleeding events, all requiring conversion to open surgery.[33] In the meta-analysis by Viñuela and colleagues,[20] 63% of the conversions to open gastrectomy were due to intraoperative bleeding. The right gastroepiploic vessels during the dissection of the infrapyloric area and common hepatic and splenic arteries during lymphadenectomy are the most common sources of bleeding reported.[32,33] Another reason for conversion is suspected injuries to the pancreas while performing lymph node dissection or lacerations of the distal esophagus during laparoscopic total gastrectomy.

Approximately 1% of patients experience postoperative hemorrhage after laparoscopic gastrectomy.[9] Most of the time, bleeding from staple or suture lines can be managed nonoperatively. For any laparoscopic procedure, bleeding from the port sites must be considered, in particular the specimen extraction site. Postoperative pseudoaneurysms are rare events in both open and laparoscopic approaches; however, they can be sources of major bleeding and sometimes only confirmed by angiography. In such cases, the treatment of choice is selective embolization in general but the surgeon should also have a low threshold for re-exploration if clinically indicated.

Wound complications in the laparoscopic setting are uncommon and occur in approximately 2% of patients. The extraction site is the wound most frequently affected by an infection. As with any surgical procedure, administration of appropriate preoperative antibiotics is recommended. To decrease further potential contamination, preventive measures can be used, including using an extraction bag for the specimen and wound protective sheaths.

Across the literature, incisional hernia rates have been reported less frequent for patients undergoing a laparoscopic approach compared with open techniques. In a systemic review and meta-analysis, Kössler-Ebs and colleagues[34] evaluated 24 randomized controlled trials with 3490 patients comparing incisional hernia rates after laparoscopic versus open abdominal surgery. In their analysis, incisional hernias were significantly reduced in the laparoscopic group (4.3%) compared with the open group (10.1%, $P = .0002$). Moreover, laparoscopically assisted procedures did not show a significant reduction of incisional hernias compared with open surgery.

In the authors' experience, adequate technique of fascial closure is the single most important preventive measure to avoid port-site hernias. Closure of the larger port sites (>12 mm) using a fascia closure device is recommended.

Long-term Complications and Outcomes

As discussed previously, the safety of laparoscopic gastrectomy has been well established in the literature. Okabe and colleagues[35] most recently evaluated various surgical techniques for laparoscopic esophagojejunostomy and established that there was no superiority of any particular method (circular or linear staplers). The incidence of anastomosis-related complications varied among studies and the overall complication rate of laparoscopic gastrectomy was similar to that of the open procedure.

Similar findings have been described regarding the effectiveness and oncologic results of the laparoscopic technique. In a recent review by Son and colleagues, cumulative results from multiple trials did not show significant differences in terms of survival rate or recurrence after surgery based on long-term follow-up evaluation. Although multiple trials and review articles have shown that the number of lymph nodes retrieved were equivalent in the 2 groups,[36–39] some studies have demonstrated a higher lymph node count. The clinical significance of that difference remains unclear, however, given the same oncologic and survival outcomes.

As reported by the authors' recent meta-analysis, postoperative mortality after laparoscopic gastrectomy is less than 1% and comparable after the open technique. This has been confirmed by various other studies.[5,9,21,40,41] Moreover, the authors demonstrated in a meta-analysis that the odds of developing serious complications after laparoscopic gastrectomy were observed similar to that of the open procedure.[31] Major features of the surgical procedure that encompass the main source of possible postoperative morbidity (extent of gastric resection, lymphadenectomy, and reconstruction) have all been described as similar in both techniques.

One long-term complication that has been reported as slightly different is potential for reduced incidence of adhesive ileus after a laparoscopic approach. This finding has been attributed to the less inflammatory and immunologic peritoneal reaction induced by laparoscopic surgery.[42,43] A recent systematic study of more than 400,000 patients followed after abdominal surgery demonstrated an incidence of bowel obstruction for cholecystectomy, gynecologic procedures, and colorectal surgery.[44] These results can likely be extrapolated to other laparoscopically performed abdominal procedures, including gastrectomies. A reduced incidence of obstructive adhesions associated with laparoscopic gastrectomy specifically has also been reported in a few smaller comparative studies, although the evidence is still somewhat controversial.

QUALITY OF LIFE

Minimally invasive techniques have been applied with the goal of enhanced recovery and improved quality of life for patients. True quality of life is challenging to measure and report and is influenced by many factors, both objective and subjective. The quality of life after gastrectomy may further be influenced by the extent of resection, incidence of complications, or disease recurrence, which may not vary with the approach used. There is, however, evidence of improvements in quality of life when minimally invasive approaches are applied to selected patients. A randomized controlled trial performed in South Korea assessed quality of life in patients with early gastric cancer randomized to either open or laparoscopic distal gastrectomy.[8] Validated questionnaires were administered up to 3 months after surgery. In the laparoscopic arm, quality-of-life scores were better in multiple domains, including physical, emotional, social, and global. Pain, sleep, appetite, diet, and body image were also improved with laparoscopic resection compared with open gastrectomy.

TECHNICAL CONSIDERATIONS FOR LAPAROSCOPIC GASTRECTOMY

The technique of laparoscopic gastrectomy has been well described.[18,22,32] The patient is placed supine on the operating table. Pneumoperitoneum can be established in the standard fashion, either by Veress needle or Hasson technique. In general, 5 ports are used, with a 12-mm trocar in the right upper quadrant 4 additional 5-mm trocars as shown in Fig. 1. The patient should be placed in steep reverse Trendelenburg position, which may be safely done with the use of a footboard on the bed. Energy

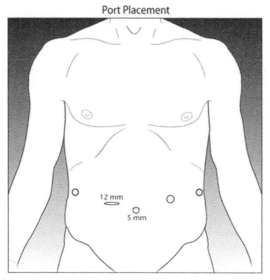

Fig. 1. Surgical field and trocar placement for laparoscopic gastrectomy. (*From* Strong VE, Devaud N, Allen PJ, et al. Laparoscopic versus open subtotal gastrectomy for adenocarcinoma: a case-control study. Ann Surg Oncol 2009;16(6):1509; with permission.)

sealing devices may be used to facilitate the dissection. Linear staplers introduced via the 12-mm port may be used to divide the bowel, stomach, or esophagus, as dictated by the anatomic location of the tumor.

Reconstruction of gastrointestinal continuity may be established using a variety of techniques.[35] These include both intracorporeal hand-sewn anastomoses, which may be technically challenging, and stapler devices. In particular, an esophagojejunostomy may be created either with linear staplers or by using a transoral anvil device and circular stapler.[45] Gastrojejunostomy and jejunojejunostomy, if Roux-en-Y reconstruction is chosen, are readily performed with a linear dividing stapler. Intracorporeal hand-sewn closure of the anastomotic gap left by the stapler is typically performed.

LEARNING CURVE FOR LAPAROSCOPIC GASTRECTOMY

Many factors influence the learning curve for laparoscopic gastrectomy. The technical challenges of laparoscopic gastrectomy, although real, are only 1 consideration. Surgeon training, experience, and volume may affect the time to proficiency, and hospital support for and experience with laparoscopic surgery programs may also influence the learning curve. Additionally, the different types of gastric resection, ranging from distal gastrectomy to total gastrectomy, pose a range of technical challenges. For example, a stapled gastrojejunostomy is less technically demanding than esophagojejunostomy.

Few publications address the learning curve for laparoscopic gastrectomy in a systematic way. Furthermore, most of the literature has been generated in Eastern countries, where the incidence of gastric cancer is greater than in the United States. One study reported the outcomes of the first series of laparoscopic distal gastrectomies performed by a single surgeon in South Korea who previously had extensive experience with open gastrectomy[46]; 177 patients with early gastric cancer undergoing distal gastrectomy were included in the study, with 102 in the laparoscopic group and 71 in the open group. The laparoscopic cases were divided into early (n = 50) and late (n = 52) groups. In the late group, mean operative time was shorter than in the early group (190 vs 230 minutes) and mean lymph node retrieval was greater (30 vs 45 nodes). The open group had the fastest mean operative time (154 minutes) and the greatest mean lymph node retrieval of 38 nodes.

Another series of 100 patients who underwent laparoscopic gastrectomy was divided into 5 groups of 20 patients according to the surgeon's level of experience.[47] For surgeons with laparoscopic experience of more than 60 cases, there were no conversions to open and the operative time approached that of a comparison group of 67 open gastrectomies (227 vs 232 minutes). Hospital length of stay was also shorter for surgeons with experience of at least 60 cases. Blood loss was decreased after an experience of 20 cases.

Similar studies also suggest a learning curve to proficiency of approximately 50 to 60 laparoscopic gastrectomies. These studies, however, included only early gastric cancers in selected patients.[48–50] The learning curve may be more difficult to overcome in unselected patients with advanced disease, in particular those requiring extended lymphadenectomy.[49] Surgeons should be aware of their level of proficiency when selecting patients for minimally invasive approaches. The learning curve for robotic-assisted gastrectomy may require fewer cases to achieve proficiency (discussed later).

ROBOTIC-ASSISTED GASTRECTOMY

Robotic-assisted gastrectomy is the newest approach to curative-intent gastric surgery. Use of the robotic platform for gastric cancer treatment was first described in

2003,[51,52] with the first report from the United States appearing in 2007.[53] In addition to the advantages of general minimally invasive techniques, including reduced hospital lengths of stay and postoperative discomfort, the robotic approach has technical advantages over traditional laparoscopic surgery. The robotic camera provides 3-D visualization and magnification that aid in fine dissection during gastrectomy. Articulating instruments provide much-improved dexterity and finer control, which is advantageous for precision.

SELECTIVE USE OF ROBOT-ASSISTED APPROACHES

Although robot-assisted gastrectomy may offer many advantages to both open and laparoscopic approaches, thoughtful patient selection is vital. In particular, robotic-assisted gastrectomy has the longest operative times of the 3 approaches,[54] and the increased duration of anesthetic must be considered when selecting patients. This is especially true early in a surgeon's learning curve, when operative times may be significantly longer. Patients with significant cardiopulmonary or other serious comorbidities are potentially poor candidates. Morbid obesity or dense intra-abdominal adhesions can create difficulties with safe visualization and technical performance of the operation. Large tumors, and those with known invasion into adjacent organs, may limit the utility of robotic approaches. With gastric cancer of diffuse histology, the proximal and distal extent of the tumor is difficult to predict preoperatively, and, therefore, tactile feedback during the operation plays a more important role in achieving an oncologically appropriate resection in confirming grossly normal tissue by palpation.

Therefore, ideal candidates for robotic-assisted gastrectomy early in a surgeon's experience are those with minimal medical problems, low body mass index, and small intestinal type tumors. There are no absolute contraindications for robotic-assisted gastrectomy, however, and inclusion criteria can be expanded as experience with the approach increases.

Patients with hereditary diffuse gastric cancer syndrome associated with CDH1 mutation are candidates for prophylactic total gastrectomy. These patients are typically excellent candidates for the robotic approach. Although these patients often have foci of high-grade dysplasia or intramucosal carcinoma in the specimen, this prophylactic operation requires only a D1 lymphadenectomy at most. Importantly, the proximal and distal margins of the specimen must be confirmed free of gastric mucosa by intraoperative frozen section, but this does not limit the applicability of the robotic approach.

Institutional experience with robotic techniques is another important consideration. To conduct safe robotic surgery at any anatomic site, all team members in the operating room, including the nursing and technical staff, must be familiar with the setup, instrumentation, safety procedures, and emergency plans unique to the approach. Institutional support for personnel and training is a critical component.

OUTCOMES OF ROBOTIC-ASSISTED GASTRECTOMY

Many retrospective series and nonrandomized prospective studies have been published regarding robotic-assisted gastrectomy.[51–53,55–61] **Table 2** shows the major findings of many series. A recent meta-analysis compares short-term outcomes in robotic, laparoscopic, and open gastrectomy.[62] Based on 7 studies that include a total of 1967 patients, robotic-assisted gastrectomy was associated with shorter hospital length of stay by a mean of 2.92 days when compared with open gastrectomy but longer operative time by a mean of 95 minutes. Blood loss was less in the

Table 2
Summary of nonrandomized clinical trials comparing robotic, laparoscopic, and open gastrectomy

Reference, Year	Study Design	Type of Approach	Type of Surgery (Total Gastrectomy/Subtotal Gastrectomy)	Operative Time (minutes)	Estimated Blood Loss (mL)	Retrieval No. of Lymph Nodes	Conversion (%)	Morbidity (%)	Mortality (%)
Pugliese et al,[74] 2010	Nonrandomized	R 18	0/18	344	90	25	2	6	6.2
	Retrospective	L 52	0/52	235	148	31	3	12.5	2
Kim et al,[75] 2009	Nonrandomized	R 16	0/16	259.2	30.3	41.1	0	0	0
	Retrospective	L 11	0/11	203.9	44.7	37.4	0	9	0
		O 12	0/12	126.7	78.8	43.3	—	16	—
Caruso et al,[76] 2011	Nonrandomized	R 29	12/17	290	197.6	28.0	—	41.4	0
	Retrospective	O 120	37/83	222	386.1	31.7	—	42.5	3.3
Woo et al,[77] 2011	Nonrandomized	R 236	62/172	219.5	91.6	39.0	0	11	0.3
	Retrospective	L 591	108/481	170.7	147.9	37.4	0	13.7	0.4
Eom et al,[78] 2012	Nonrandomized	R 30	0/30	229.1	152.8	30.2	0	13	0
	Retrospective	L 62	0/62	189.4	88.3	33.4	0	6	0
Kang et al,[79] 2012	Nonrandomized	R 100	16/84	202	93.2	—	—	14.0	0
	Retrospective	L 282	37/245	173	173.4	—	—	10.3	0
Yoon et al,[80] 2012	Nonrandomized	R 36	36/0	305.8	214.2	42.8	0	16.7	0
	Retrospective	L 65	65/0	210.2	150.3	39.4	0	15.4	0
Huang et al,[70] 2012	Nonrandomized	R 39	7/32	430	50	32	—	15.4	—
	Retrospective	L 64	7/57	350	100	26	—	15.6	—
		O 586	179/407	320	400	34	—	14.7	—
Kim et al,[81] 2012	Nonrandomized	R 436	109/327	226	85	40.2	—	10.1	0.5
	Retrospective	L 861	158/703	176	112	37.6	—	9.4	0.3
		O 4542	1232/3309	158	192	40.5	—	10.7	0.5

Study	Type	R/L								
Park et al,[82] 2012	Nonrandomized Prospective	R 30	0/30	218	75	34	0	5	0
		L 120	0/120	140	60	35	0	9	0
Uyama et al,[83] 2012	Nonrandomized Retrospective	R 25	0/25	361	51.8	44.3	0	11.2	0
		L 225	0/225	345	81.0	43.2	0	16.9	0
Hyun et al,[84] 2012	Nonrandomized Retrospective	R 38	9/29	234.4	131.3	32.8	0	47.3	0
		L 83	18/65	220.0	130.5	32.6	0	38.5	0
Suda et al,[85] 2014	Nonrandomized Retrospective	R 88	30/58	381	46	40	0	2.3	1.1
		L 438	136/302	361	34	38	0	11.4	0.2
Son et al,[86] 2014	Nonrandomized Retrospective	R 51	51/0	264.1	163.4	47.2	0	15.7	2.0
		L 58	58/0	210.3	210.7	42.8	—	22.4	0
Noshiro et al,[87] 2014	Nonrandomized Retrospective	R 21	0/21	439	96	44	0	9.5	0
		L 161	0/160	315	115	40	0	10.0	0
Junfeng et al,[88] 2014	Nonrandomized Retrospective	R 120	26/92 (PG:2)	234.8	118.3	34.6	0	5.8	—
		L 394	118/261 (PG:15)	221.3	137.6	32.7	0	4.3	—
Huang et al,[89] 2014	Nonrandomized Retrospective	R 72	8/64	357.9	79.6	30.6	—	12.5	1.4
		L 73	10/63	319.8	116.0	28.1	—	—	—

Abbreviations: L, laparoscopic gastrectomy; O, open gastrectomy; PG, proximal subtotal gastrectomy; R, robotic gastrectomy.

From Obama K, Sakai Y. Current status of robotic gastrectomy for gastric cancer. Surg Today 2016;46(5):530; with permission.

robotic-assisted group but not significantly so. Number of lymph nodes harvested was similar, as were overall complications. Compared with laparoscopic gastrectomy, robotic-assisted gastrectomy was associated with significantly less intraoperative blood loss but longer operative times. Length of stay was equivalent between the 2 minimally invasive approaches. Morbidity seems equivalent regardless of approach as does lymph node retrieval.

Nakauchi and colleagues[63] compared long-term oncologic outcomes between robotic-assisted gastrectomy and laparoscopic gastrectomy in 521 consecutive patients. At a single institution, 84 patients underwent robotic-assisted gastrectomy and 437 patients underwent laparoscopic gastrectomy between 2009 and 2012; 3-year overall survival and 3-year recurrence-free survival were identical between the 2 nonrandomized groups. Among patients who developed recurrence, the most common site of recurrence was peritoneal, occurring in 7.1% of those who underwent robotic gastrectomy and 7.6% of those who underwent laparoscopic gastrectomy. There were no local or regional lymph node recurrences in the robotic gastrectomy group, whereas in the laparoscopic group 1 patient had local recurrence and 1 patient had regional lymph node recurrence. The investigators also compared outcomes between surgeons considered "expert" (those with extensive experience in minimally invasive surgery) and those considered "nonexpert" (all others). Long-term oncologic outcomes were equivalent as were short-term complications.

POSTOPERATIVE COMPLICATIONS WITH ROBOTIC-ASSISTED GASTRECTOMY

The potential complications of robotic-assisted gastrectomy mirror those of traditional open gastrectomy and laparoscopic gastrectomy.[62–64] Specifically, in a multicenter prospective study, the incidence of overall complications in 223 patients undergoing robotic gastrectomy was 11.9% and similar to a laparoscopic comparison group.[64] Major complications occurred in 1.1% of the robotic group. Anastomotic leak occurred in 1.1%, fluid collection in 2.2%, ileus in 1.6%, intraluminal bleeding in 0.5%, intra-abdominal bleeding in 0.5%, obstruction in 0.5%, and anastomotic stenosis in 0.5%.

COST

The cost associated with robotic-assisted gastrectomy is not frequently reported. Robotic surgery in general is more expensive than laparoscopic and open surgery.[65,66] In a multicenter prospective study of robotic versus laparoscopic gastrectomy, total hospital cost was considered.[64] Although performed in the Korean health care system, a conversion to US dollars was used. The cost for robotic-assisted gastrectomy was estimated at $13,432, whereas the laparoscopic approached was estimated to cost $8090. Although the absolute values are difficult to interpret in the context of the complex US health care system, it is likely that robotic-assisted approaches will continue to be more expensive than the other surgical options. If this upfront cost is associated with more precise operation and fewer complications as a result, however, then long-term costs and outcomes may be favorable. These are issues that have not yet been resolved.

TECHNICAL CONSIDERATIONS

In positioning a patient for robotic gastrectomy, the arms may either be tucked at the patient's side or outstretched on arm boards, with appropriate padding of pressure points in either position (Fig. 2). As with laparoscopic gastric surgery, the patient must be placed in steep reverse Trendelenburg position with an angle of at least 45°. A footboard is

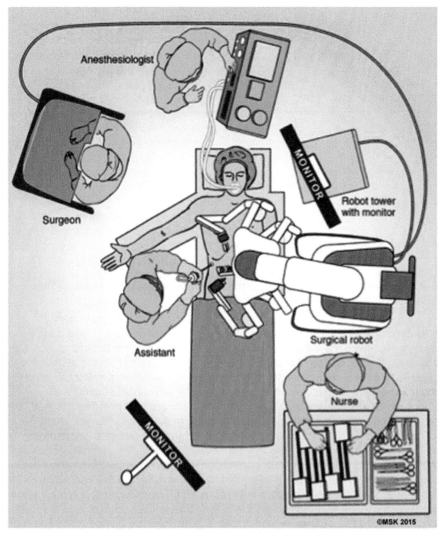

Fig. 2. Position for a patient undergoing robotic total gastrectomy. The operation is generally performed in steep reverse Trendelenburg position and the patient must be positioned prior to docking the robot. (Copyright ©2015, Memorial Sloan Kettering Cancer Center.)

commonly used, and the patient must be adequately secured to the table at the knees, hips, and shoulders. An important distinction between robotic-assisted and laparoscopic approaches is the inability to reposition the patient once the robot is docked; therefore, meticulous attention to position is required before the robot can be deployed.

Port placement is of critical importance. Although there may be several variations in appropriate port placement, in general the camera port should be 15 cm to 20 cm from the stomach. Additional ports are placed as shown in Fig. 3. The ports should be a minimum of 8 cm apart.

Pneumoperitoneum is initiated via Veress needle in the left upper quadrant or via the umbilical port site or another port site after placement. The remaining ports are placed

Port Placement

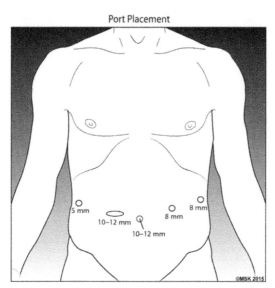

Fig. 3. Port placement for robotic total gastrectomy. (Copyright ©2015, Memorial Sloan Kettering Cancer Center.)

under direct visualization with the laparoscope. In addition to the umbilical port, 8-mm ports are placed on the left side at the midclavicular line and the anterior axillary line, as shown in **Fig. 3**. On the right side, a 10-mm to 12-mm port is placed at the midclavicular line and a 5-mm assistant port is placed at the anterior axillary line. A liver retractor can be deployed via a left upper quadrant subxiphoid stab incision.

Once adequate pneumoperitoneum and port access has been established, the abdomen should be explored laparoscopically to make an assessment of the technical and oncologic feasibility of proceeding with robotic-assisted gastrectomy. In the absence of prohibitive intra-abdominal adhesions and radiographically occult peritoneal disease, robotic surgery may commence. A judgment should be made if the tumor is found unexpectedly locally advanced as to whether or not it is resectable via the robotic approach. If proceeding, the patient should be placed in step reverse Trendelenburg position, as previously discussed. The robot is then docked, and the instruments deployed. In general, a fenestrated bipolar forceps, grasping forceps, and monopolar scissors or an energy sealing device are useful instruments.

Once the setup is achieved, the standard steps of gastrectomy are carried out via the robotic approach. Vessels can be ligated and divided using the energy sealing device. The proximal duodenum can be divided with a linear stapler introduced via the 10-mm to 12-mm port. The stomach can be divided in a similar fashion once the oncologically appropriate location is determined. The specimen is placed in a specimen bag and reconstruction can begin in the desired fashion.

Options for reconstruction of gastrointestinal continuity vary depending on type of gastrectomy and anatomic considerations. Linear staplers may be used for gastrojejunostomy, esophagojejunostomy, and/or jejunojejunostomy, if Roux-en-Y reconstruction is performed. A transoral anvil device is another option for esophagojejunostomy after total gastrectomy.[45] As a benefit of articulating robotic instruments, hand-sewn anastomoses may also be considered. A randomized trial of intracorporeal robotic-sewn anastomosis compared with standard open hand-sewn anastomosis was reported by Wang and colleagues[67]; 311 patients were randomized and were well matched. The incidence anastomotic leak was similar between the groups. Other reported complications, including surgical site infection, postoperative bleeding, abscess, and pneumonia were also similar between groups. As reported in other studies, the number of lymph nodes harvested was the same, and although duration of operation was longer in the robotic group, hospital length of stay was shorter. Blood loss was less in the robotic group. This study demonstrates that experienced surgeons can achieve excellent technical results with robotic-assisted gastric surgery.

As discussed previously, lymph node yield has been shown in several studies to be similar, regardless of the operative approach.[62] D2 lymphadenectomy is feasible with the robotic approach[55] and may be technically easier than with the laparoscopic approach, given the advanced articulation available with robotic instruments.[68]

As with any minimally invasive approach, appropriate threshold for conversion to open must be based on the level of proficiency and the clinical judgment of the operating surgeon. The operating room team should be oriented to standardized procedure in the event that the operation must be emergently converted, and roles of each team member should be specified in advance during the time-out.

LEARNING CURVE FOR ROBOTIC GASTRECTOMY

There is evidence to suggest that surgeons may more quickly become proficient with robotic-assisted gastrectomy than with laparoscopic gastrectomy. A comparison of outcomes from 20 early-experience laparoscopic gastrectomies compared with 20 late-experience laparoscopic gastrectomies and 20 robotic gastrectomies by a single surgeon showed that early-phase robotic gastrectomies had similar outcomes to late-phase laparoscopic gastrectomies. In particular, early-phase robotic operations had better outcomes in terms of blood loss, hospital length of stay, initiation of diet, and lymph node yield than did early-phase laparoscopic gastrectomies.[69] The learning curve for robotic surgery is facilitated by preexisting comfort with laparoscopic techniques. Other reports, although based on patient cohorts not matched for clinicopathologic characteristics, nevertheless suggest a learning curve to proficiency of approximately 20 to 25 robotic-assisted gastrectomies in surgeons already proficient with advanced laparoscopy.[70,71]

SUMMARY

Minimally invasive techniques are emerging as a preferred approach in the treatment of well-selected patients with gastric cancer and have a role in definitive staging, curative resection, and lymphadenectomy. Although these approaches require careful patient selection, especially in the early stages of a surgeon's learning curve, there are advantages for the patient. These include less intraoperative blood loss, faster recovery time, decreased hospital length of stay, and reduced pain. Complications are considered to occur with equal frequency compared with open techniques. It has become clear that laparoscopic and robotic-assisted gastrectomy provide equivalent surgical and oncologic outcomes in patients selected for this approach, especially in patients with early disease. Over time, as data are generated on the application of minimally invasive techniques to those with more advanced disease, the indications are likely to expand.

REFERENCES

1. Strong VE, Song KY, Park CH, et al. Comparison of gastric cancer survival following R0 resection in the United States and Korea using an internationally validated nomogram. Ann Surg 2010;251(4):640–6.

2. Torre LA, Bray F, Siegel RL, et al. Global cancer statistics, 2012. CA Cancer J Clin 2015;65(2):87–108.

3. Anderson WF, Camargo MC, Fraumeni JF, et al. Age-specific trends in incidence of noncardia gastric cancer in US adults. JAMA 2010;303(17):1723–8.

4. Kim W, Kim H-H, Han S-U, et al. Decreased morbidity of laparoscopic distal gastrectomy compared with open distal gastrectomy for stage i gastric cancer: short-term outcomes from a multicenter randomized controlled trial (KLASS-01). Ann Surg 2016;263(1):28–35.

5. Kitano S, Shiraishi N, Fujii K, et al. A randomized controlled trial comparing open vs laparoscopy-assisted distal gastrectomy for the treatment of early gastric cancer: an interim report. Surgery 2002;131(1 Suppl):S306–11.

6. Lee J-H, Han H-S, Lee J-H. A prospective randomized study comparing open vs laparoscopy-assisted distal gastrectomy in early gastric cancer: early results. Surg Endosc 2005;19(2):168–73.

7. Huscher CGS, Mingoli A, Sgarzini G, et al. Laparoscopic versus open subtotal gastrectomy for distal gastric cancer: five-year results of a randomized prospective trial. Ann Surg 2005;241(2):232–7.

8. Kim Y-W, Baik YH, Yun YH, et al. Improved quality of life outcomes after laparoscopy-assisted distal gastrectomy for early gastric cancer: results of a prospective randomized clinical trial. Ann Surg 2008;248(5):721–7.

9. Kim H-H, Hyung WJ, Cho GS, et al. Morbidity and mortality of laparoscopic gastrectomy versus open gastrectomy for gastric cancer: an interim report–a phase III multicenter, prospective, randomized Trial (KLASS Trial). Ann Surg 2010; 251(3):417–20.

10. Sarela AI, Lefkowitz R, Brennan MF, et al. Selection of patients with gastric adenocarcinoma for laparoscopic staging. Am J Surg 2006;191(1):134–8.

11. Power DG, Schattner MA, Gerdes H, et al. Endoscopic ultrasound can improve the selection for laparoscopy in patients with localized gastric cancer. J Am Coll Surg 2009;208(2):173–8.

12. Bando E, Yonemura Y, Takeshita Y, et al. Intraoperative lavage for cytological examination in 1,297 patients with gastric carcinoma. Am J Surg 1999;178(3):256–62.

13. Bentrem D, Wilton A, Mazumdar M, et al. The value of peritoneal cytology as a preoperative predictor in patients with gastric carcinoma undergoing a curative resection. Ann Surg Oncol 2005;12(5):347–53.

14. Bonenkamp JJ, Songun I, Hermans J, et al. Prognostic value of positive cytology findings from abdominal washings in patients with gastric cancer. Br J Surg 1996; 83(5):672–4.

15. Burke EC, Karpeh MS, Conlon KC, et al. Peritoneal lavage cytology in gastric cancer: an independent predictor of outcome. Ann Surg Oncol 1998;5(5):411–5.

16. Kodera Y, Yamamura Y, Shimizu Y, et al. Peritoneal washing cytology: prognostic value of positive findings in patients with gastric carcinoma undergoing a potentially curative resection. J Surg Oncol 1999;72(2):60–4 [discussion: 64–5].

17. Fukagawa T, Katai H, Saka M, et al. Significance of lavage cytology in advanced gastric cancer patients. World J Surg 2010;34(3):563–8.

18. Kitano S, Iso Y, Moriyama M, et al. Laparoscopy-assisted Billroth I gastrectomy. Surg Laparosc Endosc 1994;4(2):146–8.

19. Deng Y, Zhang Y, Guo TK. Laparoscopy-assisted versus open distal gastrectomy for early gastric cancer: A meta-analysis based on seven randomized controlled trials. Surg Oncol 2015;24(2):71–7.

20. Viñuela EF, Gonen M, Brennan MF, et al. Laparoscopic versus open distal gastrectomy for gastric cancer. Ann Surg 2012;255:446–56.

21. Hayashi H, Ochiai T, Shimada H, et al. Prospective randomized study of open versus laparoscopy-assisted distal gastrectomy with extraperigastric lymph node dissection for early gastric cancer. Surg Endosc 2005;19(9):1172–6.
22. Strong VE, Devaud N, Allen PJ, et al. Laparoscopic versus open subtotal gastrectomy for adenocarcinoma: a case–control study. Ann Surg Oncol 2009;16(6): 1507–13.
23. Adachi Y, Shiraishi N, Shiromizu A, et al. Laparoscopy-assisted Billroth I gastrectomy compared with conventional open gastrectomy. Arch Surg 2000;135(7):806–10.
24. Yano H, Monden T, Kinuta M, et al. The usefulness of laparoscopy-assisted distal gastrectomy in comparison with that of open distal gastrectomy for early gastric cancer. Gastric Cancer 2001;4(2):93–7.
25. Mochiki E, Kamiyama Y, Aihara R, et al. Laparoscopic assisted distal gastrectomy for early gastric cancer: five years' experience. Surgery 2005;137(3):317–22.
26. Kim M-C, Kim K-H, Kim H-H, et al. Comparison of laparoscopy-assisted by conventional open distal gastrectomy and extraperigastric lymph node dissection in early gastric cancer. J Surg Oncol 2005;91(1):90–4.
27. Ziqiang W, Feng Q, Zhimin C, et al. Comparison of laparoscopically assisted and open radical distal gastrectomy with extended lymphadenectomy for gastric cancer management. Surg Endosc 2006;20(11):1738–43.
28. Tanimura S, Higashino M, Fukunaga Y, et al. Respiratory function after laparoscopic distal gastrectomy–an index of minimally invasive surgery. World J Surg 2006;30(7):1211–5.
29. Song KY, Kim SN, Park CH. Laparoscopy-assisted distal gastrectomy with D2 lymph node dissection for gastric cancer: technical and oncologic aspects. Surg Endosc 2008;22(3):655–9.
30. Kim MC, Kim W, Kim HH, et al. Risk factors associated with complication following laparoscopy-assisted gastrectomy for gastric cancer: a large-scale korean multicenter study. Ann Surg Oncol 2008;15(10):2692–700.
31. Li H-Z, Chen J-X, Zheng Y, et al. Laparoscopic-assisted versus open radical gastrectomy for resectable gastric cancer: systematic review, meta-analysis, and trial sequential analysis of randomized controlled trials. J Surg Oncol 2016;113(7): 756–67.
32. Kim M-C, Choi H-J, Jung G-J, et al. Techniques and complications of laparoscopy-assisted distal gastrectomy (LADG) for gastric cancer. Eur J Surg Oncol 2007;33(6):700–5.
33. Ryu KW, Kim Y-W, Lee JH, et al. Surgical complications and the risk factors of laparoscopy-assisted distal gastrectomy in early gastric cancer. Ann Surg Oncol 2008;15(6):1625–31.
34. Kössler-Ebs JB, Grummich K, Jensen K, et al. Incisional hernia rates after laparoscopic or open abdominal surgery-a systematic review and meta-analysis. World J Surg 2016;40(10):2319–30.
35. Okabe H, Tsunoda S, Tanaka E, et al. Is laparoscopic total gastrectomy a safe operation? A review of various anastomotic techniques and their outcomes. Surg Today 2014;45(5):549–58.
36. Cai J, Wei D, Gao CF, et al. A prospective randomized study comparing open versus laparoscopy-assisted D2 radical gastrectomy in advanced gastric cancer. Dig Surg 2011;28(5–6):331–7.
37. Sakuramoto S, Yamashita K, Kikuchi S, et al. Laparoscopy versus open distal gastrectomy by expert surgeons for early gastric cancer in Japanese patients: short-term clinical outcomes of a randomized clinical trial. Surg Endosc 2013; 27(5):1695–705.

38. Macdonald JS, Smalley SR, Benedetti J, et al. Chemoradiotherapy after surgery compared with surgery alone for adenocarcinoma of the stomach or gastroesophageal junction. N Engl J Med 2001;345(10):725–30.

39. Ohgami M, Otani Y, Kumai K, et al. Curative laparoscopic surgery for early gastric cancer: five years experience. World J Surg 1999;23(2):187–92 [discussion 192–3].

40. Haverkamp L, Weijs TJ, van der Sluis PC, et al. Laparoscopic total gastrectomy versus open total gastrectomy for cancer: a systematic review and meta-analysis. Surg Endosc 2013;27(5):1509–20.

41. Fujii K, Sonoda K, Izumi K, et al. T lymphocyte subsets and Th1/Th2 balance after laparoscopy-assisted distal gastrectomy. Surg Endosc 2003;17(9):1440–4.

42. Jung I-K, Kim M-C, Kim K-H, et al. Cellular and peritoneal immune response after radical laparoscopy-assisted and open gastrectomy for gastric cancer. J Surg Oncol 2008;98(1):54–9.

43. Saba AA, Kaidi AA, Godziachvili V, et al. Effects of interleukin-6 and its neutralizing antibodies on peritoneal adhesion formation and wound healing. Am Surg 1996;62(7):569–72.

44. Barmparas G, Branco BC, Schnüriger B, et al. The incidence and risk factors of post-laparotomy adhesive small bowel obstruction. J Gastrointest Surg 2010; 14(10):1619–28.

45. LaFemina J, Viñuela EF, Schattner MA, et al. Esophagojejunal reconstruction after total gastrectomy for gastric cancer using a transorally inserted anvil delivery system. Ann Surg Oncol 2013;20(9):2975–83.

46. Yoo CH, Kim HO, Hwang SI, et al. Short-term outcomes of laparoscopic-assisted distal gastrectomy for gastric cancer during a surgeon's learning curve period. Surg Endosc 2009;23(10):2250–7.

47. Kunisaki C, Makino H, Yamamoto N, et al. Learning curve for laparoscopy-assisted distal gastrectomy with regional lymph node dissection for early gastric cancer. Surg Laparosc Endosc Percutan Tech 2008;18(3):236–41.

48. Zhang X, Tanigawa N. Learning curve of laparoscopic surgery for gastric cancer, a laparoscopic distal gastrectomy-based analysis. Surg Endosc 2009;23(6):1259–64.

49. Jin S-H, Kim D-Y, Kim H, et al. Multidimensional learning curve in laparoscopy-assisted gastrectomy for early gastric cancer. Surg Endosc 2007;21(1):28–33.

50. Kim M-C, Jung G-J, Kim H-H. Learning curve of laparoscopy-assisted distal gastrectomy with systemic lymphadenectomy for early gastric cancer. World J Gastroenterol 2005;11(47):7508–11.

51. Hashizume M, Sugimachi K. Robot-assisted gastric surgery. Surg Clin North Am 2003;83(6):1429–44.

52. Giulianotti PC, Coratti A, Angelini M, et al. Robotics in general surgery: personal experience in a large community hospital. Arch Surg 2003;138(7):777–84.

53. Anderson C, Ellenhorn J, Hellan M, et al. Pilot series of robot-assisted laparoscopic subtotal gastrectomy with extended lymphadenectomy for gastric cancer. Surg Endosc 2007;21(9):1662–6.

54. Kelly KJ, Selby L, Chou JF, et al. Laparoscopic versus open gastrectomy for gastric adenocarcinoma in the west: a case-control study. Ann Surg Oncol 2015;22(11):3590–6.

55. Patriti A, Ceccarelli G, Bellochi R, et al. Robot-assisted laparoscopic total and partial gastric resection with D2 lymph node dissection for adenocarcinoma. Surg Endosc 2008;22(12):2753–60.

56. Song J, Oh SJ, Kang WH, et al. Robot-assisted gastrectomy with lymph node dissection for gastric cancer: lessons learned from an initial 100 consecutive procedures. Ann Surg 2009;249(6):927–32.

57. Isogaki J, Haruta S, Man-I M, et al. Robot-assisted surgery for gastric cancer: experience at our institute. Pathobiology 2011;78(6):328–33.
58. D'Annibale A, Pende V, Pernazza G, et al. Full robotic gastrectomy with extended (D2) lymphadenectomy for gastric cancer: surgical technique and preliminary results. J Surg Res 2011;166(2):e113–20.
59. Lee HH, Hur H, Jung H, et al. Robot-assisted distal gastrectomy for gastric cancer: initial experience. Am J Surg 2011;201(6):841–5.
60. Park JY, Kim Y-W, Ryu KW, et al. Emerging role of robot-assisted gastrectomy: analysis of consecutive 200 cases. J Gastric Cancer 2013;13(4):255–62.
61. Tokunaga M, Sugisawa N, Kondo J, et al. Early phase II study of robot-assisted distal gastrectomy with nodal dissection for clinical stage IA gastric cancer. Gastric Cancer 2014;17(3):542–7.
62. Marano A, Choi YY, Hyung WJ, et al. Robotic versus laparoscopic versus open gastrectomy: a meta-analysis. J Gastric Cancer 2013;13(3):136–48.
63. Nakauchi M, Suda K, Susumu S, et al. Comparison of the long-term outcomes of robotic radical gastrectomy for gastric cancer and conventional laparoscopic approach: a single institutional retrospective cohort study. Surg Endosc 2016. [Epub ahead of print].
64. Kim H-I, Han S-U, Yang H-K, et al. Multicenter prospective comparative study of robotic versus laparoscopic gastrectomy for gastric adenocarcinoma. Ann Surg 2016;263(1):103–9.
65. Higgins RM, Frelich MJ, Bosler ME, et al. Cost analysis of robotic versus laparoscopic general surgery procedures. Surg Endosc 2016. [Epub ahead of print].
66. Silva-Velazco J, Dietz DW, Stocchi L, et al. Considering value in rectal cancer surgery: an analysis of costs and outcomes based on the open, laparoscopic, and robotic approach for proctectomy. Ann Surg 2016. [Epub ahead of print].
67. Wang G, Jiang Z, Zhao J, et al. Assessing the safety and efficacy of full robotic gastrectomy with intracorporeal robot-sewn anastomosis for gastric cancer: a randomized clinical trial. J Surg Oncol 2016;113(4):397–404.
68. Obama K, Sakai Y. Current status of robotic gastrectomy for gastric cancer. Surg Today 2016;46(5):528–34.
69. Song J, Kang WH, Oh SJ, et al. Role of robotic gastrectomy using da Vinci system compared with laparoscopic gastrectomy: initial experience of 20 consecutive cases. Surg Endosc 2009;23(6):1204–11.
70. Huang K-H, Lan Y-T, Fang W-L, et al. Initial experience of robotic gastrectomy and comparison with open and laparoscopic gastrectomy for gastric cancer. J Gastrointest Surg 2012;16(7):1303–10.
71. Park S-S, Kim M-C, Park MS, et al. Rapid adaptation of robotic gastrectomy for gastric cancer by experienced laparoscopic surgeons. Surg Endosc 2012;26(1):60–7.
72. Takiguchi S, Fujiwara Y, Yamasaki M, et al. Laparoscopy-assisted distal gastrectomy versus open distal gastrectomy. A prospective randomized single-blind study. World J Surg 2013;37(10):2379–86.
73. Aoyama T, Yoshikawa T, Hayashi T, et al. Randomized comparison of surgical stress and the nutritional status between laparoscopy-assisted and open distal gastrectomy for gastric cancer. Ann Surg Oncol 2014;21(6):1983–90.
74. Pugliese R, Maggioni D, Sansonna F, et al. Subtotal gastrectomy with D2 dissection by minimally invasive surgery for distal adenocarcinoma of the stomach: results and 5-year survival. Surg Endosc 2010;24(10):2594–602.
75. Kim M-C, Heo G-U, Jung G-J. Robotic gastrectomy for gastric cancer: surgical techniques and clinical merits. Surg Endosc 2009;24(3):610–5.

76. Caruso S, Patriti A, Marrelli D, et al. Open vs robot-assisted laparoscopic gastric resection with D2 lymph node dissection for adenocarcinoma: a case-control study. Int J Med Robot 2011;7(4):452–8.

77. Woo Y, Hyung WJ, Pak K-H, et al. Robotic gastrectomy as an oncologically sound alternative to laparoscopic resections for the treatment of early-stage gastric cancers. Arch Surg 2011;146(9):1086–92.

78. Eom BW, Yoon HM, Ryu KW, et al. Comparison of surgical performance and short-term clinical outcomes between laparoscopic and robotic surgery in distal gastric cancer. Eur J Surg Oncol 2012;38(1):57–63.

79. Kang BH, Xuan Y, Hur H, et al. Comparison of surgical outcomes between robotic and laparoscopic gastrectomy for gastric cancer: the learning curve of robotic surgery. J Gastric Cancer 2012;12(3):156–63.

80. Yoon HM, Kim Y-W, Lee JH, et al. Robot-assisted total gastrectomy is comparable with laparoscopically assisted total gastrectomy for early gastric cancer. Surg Endosc 2012;26(5):1377–81.

81. Kim KM, An JY, Kim HI, et al. Major early complications following open, laparoscopic and robotic gastrectomy. Br J Surg 2012;99(12):1681–7.

82. Park JY, Jo MJ, Nam B-H, et al. Surgical stress after robot-assisted distal gastrectomy and its economic implications. Br J Surg 2012;99(11):1554–61.

83. Uyama I, Kanaya S, Ishida Y, et al. Novel integrated robotic approach for suprapancreatic D2 nodal dissection for treating gastric cancer: technique and initial experience. World J Surg 2012;36(2):331–7.

84. Hyun M-H, Lee C-H, Kwon Y-J, et al. Robot versus laparoscopic gastrectomy for cancer by an experienced surgeon: comparisons of surgery, complications, and surgical stress. Ann Surg Oncol 2012;20(4):1258–65.

85. Suda K, Man-I M, Ishida Y, et al. Potential advantages of robotic radical gastrectomy for gastric adenocarcinoma in comparison with conventional laparoscopic approach: a single institutional retrospective comparative cohort study. Surg Endosc 2014;29(3):673–85.

86. Son T, Lee JH, Kim YM, et al. Robotic spleen-preserving total gastrectomy for gastric cancer: comparison with conventional laparoscopic procedure. Surg Endosc 2014;28(9):2606–15.

87. Noshiro H, Ikeda O, Urata M. Robotically-enhanced surgical anatomy enables surgeons to perform distal gastrectomy for gastric cancer using electric cautery devices alone. Surg Endosc 2014;28(4):1180–7.

88. Junfeng Z, Yan S, Bo T, et al. Robotic gastrectomy versus laparoscopic gastrectomy for gastric cancer: comparison of surgical performance and short-term outcomes. Surg Endosc 2014;28(6):1779–87.

89. Huang K-H, Lan Y-T, Fang W-L, et al. Comparison of the operative outcomes and learning curves between laparoscopic and robotic gastrectomy for gastric cancer. PLoS One 2014;9(10):e111499.

The Asian Perspective on the Surgical and Adjuvant Management of Esophagogastric Cancer

Yukinori Kurokawa, MD, PhD[a], Mitsuru Sasako, MD, PhD[b],*

KEYWORDS

- Gastric cancer • Esophagogastric junctional cancer • D2 dissection
- Adjuvant chemotherapy • Neoadjuvant chemotherapy • Multidisciplinary treatment

KEY POINTS

- D2 dissection without splenectomy has become the global standard for curable advanced gastric cancer except those invading the greater curvature of the upper body.
- Postoperative adjuvant chemotherapy improves overall survival (OS) in East Asia, where high-quality D2 dissection is routinely performed.
- Neoadjuvant chemotherapy is preferred for borderline resectable cases or linitis plastica. Conversion surgery for stage IV tumors remains under active investigation.

INTRODUCTION

Gastric cancer showed a long-term decreasing trend for both incidence and mortality in Japan, mainly due to decreased incidence of *Helicobacter pylori* infection and a Westernized diet of less salty food.[1] The Intergroup Study 0116 was one of the earliest positive adjuvant therapy trials in gastric cancer, proving the efficacy of postoperative chemoradiation therapy.[2] Its subgroup analysis, together with a small study comparing D1 versus D2 resection, ended the argument that advanced gastric cancer is already a systemic disease and does not benefit from adjuvant therapy.[3,4] Now it is widely accepted that a good local control is essential to cure gastric cancer. In the guidelines of the Japan Gastric Cancer Association (JGCA), standard surgery for

Dr M. Sasako received lecture fees from Taiho, Chugai, Lilly, Otsuka, Yakult, Medtronic, Olympus, and Johnson and Johnson. Dr Y. Kurokawa has nothing to disclose.
[a] Department of Gastrointestinal Surgery, Osaka University Graduate School of Medicine, 2-2, Yamadagaoka, Suita, Osaka Prefecture 565-0871, Japan; [b] Department of Multidisciplinary Surgical Oncology, Hyogo College of Medicine, 1-1, Mukogawacho, Nishinomiya, Hyogo Prefecture 663-8501, Japan
* Corresponding author.
E-mail address: msasako@hyo-med.ac.jp

Surg Oncol Clin N Am 26 (2017) 213–224
http://dx.doi.org/10.1016/j.soc.2016.10.011

resectable gastric cancer is defined as resection of at least two-thirds of the stomach with a D2 lymph node dissection.[5] Thus, a high degree of local control is achieved by surgery in East Asian countries.[6] After D2 surgery, the 5-year survival rates for pathologic stage IA and stage IB according to the JGCA classification (13th edition) were 92.3% and 84.7%, respectively.[7] Contrary to these high survival rates, those for pathologic stages II, IIIA, and IIIB were not adequate—72.1%, 52.8%, and 31.0%, respectively. Thus, patients with stages II–III gastric cancer often have recurrence even after curative surgery, which indicates additional treatment is warranted to improve the prognosis of these patients. This review outlines the Eastern perspective on the surgical and adjuvant management of gastric cancer.

STANDARD SURGERY FOR RESECTABLE GASTRIC CANCER IN THE EAST

In Japan, the standard surgery for resectable gastric cancer has been gastrectomy with a D2 lymph node dissection. Although the Dutch randomized controlled trial (RCT) comparing D1 and D2 dissection could not show a significant survival benefit of D2 dissection in the primary analysis,[8] it demonstrated a significant reduction in the locoregional recurrence rate and cancer-related deaths after long-term follow-up.[9] In addition, a Taiwanese RCT demonstrated a significant survival benefit of D2 or more extensive lymph node dissection compared with D1 dissection.[4] These findings led to the recent revision of the European Society for Medical Oncology guidelines for gastric cancer and the National Comprehensive Cancer Network guidelines for gastric cancer, and they now recommend D2 lymph node dissection for resectable gastric cancer similar to the JGCA guidelines.[5,10,11] The Japan Clinical Oncology Group (JCOG) conducted a phase III trial (JCOG9501) to investigate the survival benefit of para-aortic nodal dissection (D3 dissection) compared with standard D2 for cT2b-T4 gastric cancer.[12] A total of 523 patients were randomly assigned to either D2 or D3 dissection. D2 plus para-aortic nodal dissection was associated with a longer operation time ($P<.001$), greater blood loss ($P<.001$), and a significant increase in minor complications ($P<.001$). Nevertheless, there was no significant difference in OS and recurrence-free survival (RFS) between the 2 groups. Thus, a clinical benefit of prophylactic para-aortic lymph node dissection for resectable gastric cancer was not shown. Therapeutic para-aortic lymph node dissection for patients with clinically involved para-aortic node metastasis is still considered a recommended surgery in Japan.[13]

In a total gastrectomy with D2 lymph node dissection, the role of splenectomy has been an important topic of debate. A phase III trial (JCOG0110) was conducted to compare D2 with and without splenectomy for proximal gastric cancer that did not invade the greater curvature.[14] The reason for exclusion of tumors invading the great curvature is possible microscopic invasion into the gastrosplenic ligament and 3 times higher incidence of nodal metastasis in the splenic hilum.[15] A total of 505 patients were randomly assigned to either the splenectomy or spleen preservation group. The splenectomy group had higher morbidity ($P<.01$) and larger blood loss ($P = .025$) than the spleen preserving group. The 5-year OS rates were 75.1% and 76.4% in the splenectomy and spleen preservation groups, respectively, and the noninferiority of spleen preservation was demonstrated ($P = .025$). Based on these results, splenectomy should be avoided in total gastrectomy for proximal gastric cancer that does not invade the greater curvature even in Japan.

EVIDENCE FOR POSTOPERATIVE ADJUVANT THERAPY IN THE EAST

Postoperative adjuvant therapy aims to eradicate micrometastasis that exists even after surgery. Accurate staging before surgery in gastric cancer is impossible, whereas the postoperative strategy can select only patients who have high risk of recurrence based on an accurate pathologic diagnosis. This, together with a high incidence of early-stage disease, limits the broader application of neoadjuvant treatment in Korea and Japan. On the other hand, the biggest drawback of adjuvant therapy is drug compliance, which is decreased by surgical morbidity and sequelae after gastrectomy, such as body weight loss or malnutrition.[16] Therefore, the development of adjuvant therapy needs both the consideration of the intensity of the regimen required and the ability to achieve drug compliance.

Several RCTs investigating the efficacy and safety of adjuvant chemotherapy for gastric cancer have been conducted in the East since the 1990s (Table 1). In the 1990s, the JCOG9206-1 trial investigated adjuvant chemotherapy using mitomycin, 5-fluorouracil (5-FU), and cytarabine followed by oral 5-FU for 18 months.[17] A total of 252 patients with clinically serosa-negative gastric cancer after curative surgery (except for clinical T1N0 tumor) were randomly assigned to either adjuvant chemotherapy or surgery alone. Although RFS tended to be better in the adjuvant chemotherapy group than the surgery-alone group (5-year RFS rates, 88.8% vs 83.7%, respectively; $P = .14$), this trial did not show statistical significance due to small sample size. The JCOG9206-2 trial focused on clinically serosa-positive gastric cancer and investigated adjuvant chemotherapy using a combination of intraperitoneal injection of cisplatin soon after abdominal closure, postoperative intravenous injection of cisplatin and 5-FU, and oral administration of uracil-tegafur (UFT) for 12 months.[18] A total of 268 patients were randomly assigned to either adjuvant chemotherapy or surgery alone. Due to the toxicity or progressive disease, 61.5% of the patients in the adjuvant chemotherapy group discontinued the treatment. In results, this study failed to show survival benefit of adjuvant chemotherapy compared with surgery alone (5-year OS rates, 62.0% vs 60.9%, respectively; $P = .48$).

In 1990s, an RCT (Intergroup Study 0116) was conducted to evaluate the survival benefit of adjuvant chemoradiotherapy using 5-FU plus leucovorin after R0 lymph node dissection in the United States.[2] A total of 556 patients with resected adenocarcinoma of the stomach or gastroesophageal junction were randomly assigned to either chemoradiotherapy or surgery alone. Chemoradiotherapy reduced local recurrence by 10%, and the chemoradiotherapy group achieved a significant improvement in OS ($P = .005$) if patients underwent D0 or D1 surgery. The clinical benefit of chemoradiotherapy after D2 dissection, however, had not been investigated, so the Adjuvant Chemoradiation Therapy in Stomach Cancer (ARTIST) trial was conducted in a Korean single institution to evaluate the clinical benefit of the addition of radiation therapy to adjuvant chemotherapy after D2 surgery.[19,20] A total of 458 gastric cancer patients with pathologic stages IB–IV (except for M1 lymph node or distant metastases) were randomized to either the adjuvant chemotherapy group using capecitabine plus cisplatin or the adjuvant chemoradiotherapy group using capecitabine plus cisplatin. The final analysis showed similar disease-free survival (DFS) and OS between the 2 groups ($P = .092$ and $P = .527$, respectively). This trial demonstrated that adjuvant chemoradiotherapy is not effective in the East, where good local control of tumor can be achieved by D2 lymph node dissection.

In the 2000s, more feasible regimens using oral fluoropyrimidines were applied to adjuvant therapy. The National Surgical Adjuvant Study Group for Gastric Cancer (NSAS-GC) trial compared OS between adjuvant chemotherapy using UFT for 16 months and surgery alone for patients with pathologic T2 N1-2 tumor.[21] Because the accrual speed was slower than expected, it was terminated at the time of the registration of 190 patients (38% of the projected sample size). Although 7% of the patients in the adjuvant chemotherapy group experienced recurrence by 16 months, 51% of the patients could

Table 1
Clinical trials of adjuvant therapy for gastric cancer in East Asia

Trial	Country	Eligibility	Primary Endpoint	Treatment Regimen	Number of Enrolled Patients	5-y Overall Survival Rate Log-Rank P Value
JCOG9206-1	Japan	Clinically serosa-negative (except for cT1N0[a])	RFS	Mitomycin + 5-FU + cytarabine followed by oral 5-FU vs surgery alone	252	91.2% vs 86.1% $P = .13$
JCOG9206-2	Japan	Clinically serosa-positive	OS	Cisplatin (intraperitoneal and intravenous) + 5-FU followed by UFT vs surgery alone	268	62.0% vs 60.9% $P = .482$
NSAS-GC	Japan	pT2N1-2[a]	OS	UFT vs surgery alone	190	86% vs 73% $P = .017$
ACTS-GC	Japan	pStages II-IIIB[a] (except for pT1)	OS	S-1 vs surgery alone	1059	71.7% vs 61.1% $P = .002$[d]
SAMIT	Japan	cT4a or cT4b[b]	DFS	Paclitaxel followed by UFT vs paclitaxel followed by S-1 vs UFT vs S-1	1495	Sequential 59.3%[e] vs monotherapy 55.8%[e], $P = .273$; UFT 54.3%[e] vs S-1 60.7%[e], $P = .0048$
CLASSIC	Korea, China, Taiwan	pStages II-IIIB[c]	DFS	Capecitabine + oxaliplatin vs surgery alone	1035	78% vs 69% $P = .0029$
ARTIST	Korea	pStages IB(N1)-IV(M0)[b]	DFS	Capecitabine + cisplatin + radiotherapy vs capecitabine + cisplatin	458	75% vs 73% $P = .484$

[a] Japanese Classification of Gastric Carcinoma, 2nd English Edition. Ref: Japanese Gastric Cancer Association. Japanese Classification of Gastric Cancer (2nd English Edition) Response assessment of chemotherapy and radiotherapy for gastric carcinoma: clinical criteria. Gastric Cancer 2001; 4:1–8.

[b] American Joint Committee on Cancer/Union Internationale Contre le Cancer, 7th edition. Edge SB, Brd DR, Compton CC et al. AJCC/UICC cancer staging manual. New York, Springer-Verlag; 2010.

[c] American Joint Committee on Cancer/Union Internationale Contre le Cancer, 6th edition. Sobin LH and Wittekind Ch. TNM Classification of Malignant Tumours. New York, Wiley-Liss; 2002.

[d] Based on the interim analysis.

[e] 3-Year OS rate.

complete adjuvant chemotherapy using UFT for 16 months. OS was significantly better in the adjuvant chemotherapy group than the surgery-alone group (5-year OS rates, 86% vs 73%, respectively; P = .017). Although the efficacy of UFT for moderately locally advanced gastric cancer patients was demonstrated in this trial, further confirmatory studies were needed because of the small number of enrolled patients and poor OS of the control arm compared with Japanese standard results in that period.

After the NSAS-GC trial, the Adjuvant Chemotherapy for Gastric Cancer with S-1 (ACTS-GC) trial was conducted to investigate the efficacy and safety of adjuvant chemotherapy using an oral fluoropyrimidine agent that combines tegafur, gimeracil, and oteracil (S-1). A total of 1059 patients with pathologic stages II–III gastric cancer (except for pathologic T1 tumor) were randomly assigned to either S-1 for 1 year or surgery alone. On the adjuvant chemotherapy arm, 65.8% of the patients completed S-1 for 1 year. In the interim analysis, OS was significantly better in the adjuvant chemotherapy group than the surgery-alone group (3-year OS rates, 80.1% vs 70.1%, respectively; P = .003).[22] The survival difference was maintained after long-term follow-up period (5-year OS rates, 71.7% vs 61.1%, respectively).[23] Based on these results, adjuvant chemotherapy using S-1 for 1 year after D2 dissection was established as the standard treatment of stages II–III gastric cancer patients in Japan.

To develop more effective treatments, the significance of sequential agents was also investigated in a large-scale RCT. The Stomach Cancer Adjuvant Multi-Institutional Group Trial (SAMIT) compared DFS between adjuvant chemotherapy with sequential combination (paclitaxel for 11 weeks followed by UFT or S-1 for 36 weeks) and monotherapy (UFT or S-1 for 48 weeks) for clinically T4a or T4b gastric cancer after D2 dissection.[24] This trial also investigated the noninferiority of UFT compared with S-1 in a 2-by-2 factorial design. A total of 1495 patients were randomly assigned to 1 of 4 treatment groups. Comparing DFS between the sequential group and the monotherapy group, the 3-year DFS rate was 57.2% in the sequential group and 54.0% in the monotherapy group, which did not show statistical significance (P = .27). In comparison between the UFT group and the S-1 group, DFS was significantly better in the S-1 group than in the UFT group (3-year DFS rates, 58.2% vs 53.0%, respectively; P = .0048). This result demonstrated that adjuvant chemotherapy using sequential agents did not improve DFS and that S-1 was better than UFT as the monotherapy regimen for resectable gastric cancer.

Another large-scale RCT of adjuvant chemotherapy was conducted in East Asia outside Japan. The Capecitabine and Oxaliplatin Adjuvant Study in Gastric Cancer (CLASSIC) trial investigated adjuvant chemotherapy using capecitabine plus oxaliplatin for 6 months.[25,26] A total of 1035 patients with pathologic stages II–III gastric cancer after D2 dissection were enrolled from Korea, China, and Taiwan and randomly assigned to either adjuvant chemotherapy or surgery alone. On the adjuvant chemotherapy arm, 66.5% of the patients completed the treatment. The interim analysis showed a significant improvement in DFS in the adjuvant chemotherapy group compared with the surgery-alone group (3-year DFS rates, 74% vs 59%, respectively; P<.0001). In the updated results, the OS was also significantly better in the adjuvant chemotherapy group than the surgery-alone group (5-year OS rates, 78% vs 69%, respectively; P = .0029). This result indicated that adjuvant chemotherapy with capecitabine plus oxaliplatin could be one of the standard treatments for stages II–III gastric cancer patients.

FUTURE PERSPECTIVE OF POSTOPERATIVE ADJUVANT THERAPY IN THE EAST

The standard treatment of pathologic stages II–III gastric cancer patients is D2 dissection followed by adjuvant chemotherapy using S-1 for 1 year in Japan. Many unresolved issues, however, remain. First is the duration of adjuvant chemotherapy. The CLASSIC trial demonstrated a survival benefit of adjuvant chemotherapy using capecitabine plus oxaliplatin for 6 months, which was shorter than the 1 year using S-1 in the ACTS-GC trial. A shorter duration of adjuvant S-1 may bring similar clinical benefit especially for patients with earlier-stage tumor. Thus, a phase III trial (JCOG1104) is now ongoing to evaluate the noninferiority of adjuvant S-1 for 6 months compared with 1 year in pathologic stage II tumor. The primary endpoint is RFS, and the planned sample size is 1000.

The second issue is the efficacy of adjuvant S-1 for stage IIIB tumor. In the subgroup analysis of ACTS-GC, the hazard ratio (HR) for death in the adjuvant S-1 group compared with the surgery-alone group was 0.86 (95% CI, 0.51–1.43) in stage IIIB tumor, which was much larger than that in stage II (HR 0.52; 95% CI, 0.36–0.75).[23] In contrast, the CLASSIC trial showed that the HR for death in the adjuvant capecitabine plus oxaliplatin group compared with the surgery-alone group was 0.67 (95% CI, 0.39–1.13) in stage IIIB tumor, not too large compared with that in stage II (HR 0.54; 95% CI, 0.34–0.87) while that in stage IIIA (HR 0.75; 95% CI, 0.52–1.10) was much larger than that in stage II.[26] Thus, a doublet regimen with oral fluoropyrimidines, such as capecitabine plus oxaliplatin, may bring a larger survival benefit than achieved with S-1 monotherapy in late stage III tumors. A phase II trial to evaluate the feasibility of adjuvant capecitabine plus oxaliplatin (130 mg/m^2) for 6 months in Japanese patients with pathologic stages II–III tumor was conducted. Although the relative dose intensities (RDIs) for capecitabine (67.2%) and oxaliplatin (73.4%) were similar to those in the CLASSIC trial, elderly patients ($\geq$65 years) or patients after total gastrectomy showed low RDIs.[27] Another phase II trial to evaluate the feasibility of adjuvant S-1 plus oxaliplatin (100 mg/m^2) for 6 months in Japanese patients with pathologic stage III tumor was also conducted. This doublet regimen had higher RDI for S-1 (77.2%) than that for capecitabine (68.2%) in the CLASSIC trial, and even elderly patients ($\geq$65 years) showed similar RDIs for both S-1 and oxaliplatin to young patients (<65 years); however, patients after total gastrectomy showed low RDIs.[28]

Another candidate of doublet regimen with favorable feasibility is S-1 plus docetaxel, which demonstrated borderline survival benefit compared with S-1 monotherapy in unresectable or recurrent gastric cancer patients.[29] A phase II trial (OGSG0604) to evaluate the feasibility of adjuvant S-1 plus docetaxel (40 mg/m^2) for 3 months and subsequent S-1 monotherapy until 1 year after surgery in the Japanese patients with pathologic stage III tumor was conducted. The completion rates were 79.2% for S-1 plus docetaxel and 64.2% for subsequent S-1 monotherapy, respectively.[30] In addition, 3-year OS rates were 85.7% for stage IIIA and 62.5% for stage IIIB, which suggested promising efficacy of adjuvant S-1 plus docetaxel. A phase III trial (START-2) is ongoing to evaluate the superiority of adjuvant S-1 plus docetaxel for 18 weeks and subsequent S-1 monotherapy until 1 year after surgery to adjuvant S-1 monotherapy for 1 year in pathologic stage III tumor. The primary endpoint is RFS, and planned sample size is 1100.

EVIDENCE OF PREOPERATIVE NEOADJUVANT THERAPY FOR PATIENTS WITH MARGINALLY RESECTABLE TUMOR IN THE EAST

As discussed previously, the standard treatment of resectable gastric cancer patients in Japan is D2 lymph node dissection followed by adjuvant chemotherapy with S-1 for 1 year. For patients with marginally resectable tumor, however, more intensive treatment is needed. Although postoperative adjuvant strategy has the limitation of drug compliance particularly for a more toxic regimen, neoadjuvant strategy can allow intensive chemotherapy, because most preoperative patients have good general condition. Furthermore, patients can receive the treatment soon after diagnosis contrary to adjuvant chemotherapy, especially if patients have postoperative complications.

Several phase II trials to investigate the efficacy and safety of neoadjuvant chemotherapy for gastric cancer have been conducted in the East since the 2000s. In Japan, the target population was limited to patients with either extensive lymph node metastasis or Borrmann type 4 or linitis plastica (or large type 3) tumors (Table 2). An initial phase II trial (JCOG0001) of neoadjuvant therapy for patients with para-aortic node and/or bulky nodal metastasis evaluated the efficacy and safety of neoadjuvant irinotecan and cisplatin.[31] The regimen was 28-day cycles of irinotecan (70 mg/m^2 on days 1 and 15) and cisplatin (80 mg/m^2 on day 1). After 2 or 3 cycles, the patients underwent gastrectomy with D2 plus para-aortic lymphadenectomy. The primary endpoints were 3-year OS rate and incidence of treatment-related death (TRD). When 55 patients were enrolled, this study was terminated due to 3 TRDs, which exceeded the 5% upper limit. The R0 resection rate and the response rate were 65% and 55%, respectively. Any degree of pathologic response rate (ratio of patients who showed pathological Grade IB or more according to the Japanese Gastric Cancer Classification among whole patients), however, was only seen in 15%, and the 3-year OS rate was 27%.

A second phase II trial (JCOG0405) for the same target population as JCOG0001 was conducted to evaluate the efficacy and safety of neoadjuvant S-1 plus cisplatin.[13] The regimen was 28-day cycles of S-1 (80 mg/m^2 on days 1–21) and cisplatin (60 mg/m^2 on day 8). After 2 or 3 cycles, gastrectomy with D2 plus para-aortic node dissection was performed. The primary endpoint was the R0 resection rate, and 53 patients were enrolled. The R0 resection rate and the response rate were 82% and 65%, respectively. The pathologic response rate (51%) was much higher than that in JCOG0001, and the 3-year OS rate reached 59%. There were no TRD cases. Based on the very positive results of this trial, S-1 plus cisplatin is considered a standard option for neoadjuvant chemotherapy for gastric cancer with extensive lymph node metastasis.

A triplet regimen was also evaluated in a subsequent phase II trial (JCOG1002) for gastric cancer with extensive lymph node metastasis.[32] Patients received 2 or 3 28-day cycles of S-1 (80 mg/m^2 on days 1–14) plus cisplatin (60 mg/m^2 on day 1) plus docetaxel (40 mg/m^2 on day 1), followed by gastrectomy with D2 plus para-aortic node dissection. The primary endpoint was the response rate, and 53 patients were enrolled. The R0 resection rate, response rate, and the pathologic response rates were 85%, 58%, and 50%, respectively. All outcomes were not superior to those in the JCOG0405 trial.

In the meantime, an initial phase II trial (JCOG0002) of neoadjuvant chemotherapy for patients with Borrmann type 4 gastric cancer evaluated the efficacy and safety of neoadjuvant S-1 monotherapy. The regimen was 6-week cycles of S-1 (80 mg/m^2 on days 1–28).[33] After 2 cycles, the patients underwent D2 dissection without any adjuvant treatment. The primary endpoint was the 2-year OS rate. Although the safety of neoadjuvant S-1 was shown, the 2-year OS rate was only 59%, which did not reach the expected rate of 60%.

A second phase II trial (JCOG0210) for patients with Borrmann type 4 or large (≥8 cm) type 3 gastric cancer was conducted to evaluate the efficacy and safety of the neoadjuvant S-1 plus cisplatin.[34] In the regimen, S-1 (80 mg/m^2 on days 1–21) and cisplatin (60 mg/m^2 on day 8) were repeated twice every 4 weeks. The primary endpoint of the treatment completion rate was 73%, which reached the expected rate of 60%. The pathologic response rate was 57%, which was greater than 27% observed in JCOG0002. Based on this result, a phase III trial (JCOG0501) is ongoing to evaluate the survival benefit of this regimen followed by

Table 2
Clinical trials of neoadjuvant therapy for marginally resectable gastric cancer in Japan

Trial	Eligibility	Primary Endpoint	Regimen	Number of Enrolled Patients	Treatment-Related Death Rate (%)	R0 Resection Rate (%)	Response Rate (%)	Pathologic Response Rate (%)*	3-y Overall Survival Rate (%)
JCOG0001	Para-aortic node and/or bulky nodal metastasis	3-y OS rate, TRD	Irinotecan + cisplatin	55	5.5	65	55	15	27
JCOG0405	Para-aortic node and/or bulky nodal metastasis	R0 resection rate	S-1 + cisplatin	53	0	82	65	51	59
JCOG1002	Para-aortic node and/or bulky nodal metastasis	Response rate	S-1 + cisplatin + docetaxel	53	0	85	58	50	NA
JCOG0002	Borrmann type 4	2-y OS rate	S-1	55	0	65	NA	27	59 (2-y OS rate)
JCOG0210	Borrmann type 4 or large (≥8 cm) type 3	Treatment completion rate, TRD	S-1 + cisplatin	50	2	63	NA	57	24.5

Abbreviation: NA, not analyzed.
* Pathologically evaluated chemotherapy Grade IB, II, III according to the Japanese Classification of Gastric Cancer.[5]

surgery and adjuvant chemotherapy with S-1 for 1 year compared with surgery with the same adjuvant S-1. The accrual was completed a few years ago and results are expected in 2019.

FUTURE PERSPECTIVE OF PREOPERATIVE NEOADJUVANT THERAPY IN THE EAST

Regarding gastric cancer with extensive lymph node metastasis, more intensive local tumor control is warranted. Trastuzumab has shown efficacy in human epidermal growth factor receptor 2 (HER2)-positive metastatic gastric cancer in combination with oral fluoropyrimidine plus cisplatin.[35,36] A potential survival benefit of a neoadjuvant triplet regimen using trastuzumab plus S-1 plus cisplatin is being investigated in an ongoing randomized phase II trial (JCOG1301) in HER2-positive patients. Another promising triplet regimen as neoadjuvant therapy for patients with extensive lymph node metastasis is docetaxel plus oxaliplatin plus S-1. A Korean phase II trial of this triplet regimen showed high pathologic complete response rate (19.5%) for clinical stages II–III patients without any TRD case.[37] A new phase II trial of neoadjuvant triplet regimen using docetaxel plus oxaliplatin plus S-1 for patients with extensive lymph node metastasis is being planned in the JCOG.

For patients with Borrmann type 4 or large type 3 gastric cancer, the control of peritoneal recurrence is a critical issue. Intraperitoneal chemotherapy, which can maintain a high concentration of the drug in the peritoneal cavity, may overcome peritoneal recurrence for those patients. In a phase II trial of the combination of intravenous and intraperitoneal paclitaxel with S-1 for patients with peritoneal metastasis, a median survival time of 22.5 months was reached.[38] As a neoadjuvant therapy, intraperitoneal docetaxel with S-1 was evaluated for patients with positive cytology or with peritoneal metastasis followed by surgery, and 14 of 18 patients (78%) showed resolution of a positive peritoneal cytology and no macroscopic peritoneal metastasis, leading to R0 resection.[39] More than half of patients with R0 resection, however, died from peritoneal recurrence. To improve the control of peritoneal recurrence, a triplet regimen of intraperitoneal docetaxel with S-1 and cisplatin was evaluated in a phase I trial.[40] Based on the result, the recommended regimen for neoadjuvant intraperitoneal therapy was decided as 20 mg/m^2 of docetaxel on days 1 and 15, with 60 mg/m^2 of intravenous cisplatin on day 1 and 80 mg/m^2 oral S-1 on days 1 to 14 of a 28-day cycle. Intraperitoneal chemotherapy could be a promising neoadjuvant therapy for patients with type 4 or large type 3 gastric cancer, and further investigation is warranted.

SUMMARY

This article introduces perioperative treatments for gastric cancer in the East. Regarding adjuvant chemotherapy after D2 lymph node dissection, S-1 monotherapy for 1 year or capecitabine plus oxaliplatin for 6 months is the standard treatment of pathologic stages II–III gastric cancer. Superiority of a doublet regimen of oral fluoropyrimidine (S-1 or capecitabine) with platinum over S-1 alone is suggested for stage IIIB patients but further study is needed to prove its benefit. As a neoadjuvant chemotherapy, the doublet regimen of S-1 plus cisplatin suggested a potential survival benefit in patients with extensive lymph node metastasis. For patients with Borrmann type 4 or large type 3 gastric cancer, the main issue is control of peritoneal recurrence. To improve the prognosis in such patients with high risk of recurrence, intensive neoadjuvant chemotherapy using triplet or an intraperitoneal regimen is now being investigated in several clinical trials in Japan.

REFERENCES

1. Katanoda K, Matsuda T, Matsuda A, et al. An updated report of the trends in cancer incidence and mortality in Japan. Jpn J Clin Oncol 2013;43:492–507.
2. Macdonald JS, Smalley SR, Benedetti J, et al. Chemoradiotherapy after surgery compared with surgery alone for adenocarcinoma of the stomach or gastroesophageal junction. N Engl J Med 2001;345:725–30.
3. Smalley SR, Benedetti JK, Haller DG, et al. Updated analysis of SWOG-Directed intergroup study 0116: A phase III trial of adjuvant radiochemotherapy versus observation after curative gastric cancer resection. J Clin Oncol 2012;30: 2327–33.
4. Wu CW, Hsiung CA, Lo SS, et al. Nodal dissection for patients with gastric cancer: a randomised controlled trial. Lancet Oncol 2006;7:309–15.
5. Japanese Gastric Cancer Association. Japanese gastric cancer treatment guidelines 2010 (ver. 3). Gastric Cancer 2011;14:113–23.
6. Kurokawa Y, Sasako M. Recent advances in chemotherapy and chemoradiotherapy for gastrointestinal tract cancers: adjuvant chemoradiotherapy for gastric cancer. Int J Clin Oncol 2008;13:479–82.
7. Nashimoto A, Akazawa K, Isobe Y, et al. Gastric cancer treated in 2002 in Japan: 2009 annual report of the JGCA nationwide registry. Gastric Cancer 2013;16:1–27.
8. Bonenkamp JJ, Hermans J, Sasako M, et al. Extended lymph-node dissection for gastric cancer. N Engl J Med 1999;340:908–14.
9. Songun I, Putter H, Kranenbarg EM, et al. Surgical treatment of gastric cancer: 15-year follow-up results of the randomised nationwide Dutch D1D2 trial. Lancet Oncol 2010;11:439–49.
10. Waddell T, Verheij M, Allum W, et al. Gastric cancer: ESMO-ESSO-ESTRO clinical practice guidelines for diagnosis, treatment and follow-up. Eur J Surg Oncol 2014;40:584–91.
11. NCCN Guidelines for gastric cancer Ver 3.2015. Available at: http://www.nccn. org/professionals/physician_gls/PDF/gastric.pdf.
12. Sasako M, Sano T, Yamamoto S, et al. D2 lymphadenectomy alone or with para-aortic nodal dissection for gastric cancer. N Engl J Med 2008;359:453–62.
13. Tsuburaya A, Mizusawa J, Tanaka Y, et al. Neoadjuvant chemotherapy with S-1 and cisplatin followed by D2 gastrectomy with para-aortic node dissection for gastric cancer with extensive lymph node metastasis. Br J Surg 2014;101: 653–60.
14. Sano T, Sasako M, Mizusawa J, et al. Randomized controlled trial to evaluate splenectomy in total gastrectomy for proximal gastric carcinoma. Ann Surg 2016;265(2):277–83.
15. Kosuga T, Ichikawa D, Okamoto K, et al. Survival benefits from splenic hilar lymph node dissection by splenectomy in gastric cancer patients : relative comparison of the benefits in subgroups of patients. Gastric Cancer 2011; 14:172–7.
16. Aoyama T, Yoshikawa T, Shirai J, et al. Body weight loss after surgery is an independent risk factor for continuation of S-1 adjuvant chemotherapy for gastric cancer. Ann Surg Oncol 2013;20:2000–6.
17. Nashimoto A, Nakajima T, Furukawa H, et al. Randomized trial of adjuvant chemotherapy with mitomycin, Fluorouracil, and Cytosine arabinoside followed by oral Fluorouracil in serosa-negative gastric cancer: Japan Clinical Oncology Group 9206-1. J Clin Oncol 2003;21:2282–7.

18. Miyashiro I, Furukawa H, Sasako M, et al. Randomized clinical trial of adjuvant chemotherapy with intraperitoneal and intravenous cisplatin followed by oral fluorouracil (UFT) in serosa-positive gastric cancer versus curative resection alone: final results of the Japan Clinical Oncology Group trial JCOG9206-2. Gastric Cancer 2011;14:212–8.

19. Lee J, Lim do H, Kim S, et al. Phase III trial comparing capecitabine plus cisplatin versus capecitabine plus cisplatin with concurrent capecitabine radiotherapy in completely resected gastric cancer with D2 lymph node dissection: the ARTIST trial. J Clin Oncol 2012;30:268–73.

20. Park SH, Sohn TS, Lee J, et al. Phase III trial to compare adjuvant chemotherapy with capecitabine and cisplatin versus concurrent chemoradiotherapy in gastric cancer: final report of the adjuvant chemoradiotherapy in stomach tumors trial, including survival and subset analyses. J Clin Oncol 2015;33:3130.

21. Nakajima T, Kinoshita T, Nashimoto A, et al. Randomized controlled trial of adjuvant uracil-tegafur versus surgery alone for serosa-negative, locally advanced gastric cancer. Br J Surg 2007;94:1468–76.

22. Sakuramoto S, Sasako M, Yamaguchi T, et al. Adjuvant chemotherapy for gastric cancer with S-1, an oral fluoropyrimidine. N Engl J Med 2007;357:1810–20.

23. Sasako M, Sakuramoto S, Katai H, et al. Five-year outcomes of a randomized phase III trial comparing adjuvant chemotherapy with S-1 versus surgery alone in stage II or III gastric cancer. J Clin Oncol 2011;29:4387–93.

24. Tsuburaya A, Yoshida K, Kobayashi M, et al. Sequential paclitaxel followed by tegafur and uracil (UFT) or S-1 versus UFT or S-1 monotherapy as adjuvant chemotherapy for T4a/b gastric cancer (SAMIT): a phase 3 factorial randomised controlled trial. Lancet Oncol 2014;15:886–93.

25. Bang YJ, Kim YW, Yang HK, et al. Adjuvant capecitabine and oxaliplatin for gastric cancer after D2 gastrectomy (CLASSIC): a phase 3 open-label, randomised controlled trial. Lancet 2012;379:315–21.

26. Noh SH, Park SR, Yang HK, et al. Adjuvant capecitabine plus oxaliplatin for gastric cancer after D2 gastrectomy (CLASSIC): 5-year follow-up of an open-label, randomised phase 3 trial. Lancet Oncol 2014;15:1389–96.

27. Fuse N, Bando H, Chin K, et al. Adjuvant capecitabine plus oxaliplatin after D2 gastrectomy in Japanese patients with gastric cancer: a phase II study. Gastric Cancer 2016;1–9.

28. Shitara K, Chin K, Yoshikawa T, et al. Phase II study of adjuvant chemotherapy of S-1 plus oxaliplatin for patients with stage III gastric cancer after D2 gastrectomy. Gastric Cancer 2015;20(1):175–81.

29. Koizumi W, Kim YH, Fujii M, et al. Addition of docetaxel to S-1 without platinum prolongs survival of patients with advanced gastric cancer: a randomized study (START). J Cancer Res Clin Oncol 2014;140:319–28.

30. Fujitani K, Tamura S, Kimura Y, et al. Three-year outcomes of a phase II study of adjuvant chemotherapy with S-1 plus docetaxel for stage III gastric cancer after curative D2 gastrectomy. Gastric Cancer 2014;17(2):348–53.

31. Yoshikawa T, Sasako M, Yamamoto S, et al. Phase II study of neoadjuvant chemotherapy and extended surgery for locally advanced gastric cancer. Br J Surg 2009;96:1015–22.

32. Ito S, Sano T, Mizusawa J, et al. A phase II study of preoperative chemotherapy with docetaxel, cisplatin, and S-1 followed by gastrectomy with D2 plus para-aortic lymph node dissection for gastric cancer with extensive lymph node metastasis: JCOG1002. Gastric Cancer 2016;1–10.

33. Kinoshita T, Sasako M, Sano T, et al. Phase II trial of S-1 for neoadjuvant chemotherapy against scirrhous gastric cancer (JCOG 0002). Gastric Cancer 2009;12: 37–42.

34. Iwasaki Y, Sasako M, Yamamoto S, et al. Phase II study of preoperative chemotherapy with S-1 and cisplatin followed by gastrectomy for clinically resectable type 4 and large type 3 gastric cancers (JCOG0210). J Surg Oncol 2013;107: 741–5.

35. Bang YJ, Van Cutsem E, Feyereislova A, et al. Trastuzumab in combination with chemotherapy versus chemotherapy alone for treatment of HER2-positive advanced gastric or gastro-oesophageal junction cancer (ToGA): a phase 3, open-label, randomised controlled trial. Lancet 2010;376:687–97.

36. Kurokawa Y, Sugimoto N, Miwa H, et al. Phase II study of trastuzumab in combination with S-1 plus cisplatin in HER2-positive gastric cancer (HERBIS-1). Br J Cancer 2014;110:1163–8.

37. Park I, Ryu MH, Choi YH, et al. A phase II study of neoadjuvant docetaxel, oxaliplatin, and S-1 (DOS) chemotherapy followed by surgery and adjuvant S-1 chemotherapy in potentially resectable gastric or gastroesophageal junction adenocarcinoma. Cancer Chemother Pharmacol 2013;72:815–23.

38. Ishigami H, Kitayama J, Kaisaki S, et al. Phase II study of weekly intravenous and intraperitoneal paclitaxel combined with S-1 for advanced gastric cancer with peritoneal metastasis. Ann Oncol 2010;21:67–70.

39. Fujiwara Y, Takiguchi S, Nakajima K, et al. Intraperitoneal docetaxel combined with S-1 for advanced gastric cancer with peritoneal dissemination. J Surg Oncol 2012;105:38–42.

40. Kurokawa Y, Hamakawa T, Miyazaki Y, et al. Preoperative systemic and intraperitoneal chemotherapy consisting of S-1, cisplatin and docetaxel in patients with marginally resectable gastric cancer. Anticancer Res 2015;35:2223–8.

Current Progress in the Adjuvant Treatment of Gastric Cancer

David H. Ilson, MD, PhD

KEYWORDS

- Gastric cancer • D2 resection • Adjuvant chemotherapy • S-1 • Capecitabine
- Cisplatin • Oxaliplatin • Infusional 5-FU

KEY POINTS

- Staging of gastric cancer should include laparoscopy.
- Perioperative chemotherapy improves survival in addition to surgery.
- Postoperative chemotherapy after D2 resection improves survival after surgery.
- After less than a D1 resection adjuvant chemotherapy and radiation therapy improve survival.
- For gastroesophageal junction cancers, combined chemotherapy and radiation therapy may be needed to improve R0 resection rates.

Gastric cancer is a leading global health problem and accounts for the third most common cause of cancer-related death.[1] In the United States in 2016 there will be an estimated 26,370 new cases and 10,730 deaths, accounting for 1.6% of new cancer diagnoses.[2] The disease is most common in East Asia, and China accounts for more than half the of world's gastric cancer burden. *Helicobacter pylori* infection, which is the cause of a substantial portion of gastric cancer globally, is declining in incidence and may account in large part for the steep reduction in cases of gastric cancer in the West over the past century.[3] Progress has been made in the surgical management of locally advanced disease, and trials have established a clear role for combing systemic chemotherapy in the adjuvant or neoadjuvant setting with surgery. The application of adjuvant radiotherapy is shifting in utilization with the increasing use of preoperative and postoperative chemotherapy, and its relative benefit may be a function of the adequacy of surgical management performed.

The author has nothing to disclose.
Gastrointestinal Oncology Service, Memorial Sloan Kettering Cancer Center, 300 E. 66th Street, New York, NY 10065, USA
E-mail address: ilsond@MSKCC.ORG

Surg Oncol Clin N Am 26 (2017) 225–239
http://dx.doi.org/10.1016/j.soc.2016.10.008
1055-3207/17/© 2016 Elsevier Inc. All rights reserved.

surgonc.theclinics.com

STAGING AND SURGICAL MANAGEMENT OF GASTRIC CANCER

In the West, there is no effective screening for gastric cancer, given the relative rarity of the disease compared with diseases like breast and colorectal cancer, which have active screening programs. As a consequence, most patients diagnosed with gastric cancer present with locally advanced and often symptomatic disease, and up to 40% of patients present with overt metastatic disease. In high-incidence countries, such as Korea and Japan, there are population-wide screening programs leading to earlier stage at diagnosis. Stage for stage, survival outcomes appear superior in Japan and Korea, which may reflect inherent biologic differences in gastric cancer in the East and West.[4] Recent genomic profiling studies indicate similar molecular subtypes of gastric cancers between Eastern and Western patients with gastric cancer, but immune signatures may differ.[5–7]

The standards for surgical staging and management of gastric cancer have been developed largely in Asia. The American Joint Committee on Cancer has recently updated the staging of gastric cancer, using nodal count to reflect N substage and in an attempt to harmonize with Eastern staging systems.[8] After diagnosis with upper endoscopic assessment and biopsy confirmation, gastric cancer staging includes imaging with a computed tomography (CT) scan of the chest, abdomen, and pelvis. If metastatic disease is revealed on imaging, biopsy confirmation of metastatic disease may be required, as clinically indicated, before consideration for primary treatment with palliative chemotherapy. PET with fludeoxyglucose (FDG-PET) imaging is not yet routinely accepted as part of staging, but recent studies suggest that up to 15% of patients may have occult metastatic disease identified on FDG-PET scan that is not seen on CT imaging,[9] indicating an ability independently to upstage patients to metastatic disease. Diffuse gastric cancers, however, appear to have a high proportion of FDG-PET scan nonavidity. If no metastatic disease is seen on CT scan imaging, endoscopic ultrasound is performed to assess T and N stage. For early T1N0 tumors, endoscopic mucosal resection and endoscopic mucosal dissection have emerged as preferred therapy options for superficial T1A mucosal lesions.[10] For more deeply penetrating T1b lesions, limited gastrectomy and assessment of sentinel lymph node involvement is also an emerging surgical strategy.[11]

Unfortunately, in the West most patients have more extensive T3 or T4a and node-positive disease. If endoscopic ultrasound identifies T2 or greater T stage or node-positive disease, staging laparoscopy is performed to assess for peritoneal disease, often poorly imaged or missed altogether on routine CT or PET scan imaging. In the absence of visible peritoneal disease, the finding of a positive cytology on peritoneal washings is also now classified as stage IV disease and should direct patients away from surgery and toward chemotherapy-based management of metastatic disease.[8]

Surgery remains the mainstay of curative treatment. There is an emerging consensus about the appropriate surgical management of locally advanced gastric cancer. In Asia, the surgical standard of care combines a subtotal or total gastrectomy with D2 lymph node resection, which encompasses greater and lesser curvature nodes taken in a D1 resection, and also includes gastrohepatic, celiac, and splenic nodes. Extending surgery to include more extensive nodal resection, including retroperitoneal nodes in a D3 resection, has not been shown to improve outcome in a randomized trial conducted in Japan comparing D2 and D3 resections.[12] Although earlier small, comparative trials of D2 versus lesser resections in the West failed to indicate a survival advantage for a D2 resection and suggested greater operative morbidity and the potential need for splenic and pancreatic resection,[13–15] more contemporary series and updates of earlier series indicate superior survival for a D2 resection.[16,17]

Already the standard surgical procedure in Asia, D2 resection is also now the standard surgical procedure to treat gastric cancer in Europe and the United States. Adequacy of surgical resection in adjuvant therapy trials has clearly influenced outcome in modern trials, and may explain the relative contributions of adjuvant chemotherapy and radiotherapy to surgical resection.

ADJUVANT CHEMOTHERAPY IN GASTRIC CANCER: PREOPERATIVE CHEMOTHERAPY

The incorporation of adjuvant chemotherapy into the surgical management of locally advanced gastric cancer has now become a global standard of care based on accumulating evidence from controlled clinical trials comparing surgery alone with or without the inclusion of systemic chemotherapy. Early individual clinical trials evaluating postoperative adjuvant chemotherapy both in Asia and the West were almost uniformly negative. Investigational use of preoperative and postoperative chemotherapy led to randomized trials of this approach, with results of contemporary phase III trials outlined in Table 1. Preoperative chemotherapy has a number of potential advantages, including better therapy tolerance and an enhanced ability to deliver preoperative versus postoperative chemotherapy. There is the potential for downstaging of the primary tumor and increasing the rate of curative resection, and the early introduction of systemic therapy to treat micrometastatic disease. Preoperative therapy also allows the potential to assess response to preoperative therapy, either on imaging or at pathologic assessment at surgery. One could argue that the delay in surgery might allow patients destined to develop early metastatic disease to declare themselves during the period of preoperative therapy, potentially sparing patients from gastric resection that may not help them. The counter argument is the risk of disease progression on ineffective preoperative therapy and missing the opportunity for curative resection. Pathologic stage determined at up-front surgery might also more accurately identify higher-risk patients most appropriate for adjuvant therapy treatment.

The seminal Medical Research Council Adjuvant Gastric Infusional Chemotherapy (MAGIC) trial of perioperative chemotherapy in gastric cancer conducted by Cunningham and colleagues[18] in the United Kingdom was first reported in 2006. Patients were eligible for this trial if they had evidence of clinical stage II or higher adenocarcinomas of the lower third of the esophagus, gastroesophageal (GE) junction, or stomach

Table 1					
Preoperative chemotherapy in gastroesophageal junction and gastric cancer					
Trial	Patient No.	Treatment	PFS or DFS	5-y OS	Reference
MAGIC	250	ECF	PFS HR 0.66	36.3%	Cunningham et al,[18] 2006
	253	Surgery		23.0%	
FNCLCC-FFCD	113	CF	5-y DFS 34%	38%	Ychou et al,[19] 2011
	111	Surgery	19%	24%	
EORTC 40954	72	CF	PFS HR 0.76	2-y OS 73%	Schuhmacher et al,[20] 2010
	72	Surgery		70%	

Abbreviations: CF, cisplatin + 5-FU; DFS, disease-free survival; ECF, epirubicin, cisplatin, and 5-FU; EORTC, European Organization for the Research and Treatment of Cancer; FNCLCC-FFCD, Federation Nationales des Centres de Lutte Contre de Cancer—Federation Francophone de Cancerologie Digestive; HR, hazard ratio; MAGIC, Medical Research Council Adjuvant Gastric Infusional Chemotherapy; OS, overall survival; PFS, progression-free survival.

based on CT imaging, ultrasonography, or laparoscopy. However, no specific pre-treatment staging was mandated nor was pretherapy clinical stage captured. Of the 503 patients enrolled in the study, most (74%) had gastric primaries and the remainder had cancers of the distal esophagus or GE junction. Patients were assigned to imme-diate surgery or treatment with 3 cycles of epirubicin, cisplatin, and continuous-infusion fluorouracil (5-FU) administered over a 3-week cycle followed by surgery, and then 3 additional cycles of epirubicin, cisplatin, and 5-FU (ECF) after surgery. Fewer patients on the preoperative chemotherapy arm went to surgery (229 patients, 92%) compared with the immediate surgery patients (244 patients, 96%) mainly due to disease progression. Comparable rates of R0 resection were reported on the preop-erative therapy arm (69%) and surgery alone arm (66%), with esophagogastrectomy or D1 resection performed in 43% to 44% and D2 resection in 40% to 42% of patients. In comparing postoperative pathologic findings, there was a suggestion of tumor down-staging with more T1-2 tumors in the chemotherapy group compared with surgery alone (52% vs 37%) and more N0-1 tumors (84% vs 72%), although similar numbers of patients had N0 disease with or without chemotherapy (31%–27%). Progression-free and overall survival were superior for the chemotherapy arm, with a 5-year overall survival improved from 23% to 36% with chemotherapy. This translated into a 25% reduction in the risk of death with preoperative therapy. Only 49% of patients who completed preoperative therapy and surgery completed postoperative chemo-therapy. There were no untoward toxicity signals observed with the use of preopera-tive therapy, and no increase in surgical complications or postoperative mortality. Based on the results of this trial, and in particular given the failure of prior studies to demonstrate a clear-cut survival benefit for postoperative adjuvant chemotherapy, preoperative and postoperative chemotherapy became a new care standard in West-ern Europe and the United States.

Supportive evidence for a survival benefit for perioperative chemotherapy was also reported by the subsequently published FNCLCC-FFCD (Federation Nationales des Centres de Lutte Contre de Cancer—Federation Francophone de Cancerologie Diges-tive) French trial in 224 patients with adenocarcinoma of the lower esophagus, GE junc-tion, or stomach.[19] Most patients on this trial (75%) had cancers of the lower esophagus or GE junction and 25% had stomach cancer. Patients were required to have resectable disease based on CT scan, but staging endoscopic ultrasound was optional. Patients were treated with 2 to 3 cycles of a preoperative 5-day infusion 5-FU with cisplatin and up to 4 cycles of postoperative chemotherapy, or surgery alone. At least 2 cycles of preoperative therapy were delivered in 87% of patients and nearly all patients went to surgery, and 50% of patients received at least 1 cycle of postoperative chemotherapy. Unlike the MAGIC trial, in this trial the rate of curative resection was improved with pre-operative chemotherapy (74%–84%). There was a trend toward a lower rate of node positivity (33% vs 20%) in patients treated with chemotherapy. Progression-free and overall survival were superior on the chemotherapy arm with improved 5-year survival for preoperative chemotherapy compared with surgery (38% compared with 24%), which led to a 31% reduction in the risk of death. This trial, although smaller and less well powered than the MAGIC trial, achieved a similar survival benefit for perioperative chemotherapy and used a regimen without the inclusion of epirubicin.

A smaller recently reported trial of preoperative 5-FU and cisplatin versus surgery alone conducted by the European Organisation for the Research and Treatment of Can-cer in an equal mixture of patients with gastric and GE junction adenocarcinoma, was closed prematurely due to poor accrual.[20] Patients were required to have staging with a CT scan of the chest, abdomen, and pelvis; endoscopic ultrasound documenting T3-4 disease; and negative findings at staging laparoscopy, and at least a D1 or D2 surgical resection was mandated. Of the 144 patients, the preoperative chemotherapy group had significantly higher rates of R0 resection (82% vs 67%), and a complete pathologic response to chemotherapy was reported in 7.1% of patients. There was no difference in progression-free survival between the 2 therapy arms, and overall survival at 2 years was similar on the surgery alone and chemotherapy arms (70% vs 73%).

Anxiously awaited are the results of the FLOT4 trial, which compares in more than 700 patients with GE junction and gastric cancer perioperative chemotherapy with ECF or a regimen combining docetaxel with infusional 5-FU and oxaliplatin (FLOT). An encouraging rate of pathologic complete response favoring the FLOT arm was reported in an early interim analysis, and final report of this trial is still pending.[21]

ADJUVANT CHEMOTHERAPY IN GASTRIC CANCER: POSTOPERATIVE CHEMOTHERAPY

Historically, postoperative adjuvant chemotherapy trials have not indicated a clear survival benefit for postoperative adjuvant chemotherapy after gastrectomy, despite positive signals from some early small, underpowered trials. The landscape changed with publication of large trials conducted in Asia with universally superior quality of surgery performed, with mandates for D2 resection in all patients entering adjuvant therapy trials. Results from these contemporary adjuvant trials are outlined in Table 2. In 2007, Sakuramoto and colleagues[22] from Japan reported results of the Adjuvant Chemotherapy for Gastric Cancer with S-1 (ACTGS) trial. More than 1000 patients post curative D2 resection of stage II or III gastric cancer were randomized to observation alone, or to 1 year of therapy with the oral agent S-1, which combines the oral 5-FU prodrug tegafur with a dihydropyrimidine dehydrogenase inhibitor gimeracil and the bowel protectant oteracil, which inhibits phosphorylation of fluorouracil in the gastrointestinal tract. Of the patients treated, 54% to 55% had T2 disease and 43% to 44% had T3 disease, and 53% to 56% were N1 and 34% to 35% were N2. Progression-free and overall survival were improved with S-1 at the first interim analysis, with a 3-year survival of 80% for S-1 compared with 70% for surgery alone. At long-term follow-up, a significant survival benefit was maintained for therapy with S-1.[23] Relapse-free survival was improved from 53% to 65% with S-1, overall survival was improved from 61% to 72%, and this resulted in a 35% reduction in the risk of death. In subgroup analyses, the greatest incremental survival benefit for S-1 was seen for patients who were node negative (hazard ratio [HR] 0.317) and a lesser but still significant benefit was seen for N1 patients (HR 0.608) and N2 patients (0.839). Rates of grade 3 and 4 toxicities were in the single digits with therapy. Only 66% of patients completed the entire year of therapy, and 78% completed at least 6 months of therapy. Given this clear validation for the use of adjuvant postoperative chemotherapy after adequate D2 surgical resection, in Japan treatment with S-1 for 1 year after gastrectomy became and continues to be a standard of care.

Table 2
Postoperative chemotherapy in gastroesophageal junction and gastric cancer

Trial	Patient No.	Treatment	5-y Disease-Free Survival, %	5-y Overall Survival, %	Reference
ACTGS	515	S-1	65	72	Sasako et al,[23]
	519	Surgery	53	61	2011
CLASSIC	520	Cape-Oxali	68	78	Noh et al,[25]
	515	Surgery	53	69	2014

Abbreviations: ACTGS, Adjuvant Chemotherapy for Gastric Cancer with S-1; Cape-Oxali, Capecitabine + Oxaliplatin; CLASSIC, Capecitabine and Oxaliplatin Adjuvant Study in Gastric Cancer.

Many investigators in the West were reluctant to accept the benefits of adjuvant chemotherapy for S-1, as Western trials of this agent in more advanced metastatic disease indicated greater toxicity in Western patients and the requirement to deliver lower doses to patients. However, supportive evidence for a benefit for adjuvant chemotherapy after D2 gastrectomy came shortly thereafter for use of a chemotherapy regimen already widely used in Western countries in the treatment of advanced gastric cancer: oral capecitabine combined with oxaliplatin. Korean investigators reported results of the Capecitabine and Oxaliplatin Adjuvant Study in Gastric Cancer (CLASSIC) trial first in 2012.[24] This trial enrolled more than 1000 patients with gastric cancer undergoing prior curative D2 gastrectomy with pathologic stage II-IIIB disease. The chemotherapy consisted of 8, 3-week cycles of oxaliplatin combined with capecitabine administered 2 of every 3 weeks. T2 disease was present in 54% to 55% and T3 disease in 44%, and N1 disease was seen in 60% and N2 disease in 29% to 31%. Three-year disease-free survival was increased from 59% to 74% with adjuvant chemotherapy and overall survival was increased from 78% to 83%, which even at early follow-up reached statistical significance. The investigators recently reported updated mature follow-up and survival data for the CLASSIC Trial.[25] Five-year overall survival with surgery alone was 69% and was increased to 78% with adjuvant chemotherapy and resulted in a 31% reduction in the risk of death. No new toxicity signals were seen with this commonly used chemotherapy regimen. In contrast to the Japanese ACTGS trial of S-1, which indicated the greatest survival benefit for N0 disease, the CLASSIC trial indicated the greatest survival benefit for N1-2 disease (HR 0.67) compared with N0 disease (0.79), and has suggested to some Asian investigators that adjuvant therapy with S-1 is appropriate for node-negative patients and combination chemotherapy with capecitabine and oxaliplatin is more appropriate for node-positive disease. Based on the positive results in these 2 trials for adjuvant chemotherapy in more than 2000 patients with gastric cancer undergoing D2 resection, Western treatment guidelines now acknowledge that postoperative adjuvant chemotherapy is an acceptable therapy option after D2 gastrectomy.

Additional support for a benefit for postoperative chemotherapy after gastrectomy also comes from a recent meta-analysis of Western adjuvant chemotherapy trials.[26] In a pooled analysis of 17 trials treating more than 3800 patients with more than 7 years of follow-up, 5-year overall survival was improved by 5.7% and resulted in 18% reduction in the risk of death with the use of postoperative adjuvant chemotherapy after gastrectomy.

ADJUVANT CHEMOTHERAPY IN GASTRIC CANCER: THE ROLE OF POSTOPERATIVE RADIOTHERAPY AND PATTERNS OF LOCAL RECURRENCE

The role of adjuvant radiotherapy combined with chemotherapy in gastric cancer has become increasingly controversial given the advent of positive data for both perioperative chemotherapy and, in patients undergoing D2 resection, postoperative adjuvant chemotherapy alone. The quality of surgery performed has also impacted on contemporary trial outcomes with the near universal adoption of a D2 gastric resection. Results from clinical trials evaluating postoperative chemotherapy and radiation therapy are outlined in Table 3. The early landmark trial reported by Macdonald and colleagues[27] in 2001 evaluated the role of postoperative 5-FU and leucovorin given in conjunction with postoperative radiotherapy after gastric cancer resection. The impetus for this trial was earlier reports of a potential long-term survival benefit in patients with locally unresectable gastric cancer achieving long-term survival with 5-FU and radiation-based therapy.[28] Patients on the INT-0116/SWOG 9008 trial were

Table 3
Postoperative chemotherapy with or without radiotherapy in gastroesophageal junction and gastric cancer

Trial	Patient No.	Treatment	Disease-Free Survival	5-y Overall Survival	Reference
INT 0116	281	5-FU/LV + RT	3-y DFS 48%	3-y OS 50%	Macdonald et al,[27] 2001
	275	Surgery	31%	41%	
ARTIST	230	Cape-Cis + RT	DFS HR 0.740	75%	Park et al,[31] 2015
	228	Cape-Cis		73%	
CRITICS	332	ECC → Cape-Cis + RT	5-y DFS 39.5%	40.9%	Verheij et al,[32] 2016
	316	ECC → ECC	38.5%	40.8%	

Abbreviations: 5-FU, 5-fluorouracil; ARTIST, Adjuvant Chemoradiation Therapy in Stomach Cancer; Cape-Cis, Capecitabine + Cisplatin; CRITICS, ChemoRadiotherapy after Induction chemotherapy in Cancer of the Stomach; DFS, disease-free survival; ECC, epirubicin, cisplatin, and capecitabine; HR, hazard ratio; LV, leucovorin; OS, overall survival; RT, radiotherapy.

randomized after curative gastric resection to observation alone, or to a regimen of adjuvant chemotherapy with bolus 5-FU and leucovorin for 3 months, with administration during months 2 to 3 of 45 Gy of radiation therapy combined with bolus 5-FU and leucovorin during weeks 1 and 5 of radiotherapy. Patients were eligible if they had curative resection of American Joint Committee on Cancer 1988 stage IB through IV M0 adenocarcinoma of the stomach or GE junction. Of the 556 patients randomized and treated, 31% were T2 and 61% to 62% were T3, 41% to 42% had 1 to 3 involved nodes and 43% had 4 or more involved nodes, and most had cancers of the corpus or antrum (77%–81%). Only 64% of patients completed all planned therapy and 17% discontinued therapy due to toxicity. Adjuvant therapy increased the median survival from 27 to 36 months and 3-year survival was improved from 41% to 50%. At long-term follow-up, a survival benefit for postoperative chemoradiotherapy was maintained, with a 24% reduction in mortality and an absolute survival improvement of 10%.[29] At the time of reporting of this trial, this was the first positive trial for the use of adjuvant chemotherapy or radiotherapy from the West in an adequately powered, controlled randomized trial. This trial established a care standard until the advent of results from perioperative and postoperative adjuvant chemotherapy trials, discussed previously, which indicted a survival benefit for the use of chemotherapy without radiotherapy. The quality of surgical resection and lymph node retrieval was relatively poor on INT-0116: only 10% underwent a formal D2 resection, most underwent a D0 resection (54%), and 36% had a D1 resection. In contrast, the more contemporary chemotherapy alone trials reported D1-D2 resection rates of 80% to 100%. More troubling is the actual impact of postoperative chemoradiotherapy: there was no impact on reduction of distant metastatic disease, and the survival improvement appeared to accrue only due to a reduction in local tumor recurrence with chemoradiotherapy. The poor quality of surgery on INT-0116 and the ability of adjuvant therapy to reduce only local recurrence led many to question the contribution, if any, of radiation therapy to adjuvant chemotherapy if better surgical quality, including the achieving of a least a D1 and preferably a D2 resection, was mandated.

More contemporary clinical trials evaluating the role of postoperative radiotherapy in conjunction with adjuvant chemotherapy and surgery have now been reported. In particular, these trials have had more rigorous surgery mandated as part of protocol therapy. The Korean Adjuvant Chemoradiation Therapy in Stomach Cancer (ARTIST) trial evaluated the addition of radiation therapy to adjuvant chemotherapy in resected gastric cancer.[30] On this trial, 458 patients underwent D2 resection of gastric cancer. Patients were assigned to adjuvant chemotherapy with capecitabine and cisplatin administered for 6, 3-week cycles, or to receive adjuvant chemoradiotherapy with 45 Gy or radiation therapy combined with concurrent daily capecitabine preceded by 2 cycles of capecitabine cisplatin and then followed by 2 cycles of capecitabine cisplatin. Most patients had stage II or IIIA disease (59%–60%), 54% to 57% had N1 disease, and 21% to 23% had N2 disease. At initial report, there was no difference in 3-year disease-free survival either with (78%) or without chemoradiotherapy (72%). At long-term follow-up,[31] there was no survival benefit at 5 years comparing chemotherapy alone (73%) with chemoradiotherapy (75%). In a subset analysis, patients with intestinal and node-positive cancers did achieve a survival benefit with the addition of radiation therapy to chemotherapy. Three-year disease-free survival was increased from 72% to 76% with the addition of radiation therapy in 396 patients with node-positive disease, and a potential greater benefit for radiation therapy added to chemotherapy in the 163 patients with intestinal tumors (83% to 94%) with no benefit seen in node-negative tumors or in diffuse cancers. Based on these results, in Korea the ARTIST 2 Trial is under way comparing adjuvant chemotherapy alone or with chemoradiotherapy after D2 gastrectomy in intestinal, node-positive cancers.

Investigators from Europe recently reported results of the ChemoRadiotherapy after Induction chemotherapy in Cancer of the Stomach (CRITICS) trial in abstract form.[32] This trial melded the approach or perioperative chemotherapy with postoperative chemoradiotherapy, with patients all treated with 3 cycles of preoperative chemotherapy with epirubicin, cisplatin, and capecitabine (ECC) followed by surgery. Patients after surgery were then randomly assigned to either complete 3 additional cycles of ECC, or receive 45 Gy of postoperative radiotherapy combined with capecitabine and cisplatin. Patients were required to have surgically resectable clinical stage Ib to IVa gastric cancer based on endoscopic ultrasound and CT scan imaging, and laparoscopic staging was optional. Most patients had mid or distal gastric cancers (62%) and only 17% had cancers of the GE junction, and roughly a third each had intestinal, diffuse, or subtype unknown gastric cancer. Chemotherapy preoperatively was completed in 81% to 85% of patients, 93% to 94% went to surgery, and 80% to 84% had an R0 resection. A D1 resection was performed in 49% and a D2 resection in 37%. All therapy was completed in 47% to 52% of patients, and 61% to 63% received at least some planned postoperative therapy. There was no difference in median overall survival with or without postoperative radiotherapy (3.3–3.5 years) and there was no difference in 5-year overall survival (41%).

Two contemporary randomized trials evaluating either preoperative or postoperative chemotherapy have now failed to show a clear survival benefit for the addition of postoperative radiotherapy when a D1 or D2 resection is performed. It is arguable given currently available data that postoperative radiation therapy should be considered primarily in patients with gastric cancer undergoing less than a D1 resection, and using either perioperative chemotherapy or postoperative adjuvant chemotherapy alone is the preferred adjuvant strategy in patients undergoing D1-2 resection. The ARTIST Trial suggests a small survival benefit in node-positive disease potentially limited to intestinal tumors, and an ongoing trial is addressing the role of postoperative radiotherapy in these patients.

Understanding the recurrence patterns in these adjuvant trials as a function of adequacy of surgical resection further clarifies the potential role for postoperative radiation therapy. INT-0116 (10% D2 resection) reported local recurrences as the first site of relapse in 29% of patients undergoing surgery alone, reduced to 19% with chemo-radiotherapy. On the MAGIC trial (42% D2 resection), local recurrence with surgery alone was reported in 20% of patients, reduced to 14% on the chemotherapy arm. On the ACTGS study (100% D2 resection), local recurrence was reported in 3% of patients receiving surgery alone and 2% receiving S-1. On the CLASSIC Trial (100% D2 resection), local recurrence with surgery alone was 8.5% reduced to 4.4% with adjuvant chemotherapy. On the ARTIST Trial (100% D2 resection), local recurrence on the chemotherapy arm occurred in 13% and was reduced to 7% with chemoradiotherapy. Local recurrences appear less common with D2 resection, and again the role of radiotherapy in node-positive, intestinal tumors will now be addressed in the ARTIST 2 Trial.

ADJUVANT CHEMOTHERAPY IN GASTRIC CANCER: ROLE OF NUMBER OF AGENTS AND THERAPY DURATION

The optimal agents to use in adjuvant or neoadjuvant chemotherapy, and the optimal duration of therapy, also have been the subject of contemporary randomized clinical trials. INT-0116 established 5-FU and leucovorin as an effective component of adjuvant chemotherapy (with radiation), and the subsequent S-1 trial from Japan reinforced a survival benefit for fluorinated pyrimidine monochemotherapy, given for a year, as adjuvant treatment after gastric resection. The CLASSIC Trial indicated a survival benefit for combined capecitabine and oxaliplatin given for only 6 months, and as discussed previously, cross-trial comparison with the S-1 trial suggested a potential benefit for combination chemotherapy versus monotherapy in node-positive disease. A follow-up trial to INT-0116, CALGB 80101, attempted chemotherapy intensification of adjuvant treatment, comparing postoperative 5-FU and leucovorin with postoperative ECF in patients also receiving infusional 5-FU and postoperative radiation therapy,[33] published in abstract form. There was no survival benefit for ECF versus 5-FU/leucovorin adjuvant chemotherapy with no difference in either median survival (37–38 months) or 3-year overall survival (41%–44%). There appeared to be no survival benefit for ECF compared with adjuvant chemotherapy with 5-FU and leucovorin. A larger trial from Korea also compared fluorinated pyrimidine–based monochemotherapy with or without the addition of cisplatin, the AMC0201 trial.[34] Patients were randomized to receive a single dose of postoperative mitomycin followed by 3 months of the oral fluorinated pyrimidine doxifluridine, versus the same treatment plus extension of treatment with doxifluridine out to 1 year and the addition of cisplatin to the first 6 months of adjuvant chemotherapy. Both intensifying therapy with cisplatin and extending therapy beyond 3 months failed to improve outcome compared with 3 months of therapy (5-year survival of 65% compared with 66%).

The addition of other agents to fluorinated pyrimidine–based chemotherapy has also been reported in 2 recent large randomized clinical trials. The Stomach cancer Adjuvant multi-Institutional group Trial (SAMIT) randomized nearly 1500 patients after D2 resection to receive 12 months of S-1 alone, UFT (tegafur and uracil) alone, or paclitaxel weekly therapy for 11 weeks followed by either 36 weeks of UFT or S-1.[35] There was no improvement for the addition of paclitaxel in 3-year overall survival (59%) compared with monotherapy (56%). The Intergroup Trial of Adjuvant Chemotherapy in Adenocarcinoma of the Stomach (ITACA-S) Trial compared adjuvant chemotherapy after gastric cancer resection with every 2 weekly infusional 5-FU and leucovorin over 4 months, or to a sequencing of therapy first with infusional 5-FU, leucovorin, and irinotecan for 4 cycles followed by docetaxel combined with cisplatin for 3 cycles.[36] In more than 1100 patients treated in this trial, no difference in 5-year survival was seen for infusional 5-FU versus sequential therapy (45%). These trial results indicated that introduction of either a taxane or irinotecan in sequence with fluorinated pyrimidine chemotherapy failed to improve outcome. These trials also indicate uncertain benefits for 3 months versus 6 months versus 1 year of adjuvant chemotherapy. The ARTIST 2 Trial, in addition to evaluating the contribution of radiation therapy to postoperative chemotherapy, also will include a comparison of the standards of 12 months of S-1 chemotherapy versus 6 months of capecitabine/platinum-based chemotherapy.

ALTERNATIVE ADJUVANT APPROACHES IN GASTRIC CANCER

In addition to study of perioperative chemotherapy, postoperative chemotherapy, and postoperative chemotherapy and radiation therapy, investigational trials have evaluated the inclusion of regional treatment by intraperitoneal (IP) administration of chemotherapeutic agents. The rationale for this approach includes the risk of peritoneal recurrence after gastric cancer resection, and the potential of the IP route of administration to escalate dose exposure to chemotherapeutic agents. The data for some of the smaller, underpowered studies have been conflicting, and there is no confirmed trial affirming a benefit for the use of IP chemotherapy. One of the larger contemporary trials conducted in Korea, AMC0101, randomized 521 patients at the time of surgery for gastric cancer to receive a single dose of IP cisplatin followed by systemic adjuvant chemotherapy versus adjuvant chemotherapy alone.[37] Patients were eligible intraoperatively if they had evidence of serosal penetrating gastric cancer, and who underwent D2 resection. The 2 groups, however, received different postoperative adjuvant regimens, with the IP cisplatin group going on to receive one dose of mitomycin followed by 12 months of doxifluridine combined with 6 months of cisplatin, and the non IP group received one dose of mitomycin and only 3 months of doxifluridine. Relapse-free survival was increased from 50% to 60% on the IP chemotherapy arm with a corresponding increase in overall survival from 60% to 71%. Interpretation of the impact of IP chemotherapy is confounded by the shorter duration of chemotherapy administered on the control arm, as well as the addition of cisplatin and prolonged administration of chemotherapy on the IP experimental arm. It is unclear whether or not further evaluation of IP chemotherapy will continue in Korea based on these results.

Pilot studies have evaluated the combination of chemotherapy and radiotherapy as preoperative treatment in more distal gastric cancers. Ajani and colleagues[38] reported feasibility of combining chemotherapy and radiation therapy in resectable gastric cancer in single-institution series and a pilot trial conducted through the Radiation Therapy Oncology Group. Induction chemotherapy with infusional 5-FU plus cisplatin was followed by radiation therapy combined with infusional 5-FU and paclitaxel followed by surgery in 43 evaluable patients. An encouraging rate of pathologic complete response was reported in 26% of patients and an R0 resection rate of 77% was achieved. The use of preoperative radiation therapy for gastric cancer has not been widely adopted given the increasing use of preoperative chemotherapy and given the debatable role for radiation therapy raised by contemporary randomized trials.

OUTCOMES IN GASTROESOPHAGEAL JUNCTION CANCERS

Clinical trials evaluating preoperative chemotherapy in gastric cancer have also included patients with cancer of the GE junction and sometimes of the distal esophagus. Early trials of preoperative chemotherapy for esophageal and GE junction adenocarcinoma indicated poor rates of R0 curative resection with preoperative chemotherapy ranging from 54% to 63%, with some studies showing no survival benefit for preoperative chemotherapy beyond surgery alone.[39,40] High rates of local failure even in patients achieving R0 resection were reported ranging from 27% to 32%. Increasingly the combination of chemotherapy and radiotherapy as preoperative therapy of esophageal and GE junction cancers has emerged as an international standard of care based on results reported from the contemporary Chemoradiotherapy for Esophageal Cancer followed by Surgery Study (CROSS).[41] This trial compared surgery alone with preoperative weekly carboplatin, paclitaxel, and radiotherapy followed by surgery in esophageal and GEJ adenocarcinoma and squamous cell carcinoma, although most patients treated on trial had adenocarcinoma. In addition to increasing survival with combined preoperative chemoradiotherapy, high rates of R0 resection (92%) and relatively low rates of local recurrence (14%) were reported on this trial. Concern about the adequacy of preoperative chemotherapy alone in these patients has been underscored by reports even in contemporary trials of persistently poor rates of R0 resection for esophageal and GE junction cancers, despite careful preoperative staging with endoscopic ultrasound, PET scan, and laparoscopy. Two trials from the United Kingdom recently reported in abstract form evaluating preoperative chemotherapy in 1900 patients, including 1600 patients with esophageal and GE junction cancers, reported R0 resection rates of 57% to 67% with preoperative chemotherapy,[42,43] despite endoscopic ultrasound, laparoscopic, and PET scan staging. These alarming results question the adequacy of preoperative chemotherapy without radiation therapy, and indicate the potential need to include preoperative radiation therapy to ensure at least a curative resection in patients with tumors involving the esophagus and GE junction. One ongoing trial in GE junction and gastric cancer, TOP-GEAR, is evaluating the use or perioperative chemotherapy with ECF with or without preoperative radiotherapy (NCT01924819).

NEW DIRECTIONS IN THE ADJUVANT TREATMENT OF GASTRIC CANCER

The benefits of any adjuvant treatment of gastric cancer have been modest, and the impact of such therapy translates into relatively small incremental survival benefits of 9% to 15%. In the West, most patients with resected gastric cancer still die of their disease.

Recent clinical trials have introduced novel targeted agents into adjuvant therapy. The large MAGIC 2 trial evaluated the contribution of the vascular endothelial growth factor-A ligand targeted agent bevacizumab combined with perioperative chemotherapy in resectable gastric cancer. The trial was undertaken before publication of negative results indicating a failure of bevacizumab to improve survival in metastatic gastric cancer when added to chemotherapy.[44] Results from the UK Medical Research Council ST03 trial were recently reported in abstract from.[43] The addition of bevacizumab to perioperative chemotherapy failed to improve survival compared with chemotherapy alone.

Genes amplified more commonly in esophagogastric cancers, which are also potentially targetable, include epidermal growth factor receptor (EGFR), MET, and human epidermal growth factor receptor 2 (HER2).[45] Trials of EGFR-targeted agents in esophagogastric cancer have failed to improve outcome in advanced disease combining agents such as cetuximab or panitumumab with chemotherapy.[46,47] Initial promise for MET-targeted agents in patients overexpressing the MET receptor ultimately led to disappointing negative results for MET-targeted agents added to chemotherapy in phase III trials.[48,49]

The HER2-targeted agent trastuzumab improved response, progression-free, and overall survival in the landmark Trastuzumab for Gastric Cancer (TOGA) trial when combined with chemotherapy in HER2-positive gastroesophageal cancer.[50] Ongoing trials are evaluating the addition of HER2-targeted agents to perioperative therapy in HER2-positive patients with esophagogastric cancer, including the INNOVATION trial in Europe evaluating the addition of trastuzumab, or dual targeting of the HER2 receptor with trastuzumab and pertuzumab, to chemotherapy (NCT02205047, NCT02581462).

Data are emerging from genomic analyses of gastric and GE junction cancers using broad genomic screening for gene mutation, amplification, and deletion. Remarkably similar genomic profiles have emerged from genomic studies evaluating Western and Asian patients with gastric cancer.[5,6] Molecular subgroups identified include genomically unstable tumors with higher rates of receptor-associated tyrosine kinase pathway gene amplification, genomically stable tumors, tumors with higher rates of gene hypermethylation leading to higher mutation burden, and tumors associated with Epstein-Barr virus infection. Stratification of patients on the basis of molecular profile will be obligatory in future adjuvant therapy trials given the potential for intrinsic biologic differences in these subsets. The identification of subsets also potentially more responsive to immunotherapy agents, including the emerging immune checkpoint inhibitors, may help guide future trial design.

Imaging during induction chemotherapy with PET scan may identify patients with early PET response who appear to have better clinical outcomes than PET nonresponders, with higher rates of pathologic response, R0 resection, and potentially improved survival. The use of PET scan to identify potential early response to induction chemotherapy in gastric cancer, and assigning PET scan nonresponding patients to alternative preoperative chemotherapy, is the subject of the ongoing Alliance trial A021302 (NCT02485834).

REFERENCES

1. Torre LA, Bray P, Siegel RL, et al. Global cancer statistics, 2012. CA Cancer J Clin 2015;65:87–108.
2. Siegel RL, Miller KD, Jemal A. Cancer statistics, 2016. CA Cancer J Clin 2016;66: 7–130.
3. Lee YC, Chiang TH, Chou CK, et al. Association between *Helicobacter pylori* eradication and gastric cancer incidence: a systematic review and meta-analysis. Gastroenterology 2016;150:1113–24.
4. Markar SR, Karthikesalingam A, Jackson D, et al. Long-term survival after gastrectomy for cancer in randomized, controlled oncological trials: comparison between East and West. Ann Surg Oncol 2013;20:2328–38.
5. Deng N, Doh LK, Wang H, et al. A comprehensive surgery of genomic alterations in gastric cancer reveals systemic patterns molecular exclusivity and co-occurrence among distinct therapeutic targets. Gut 2012;61:673–84.
6. Cancer Genome Atlas Research Network. Comprehensive molecular characterization of gastric adenocarcinoma. Nature 2014;513:202–9.
7. Lin SJ, Gagnon-Bartsch JA, Tan IB, et al. Signatures of tumour immunity distinguish Asian and non-Asian gastric adenocarcinomas. Gut 2015;64:1721–31.
8. Dikken JL, van de Velde CJ, Gönen M, et al. The New American Joint Committee on Cancer/International Union Against Cancer staging system for adenocarcinoma of the stomach: increased complexity without clear improvement in predictive accuracy. Ann Surg Oncol 2012;19:2443–51.
9. Smyth E, Schoder H, Strong VE, et al. A prospective evaluation of the utility of 2-deoxy-2-[(18) F]fluoro-D-glucose positron emission tomography and computed

tomography in staging locally advanced gastric cancer. Cancer 2012;118: 5481–8.

10. Kinami S, Funaki H, Fujita H, et al. Local resection of the stomach for gastric cancer. Surg Today 2016. [Epub ahead of print].

11. Fujimura T, Fushida S, Tsukada K, et al. A new stage of sentinel node navigation surgery in early gastric cancer. Gastric Cancer 2015;18:210–7.

12. Sasako M, Sano T, Yamamoto S, et al. D2 lymphadenectomy alone or with para-aortic nodal dissection for gastric cancer. N Engl J Med 2008;359:453–62.

13. Bonenkamp JJ, Songun I, Hermans J, et al. Randomised comparison of morbidity after D1 and D2 dissection for gastric cancer in 996 Dutch patients. Lancet 1995; 345:745–8.

14. Cuschieri A, Weeden S, Fielding J, et al. Patient survival after D1 and D2 resections for gastric cancer: long term results of the MRC randomized surgical trial. Br J Cancer 1999;79:1522–30.

15. Degiuli M, Sasako M, Ponti A. Morbidity and mortality in the Italian Gastric Study Group randomized clinical trial of D1 versus D2 resection for gastric cancer. Br J Surg 2010;97:643–9.

16. Seevaratnam R, Bocicariu A, Cardoso R, et al. A meta-analysis of D1 versus D2 lymph node dissection. Gastric Cancer 2012;15:S60–9.

17. Songun I, Putter H, Kranenbarg EMK, et al. Surgical treatment of gastric cancer: 15-year follow-up results of the randomised nationwide Dutch D1D2 trial. Lancet Oncol 2010;11:439–49.

18. Cunningham D, Allum WH, Stenning SP, et al. Perioperative chemotherapy versus surgery alone for resectable gastroesophageal cancer. N Engl J Med 2006;355: 11–20.

19. Ychou M, Boige V, Pignon JP, et al. Perioperative chemotherapy versus surgery alone for resectable gastroesophageal adenocarcinoma: an FNLCC and FFCD multicenter phase III trial. J Clin Oncol 2011;29:1715–21.

20. Schuhmacher C, Gretschel S, Lordick F, et al. Neoadjuvant chemotherapy compared with surgery alone for locally advanced cancer of the stomach and cardia: European Organisation for Research and Treatment of Cancer Randomized Trial 40954. J Clin Oncol 2010;28:5210–8.

21. Pauligk C, Tannapfel A, Meller J, et al. Pathologic response to neoadjuvant 5-FU, oxaliplatin, and docetaxel versus epirubicin, cisplatin, and 5-FU in patients with locally advanced resection gastric/esophageal junction cancer: data from the phase II part of the FLOT4 phase III study of the AIO. J Clin Oncol 2015; 33(Suppl) [abstract: 4016].

22. Sakuramoto S, Sasako M, Yamaguchi T, et al. Adjuvant chemotherapy for gastric cancer with S-1, an oral fluoropyrimidine. N Engl J Med 2007;357:1810–20.

23. Sasako M, Sakuramoto S, Katai H, et al. Five-year outcomes of a randomized phase III trial comparing adjuvant chemotherapy with S-1 versus surgery alone in stage II or III gastric cancer. J Clin Oncol 2011;29:4387–93.

24. Bang YJ, Kim YW, Yang HK, et al. Adjuvant capecitabine and oxaliplatin for gastric cancer after D2 gastrectomy (CLASSIC): a phase 3 open-label, randomised controlled trial. Lancet 2012;379:315–21.

25. Noh SH, Park SY, Yang HK, et al. Adjuvant capecitabine plus and oxaliplatin for gastric cancer after D2 gastrectomy (CLASSIC): 5-year follow-up of an open-label, randomised phase 3 trial. Lancet Oncol 2014;15:1389–96.

26. GASTRIC (Global Advanced/Adjuvant Stomach Tumor Research International Collaboration) Group, Paoletti X, Oba K, Burzykowski T, et al. Benefit of adjuvant

chemotherapy for resectable gastric cancer: a meta analysis. JAMA 2010;303: 1729–37.

27. Macdonald JS, Smalley SR, Benedetti J, et al. Chemoradiotherapy after surgery compared with surgery alone for adenocarcinoma of the stomach or gastro-esophageal junction. N Engl J Med 2001;345:725–30.

28. A comparison of combination chemotherapy and combined modality therapy for locally advanced gastric carcinoma. Gastrointestinal Tumor Study Group. Cancer 1982;49:1771–7.

29. Smalley SR, Benedetti JK, Haller DG, et al. Updated analysis of SWOG-directed Intergroup Study 0116: a phase III trial of adjuvant radiochemotherapy versus observation after curative gastric cancer resection. J Clin Oncol 2012;30: 2327–33.

30. Lee J, Lim DH, Kim S, et al. Phase III trial comparing capecitabine plus cisplatin versus capecitabine plus cisplatin with concurrent radiotherapy in completely re-sected gastric cancer with D2 lymph node dissection: the ARTIST Trial. J Clin On-col 2011;29:269–73.

31. Park SH, Sohn TS, Lee J, et al. Phase III trial to compare adjuvant chemotherapy with capecitabine and cisplatin versus concurrent chemoradiotherapy in gastric cancer: final report of the Adjuvant Chemoradiotherapy in Stomach Tumors Trial, including survival and subset analysis. J Clin Oncol 2015;33:3130–6.

32. Verheij M, Jansen EM, Annemieke Cats, et al. A multicenter randomized phase III trial of neo-adjuvant chemotherapy followed by surgery and chemotherapy or by surgery and chemoradiotherapy in resectable gastric cancer: first results from the CRITICS Study. J Clin Oncol 2016;34(suppl) [abstract: 4000].

33. Fuchs CS, Tepper JE, Niedzwiecki D, et al. Postoperative adjuvant chemoradia-tion for gastric or gastroesophageal junction adenocarcinoma using epirubicin, cisplatin, and infusional 5-FU before and after infusional 5-FU and radiotherapy compared with bolus 5-FU/LV before and after chemoradiotherapy: Intergroup Trial CALGB 80101. J Clin Oncol 2011;29(suppl) [abstract: 4000].

34. Kang YK, Chang HM, Yook YH, et al. Adjuvant chemotherapy for gastric cancer: a randomized phase 3 trial of mitomycin-C plus either short term doxifluridine or long term doxifluridine plus cisplatin after curative D2 gastrectomy (AMC0201). Br J Cancer 2013;108:1245–51.

35. Tsubuyara A, Yoshida K, Kobayashi M, et al. Sequential paclitaxel followed by te-gafur and uracil (UFT) or S-1 versus UFT or S-1 monotherapy as adjuvant chemo-therapy for T4a/b gastric cancer: a phase III factorial randomized controlled trial. Lancet Oncol 2014;15:886–93.

36. Bajetta E, Floriani I, Di Bartolomeo M, et al. Randomized trial on adjuvant treat-ment with FOLFIRI followed by docetaxel and cisplatin versus 5-fluorouracil and folinic acid for radically resected gastric cancer. Ann Oncol 2014;25:1373–8.

37. Kang YK, Yook JH, Chang HM, et al. Enhanced efficacy of postoperative adjuvant chemotherapy in advanced gastric cancer: results from a phase 3 randomized trial (AMC0101). Cancer Chemother Pharmacol 2014;73:139–49.

38. Ajani JA, Winter K, Okawara GS, et al. Phase II trial of preoperative chemoradia-tion in patients with localized gastric adenocarcinoma (RTOG 9904): quality of combined modality therapy and pathologic response. J Clin Oncol 2006;24: 3953–8.

39. Kelsen DP, Ginsberg R, Pajak TJ, et al. Chemotherapy followed by surgery compared with surgery alone for localized esophageal cancer. N Engl J Med 1998;339:1979–84.

40. Medical Research Council oesophageal Cancer Working Group. Surgical resection with or without preoperative chemotherapy in oesophageal cancer: a randomized controlled trial. Lancet 2002;359:1727–33.

41. Van Hagen P, Hulshof MC, van Lanschot JJ, et al. Preoperative chemoradiation for esophageal or junctional cancer. N Engl J Med 2012;366:2074–84.

42. Alderson D, Langley RE, Nankivell MG, et al. Neoadjuvant chemotherapy for resectable esophageal and junctional adenocarcinoma: results of the UK Medical Research Council randomized OEO5 trial. J Clin Oncol 2015;33(suppl) [abstract: 4002].

43. Cunningham D, Smyth E, Stenning S, et al. Perioperative chemotherapy +/- bevacizumab for resectable gastroesophageal adenocarcinoma: results from the UK Medical Research Council randomized STO3 trial. European Cancer Congress, Vienna (Austria), September 25–29, 2015. [abstract: 2201].

44. Ohtsu A, Shah MA, van Cutsem E, et al. Bevacizumab in combination with chemotherapy as first-line therapy in advanced gastric cancer: a randomized, double-blind placebo controlled phase III study. J Clin Oncol 2011;29:3968–76.

45. Dulak AM, Schumacher SE, van Lieshout J, et al. Gastrointestinal adenocarcinomas of the esophagus, stomach, and colon exhibit distinct patterns of genome instability and oncogenesis. Cancer Res 2012;72:4383–92.

46. Waddell T, Chau I, Cunningham D, et al. Epirubicin, cisplatin, and capecitabine with or without panitumumab for patients with previously untreated advanced esophagogastric cancer: a randomized, open-label phase III trial. Lancet Oncol 2013;14:481–9.

47. Lordick F, Kang YK, Chung HC, et al. Capecitabine and cisplatin with or without cetuximab for patients with previously untreated advanced gastric cancer (EXPAND): a randomised, open-label phase 3 trial. Lancet Oncol 2013;14:490–9.

48. Shah M, Bang YJ, Lordic F, et al. METGastric: a phase III study of onartuzumab plus mFOLFOX6 in patients with metastatic HER2-negative and MET-positive adenocarcinoma of the stomach or gastroesophageal junction. J Clin Oncol 2015;33(suppl) [abstract: 4012].

49. Cunningham D, Tebbutt N, Davidenko I, et al. Phase III, randomized, double-blind, multicenter, placebo (P)-controlled trial of rilotumumab (R) plus epirubicin, cisplatin and capecitabine (ECX) as first-line therapy in patients (pts) with advanced MET-positive (pos) gastric or gastroesophageal junction (G/GEJ) cancer: RILOMET-1 study. J Clin Oncol 2015;33(suppl) [abstract: 4000].

50. Bang YJ, van cutsem E, Feyereislova A, et al. Trastuzumab in combination with chemotherapy versus chemotherapy alone for treatment of HER2-positive advanced gastric or gastro-oesophageal junction cancer (ToGA): a phase 3, open-label, randomised controlled trial. Lancet 2010;376:687–97.

Controversies and Consensus in Preoperative Therapy of Esophageal and Gastroesophageal Junction Cancers

Geoffrey Y. Ku, MD

KEYWORDS

- Adenocarcinoma • Squamous cell carcinoma • Preoperative • Adjuvant
- Chemoradiation • Chemotherapy

KEY POINTS

- Chemoradiation is the standard of care for unresectable esophageal cancer and an option for squamous cell carcinoma (SCC); surgery reserved is for persistent/recurrent disease.
- There are limited and conflicting data supporting a role for preoperative or postoperative chemotherapy for resected SCC.
- Preoperative chemoradiation and surgery is a standard of care for esophageal/gastroesophageal junction (GEJ) adenocarcinoma.
- Other options for GEJ adenocarcinomas include perioperative chemotherapy or adjuvant chemoradiation.
- Adjuvant chemotherapy alone is an option for gastric adenocarcinoma based on Asian studies, where fewer than 10% of tumors involve the proximal stomach or GEJ.

INTRODUCTION

Esophageal cancer, an uncommon but highly virulent malignancy in the United States, will be diagnosed in 16,910 patients in 2016, with 15,690 deaths.[1] It is the seventh leading cause of death in men in the United States. In comparison with its relative rarity in the United States, esophageal cancer (predominantly squamous cell carcinoma [SCC]) is endemic in parts of East Asia, which accounts for more than one-half of the approximately 500,000 cases that develop per year (this number does not fully

The author has nothing to disclose.

Gastrointestinal Oncology Service, Department of Medicine, Memorial Sloan Kettering Cancer Center, 300 East 66th Street, Room 1035, New York, NY 10065, USA

E-mail address: kug@mskcc.org

Surg Oncol Clin N Am 26 (2017) 241–256
http://dx.doi.org/10.1016/j.soc.2016.10.009
surgonc.theclinics.com

take into account gastroesophageal or gastroesophageal junction (GEJ) tumors, which may variously be categorized as gastric cancers).[2]

SCC and adenocarcinoma account for 98% of all cases of esophageal cancer. SCCs typically occur in the proximal two-thirds of the esophagus, whereas adenocarcinomas are found in the distal one-third and at the GEJ. Although cases of SCC have declined steadily, the incidence of adenocarcinoma of the distal esophagus, GEJ and gastric cardia has increased 4% to 10% per year among US men since 1976, so that it now comprises 75% of all tumors.[3,4]

For locally advanced esophageal cancer, surgery remains the mainstay of treatment. Numerous studies—that have included both adenocarcinoma and SCC histologies and focused on tumors from the esophagus/GEJ and/or stomach—have evaluated preoperative and postoperative strategies for locally advanced disease, including chemotherapy or chemoradiation. As a whole, these studies show that some treatment in addition to surgery clearly improves outcomes. This review article discusses these studies; where relevant, we note whether these studies primarily enrolled patients with esophageal/GEJ or gastric tumors.

PREOPERATIVE CHEMOTHERAPY

A strategy of perioperative chemotherapy is the predominant approach in Europe, based primarily on the phase III MAGIC (Medical Research Council Adjuvant Gastric Infusional Chemotherapy) trial performed in the UK.[5] This trial randomized 503 patients with gastric cancer (26% of whom had tumors in the lower esophagus/GEJ) to 3 cycles (9 weeks) each of preoperative and postoperative ECF (epirubicin/cisplatin/5-fluorouracil [5-FU]) and surgery or surgery alone. Perioperative chemotherapy resulted in significant improvement in 5-year overall survival (OS; 36% vs 23%; $P = .009$), establishing this regimen as a standard of care.

A similar degree of benefit was also noted in the contemporaneous French FFCD 9703 trial of 224 patients with esophagogastric adenocarcinoma.[6] Patients were randomized to 6 cycles (18 weeks) of perioperative 5-FU/cisplatin followed by surgery versus surgery alone. Perioperative chemotherapy on this trial was associated with a significant improvement in 5-year disease-free survival (DFS; 34% vs 19%; $P = .003$) and OS (38% vs 24%; $P = .02$). Although comparisons between different clinical trials must be made cautiously, the survival benefit seen with 5-FU/cisplatin on this trial seems to be nearly identical to that seen with ECF in the MAGIC trial.

The benefit of the anthracycline—and the duration of preoperative therapy—has now been disputed definitively by the MRC OEO-5 study which has so far only been presented in abstract form.[7] This study randomized 897 patients with esophageal/GEJ adenocarcinomas to preoperative chemotherapy with either 6 weeks of 5-FU/cisplatin or 12 weeks of ECX (epirubicin/cisplatin/capecitabine) chemotherapy. Although the pathologic response rate was improved in the ECX group versus the 5-FU/cisplatin group (including a pathologic complete response [pCR] rate of 11% vs 3% in the patients who underwent surgery), there was no difference in median progression-free survival between the groups (PFS; 1.78 vs 1.53 years; $P = .058$) or OS (2.15 vs 2.02 years; $P = .86$).

The OEO-5 study has therefore also raised the provocative suggestion that as little as 6 weeks of preoperative chemotherapy conveys the same OS benefit as 12 weeks of chemotherapy. Although this may be counterintuitive based on the MAGIC and FFCD studies, as well as other studies in gastric cancer that have administered 6 to 12 months of adjuvant chemotherapy,[8,9] these results are not without precedent. As will be discussed elsewhere in this article, the CROSS study (ChemoRadiotherapy for Oesophageal cancer followed by Surgery Study) found benefit for preoperative chemoradiation, where patients received only 5 weekly treatments of carboplatin/paclitaxel as the entirety of their systemic chemotherapy.[10,11] The absolute improvement in OS seen in the CROSS study is also very much in the range of 10% to 15% seen in other positive phase III studies discussed herein.

It is also important to remember that, although the MAGIC and FFCD studies aimed to deliver 18 weeks of perioperative chemotherapy, only 50% of patients who underwent preoperative chemotherapy and surgery were able to receive or complete adjuvant chemotherapy on both studies, further suggesting that most patients derived the survival benefit of chemotherapy from receiving significantly less than 18 weeks of treatment. The generally poor ability to deliver therapy after surgery was also seen in the recently presented Dutch CRITICS study and would suggest, especially given the absence of a biological rationale to split up the same systemic treatment with surgery, that future experimental strategies should focus on exclusively preoperative approaches.

Aside from the MAGIC and FFCD studies, other phase III evaluations of preoperative or perioperative chemotherapy in esophagogastric adenocarcinomas have either been negative or had more marginal benefit. The North American Intergroup 113 trial failed to show a survival benefit for perioperative 5-FU/cisplatin in 440 patients with esophageal cancer (approximately one-half of whom had adenocarcinomas; eligibility was limited to extension of the tumor to 2 cm beyond the GEJ into the stomach).[12] The MRC OEO-2 trial, which randomized 802 patients to surgery alone versus 2 cycles of preoperative 5-FU/cisplatin, reported a modest improvement in 5-year OS with chemotherapy (23% vs 17%; $P = .03$).[13] Two-thirds of patients had adenocarcinomas and three-quarters of tumors were in the lower esophagus or gastric cardia. Most recently, the European EORTC (Eurropean Organization for Research and Treatment of Cancer) 40954 trial evaluated a strategy of preoperative 5-FU/leucovorin/cisplatin in 144 patients with GE and gastric adenocarcinoma.[14] The trial was stopped because of poor accrual, which limited the power of the study, and no differences in survival were detected.

These data are summarized in Table 1. An updated metaanalysis by Sjoquist and colleagues[15] of 10 randomized trials involving preoperative chemotherapy for esophageal and GEJ cancers suggested a 13% decreased risk of all-cause mortality for this approach in patients with adenocarcinomas versus surgery alone (hazard ratio [HR], 0.87; 95% confidence interval [CI], 0.79–0.96; $P < .005$). In this metaanalysis, both the MAGIC and EORTC 40954 trials were excluded because their outcomes were not stratified based on gastric versus GEJ tumors.

PREOPERATIVE CHEMORADIATION

The seminal phase III RTOG trial (US Radiation Therapy Oncology Group 85-01) demonstrated the superiority of chemoradiation over radiation alone.[16] This nonoperative study compared standard fractionation radiation (64 Gy) versus radiation (50 Gy) plus concurrent 5-FU/cisplatin. The trial was stopped when data from 121 patients showed an improved median OS in favor of chemoradiation (12.5 vs 8.9 months). The 2-year survival was also improved in the chemoradiation group (38% vs 10%), as was 5-year survival (21% vs 0%).[17] Although the majority of patients treated on this trial had SCC, long-term survival was also seen in the small number of adenocarcinoma patients on the trial, with 13% of patients alive at 5 years. Based on this study,

Table 1
Results of phase III preoperative or perioperative chemotherapy trials in esophageal and gastroesophageal junction cancer

Treatment	Histology	No. of Patients	R0 Resection Rate (%)	Pathologic CR Rate (%)	Survival Median	Survival Overall	Local failure (%)	Reference
Perioperative ECF + surgery	Adeno	250	69	0	**24 mo**	**5-y 36%**	14	Cunningham et al,[5] 2006
Surgery		253	66	N/A	**20 mo**	**5-y 23%**	21	
Perioperative 5FU/Cis + surgery	Adeno	109	**87**	NS	NS	**5-y 38%**	24	Ychou et al,[6] 2011
Surgery		110	**74**	N/A	NS	**5-y 24%**	26	
Preoperative ECF + surgery	Adeno	446	67	**11**	25.8	3-y 42%	NS	Alderson et al,[7] 2015
Preoperative 5FU/Cis + surgery		451	60	**3**	24.2	3-y 39%	NS	
Perioperative 5FU/Cis + surgery	Adeno (54%) + SCC	213	62	2.5	14.9 mo	3-y 23%	32	Kelsen et al,[12] 1998
Surgery		227	59	N/A	16.1 mo	3-y 26%	31	
Preoperative 5FU/Cis + surgery	Adeno (66%) + SCC	400	**60**	NS	**16.8 mo**	**5-y 23%**	19	Medical Research Council,[48] 2002; Allum et al,[13] 2009
Surgery		402	**54**	N/A	**13.3 mo**	**5-y 17%**	17	
Preoperative 5FU/LV/Cis + surgery	Adeno	72	**82**	7.1	64.6 mo	**2-y 73%**	NS	Schuhmacher et al,[14] 2010
Surgery		72	**66.7**	N/A	52.5 mo	**2-y 69.9%**	NS	

Values in bold are statistically significant.
Abbreviations: Adeno, adenocarcinoma; Cis, cisplatin; CR, complete response; ECF, epirubicin; cisplatin, 5-fluorouracil; ECX, epirubicin; cisplatin, capecitabine; LV, leucovorin; N/A, not applicable; NS, not stated; SCC, squamous cell carcinoma.

chemoradiation was established as the standard of care in the nonsurgical management of locally advanced esophageal SCC.

Since then, preoperative chemoradiation has been evaluated extensively in trials of esophageal cancer. Six contemporary randomized trials have compared preoperative chemoradiation followed by surgery versus surgery alone.[10,18–22] Of these, 3 have been positive and revealed a survival benefit for this approach. These results are summarized in Table 2.

A potential new standard of care was established by the rigorously conducted Dutch CROSS trial.[10] In this study of 366 evaluable patients with esophageal tumors (of which 75% and 65% respectively were adenocarcinomas and lymph node positive by endoscopic ultrasound [EUS]), patients were randomized to preoperative carboplatin/paclitaxel combined with 41.4 Gy of radiation versus surgery alone. Preoperative chemoradiation resulted in an improvement in R0 resection rates (92% vs 67%; P<.001), in a pCR rate of 29% (23% for adenocarcinoma and 49% for SCC) and in improved OS compared with surgery alone (median OS, 49.4 vs 24.0 months; 3-year OS, 58% vs 44%; P = .003). Preoperative therapy was also relatively well-tolerated, with mostly grade 3 toxicities noted in only 20% of patients (13% nonhematologic, 7% hematologic). There did seem to be a greater degree of benefit for patients with SCC versus adenocarcinoma histology (univariate HR for death 0.45 vs 0.73), but all patients derived benefit. Long-term follow-up of this study confirmed an OS benefit for both adenocarcinoma and SCC patients and reported a 9% reduction in distant metastases for patients who received preoperative chemoradiation.[11]

Although this study demonstrates a clear benefit for chemoradiation, it is not possible to conclude definitively that carboplatin/paclitaxel is the preferred regimen combined with radiation relative to standard 5-FU/cisplatin used in other trials. Nevertheless, the pCR rate of 49% in SCC is the highest ever reported in a phase III trial, while the pCR rate of 23% for adenocarcinomas compares favorably with other phase II and III studies. Coupled with the ease of administration and tolerability, carboplatin/paclitaxel is the new standard of care and the reference regimen for future trial design. Some insight into the relative merits of carboplatin/paclitaxel versus a 5-FU/platinum regimen may come from the ongoing CALGB (Cancer and Leukemia Group B 80803 study; discussed elsewhere in this article).

Overall, many of the other randomized trials conducted are associated with methodologic concerns (including the lack of rigorous pretherapy staging with EUS and/or laparoscopy) and are significantly smaller than randomized preoperative chemotherapy trials (eg, the positive CALGB 9781 study only enrolled 56 patients). Although the results of these trials are conflicting, they do at a minimum suggest improved curative resection rates as well as decreased local recurrence.

A benefit for preoperative chemoradiation is supported by the previously discussed metaanalysis, in which 13 randomized trials of preoperative chemoradiation (including the 5 trials discussed herein) were analyzed.[15] Preoperative chemoradiation was associated with a decreased risk of all-cause mortality of 25% (HR, 0.75; 95% CI, 0.59–0.95; P = .02) in patients with adenocarcinoma histology versus surgery alone.

PREOPERATIVE CHEMORADIATION FOR EARLY STAGE DISEASE

Although the studies discussed have focused on locally advanced tumors (which, by contemporary standards, would include staging with EUS and comprise mostly uT3-4N + tumors), the recently published French FFCD 9901 study treated 195 patients with early-stage cT1-2N$_{any}$ or cT3N0 tumors with preoperative 5-FU/cisplatin

Table 2
Results of phase III preoperative chemoradiation trials in esophageal and gastroesophageal junction cancer

Treatment	Histology	No. of Patients	R0 Resection Rate (%)	Pathologic CR Rate (%)	Survival Median	Survival Overall	Local Failure (%)	Reference
Preoperative CRT	Adeno (76%) + SCC	50	45	24	16.9 mo	3-y 30%	19	Urba et al,[20] 2001
Surgery		50	45	N/A	17.6 mo	3-y 16%	42	
Preoperative CRT	Adeno	58	NS	25	**16 mo**	3-y **32%**	NS	Walsh et al,[21] 1996
Surgery		55	NS	N/A	**11 mo**	3-y **6%**		
Preoperative CRT	SCC	143	81	26	18.6 mo	5-y 26%	NS	Bosset et al,[18] 1997
Surgery		139	69	N/A	18.6 mo	5-y 26%		
Preoperative CRT	Adeno (63%) + SCC + other	128	**80**	9	22.2 mo	NS	15	Burmeister et al,[19] 2005
Surgery		128	**59**	N/A	19.3 mo		26	
Preoperative CRT	Adeno (75%) + SCC	30	NS	40	**4.5 y**	5-y **39%**	NS	Tepper et al,[22] 2008
Surgery		26	NS	N/A	**1.8 y**	5-y **16%**		
Preoperative CRT	Adeno (74%) + SCC	178	**92**	29	**49.4 mo**	3-y **58%**	NS	Van Hagen et al,[10] 2012
Surgery		188	**69**	N/A	**24.0 mo**	3-y **44%**		

Values in bold are statistically significant.
Abbreviations: Adeno, adenocarcinoma; CR, complete response; N/A, not applicable; NS, not stated; CRT, chemoradiation; SCC, squamous cell carcinoma.

and radiation and surgery versus surgery alone.[23] Of patients on this study, 72% had SCCs and 24% and 74%, respectively, had cT1 and cN0 tumors. This study revealed a strikingly high 93% R0 resection rate in the surgery alone arm, which was not improved with preoperative chemoradiation. Similarly, median DFS and OS were not different in both arms; however, in-hospital postoperative mortality was significantly increased in the chemoradiation arm (11.1% vs 3.4%; $P = .049$).

These results are somewhat surprising; despite the lack of improvement in R0 resection rates, locoregional recurrence was reduced in the chemoradiation arm (22.1% vs 28.9%; $P = .02$); in contrast, the rate of distant recurrence was not different between the arms (22.5% vs 28.9%; $P = .31$). In addition, the unexpectedly high postoperative mortality in the chemoradiation arm—compared with 4% in both treatment arms of the CROSS study—might have obscured a small survival benefit from chemoradiation.

Nevertheless, these results are not necessarily inconsistent with other published data. An accepted approach—as discussed elsewhere in this article—is definitive chemoradiation without surgery for patients with SCC who achieve a clinical CR. Because 72% of patients on this study had SCC tumors, it arrives at the complementary conclusion that SCC patients who do undergo chemoradiation should not undergo mandatory surgery. Similarly, these results are concordant with current guidelines by the National Comprehensive Cancer Network, which recommend surgery alone for patients with cT1N0 tumors.

PREOPERATIVE CHEMORADIATION VERSUS CHEMOTHERAPY

The possible superiority of preoperative chemoradiation over preoperative chemotherapy was suggested by the German POET (PreOperative Chemotherapy or Radiochemotherapy in Esophagogastric Adenocarcinoma Trial) study, in which patients with GEJ adenocarcinomas were randomized to either 5-FU/leucovorin/cisplatin followed by surgery versus 5-FU/leucovorin/cisplatin followed by chemoradiation with cisplatin/etoposide and then surgery.[24] One hundred nineteen eligible patients were randomized before the trial was closed owing to poor accrual, limiting the power of this study to detect a difference between the treatment groups. Nevertheless, patients who received preoperative chemoradiation had a higher pCR rate (15.6% vs 2%; $P = .03$) and tumor-free lymph node status (ypN0 64.4% vs 36.7%; $P = .01$) than those who received preoperative chemotherapy. There were also trends toward an improvement in local control (76.5% vs 59%; $P = .06$) and in 3-year OS (47.4% vs 27.7%; $P = .07$) for the chemoradiation group that nearly approached statistical significance.

A similar nonsignificant trend toward improved outcomes with preoperative chemoradiation over chemotherapy was also suggested in the meta-analysis by Sjoquist and colleagues,[15] which revealed an all-cause mortality HR of 0.88 (95% CI, 0.76–1.01, $P = .07$) favoring chemoradiation.

A major benefit of preoperative chemoradiation over chemotherapy alone may stem from an improvement in R0 resection rates for tumors that involve the GEJ. For example, the R0 resection rates in the 1400 patients treated on the contemporary MAGIC and OEO-5 studies were consistently less than 70%; in the OEO-5 study, the majority of patients were assessed to be surgical candidates based on preoperative EUS and PET scan. The addition of radiation to preoperative chemotherapy in the CROSS study improved the R0 resection rate to greater than 90%.

DEFINITIVE CHEMORADIATION WITHOUT SURGERY

Two randomized European trials have compared definitive chemoradiation versus chemoradiation followed by surgery in (mostly) esophageal SCC patients.[25,26] Taken together, these studies suggest that local control is improved by subsequent surgery, but that there is no clear improvement in survival.

In the setting of definitive chemoradiation, FOLFOX (5-FU/leucovorin/oxaliplatin) also seems to be a comparable option with 5-FU/cisplatin based on the French PRO-DIGE5/ACCORD17 study, which randomized 267 patients to either regimen with radiation as definitive therapy.[27] Of the patients on this study, 85% had SCC. Survival and toxicities were comparable in both arms.

An interesting question that arises from one of these studies (the FFCD 9102 trial) is whether patients who do not respond to initial therapy benefit from subsequent surgery. In this study, patients received initial treatment with 5-FU/cisplatin and radiation; only responders were randomized subsequently to surgery versus additional chemoradiation. Of the 451 registered patients, 192 were not randomized to further protocol therapy after initial chemoradiation, primarily because of a lack of response (111 patients) but also because of medical contraindication or patient refusal.[28] Of these nonrandomized patients, 112 subsequently underwent surgery. The median OS for the nonresponding patients who underwent surgery was significantly superior to the median OS of those who did not (17.0 vs 5.5 months; P<.0001) and was comparable with the median OS of the patients who were randomized (18.9 months; P = .40). Although there are clear limitations and potential strong confounders to such an analysis, these data suggest that salvage esophagectomy may be beneficial for a subset of patients who do not respond to initial therapy.

In contrast, there are no randomized data in patients with adenocarcinomas to suggest that definitive chemoradiation is comparable with chemoradiation and surgery. However, given the significant morbidity and mortality associated with esophagectomy even at high-volume institutions, one option is to closely follow adenocarcinoma patients who achieve a clinical CR to preoperative chemoradiation—especially those who are relatively frail—with repeat endoscopy and imaging. Those patients who develop locoregional failure without distant metastases may then be evaluated for salvage esophagectomy.

A major concern about such an approach is that postoperative complications and deaths may increase significantly when surgery is delayed beyond the standard 6- to 8-week break after chemoradiation. The group at MD Anderson Cancer Center reported their experience in 65 patients with esophageal adenocarcinoma who underwent salvage esophagectomies a median of 216 days after chemoradiation.[29] When compared with matched patients who underwent planned esophagectomy after chemoradiation, postoperative complications and survival did not seem to be different.

Similar conclusions were drawn from a retrospective French review, which examined this approach in 848 patients, 540 of whom underwent esophagectomy after preoperative chemoradiation and 308 who underwent salvage surgery after chemoradiation for either persistent (234 patients) or recurrent (74 patients) cancer.[30] Although the rate of anastomotic leak and surgical infection were increased in the salvage versus immediate surgery groups, in-hospital mortality was similar and relatively high in both groups (8.4% vs 9.3%; P = .688). The 3-year DFS (39.2% vs 32.8%; P = .232) and OS (43.3% vs 40.1%; P = .542) were also similar in both groups.

In addition, the RTOG 0246 study evaluated induction chemotherapy with 5-FU/cisplatin/paclitaxel and chemoradiation with 5-FU/cisplatin in 43 patients with locally advanced esophageal cancer; salvage surgery was reserved for patients with locally persistent or recurrent disease.[31] Although the study did not meet its primary endpoint of improving 1-year survival to 77.5%, it did suggest that postoperative mortality was not increased by delaying surgery. Therefore, such an approach can be considered for select patients at institutions with significant experience in this strategy.

PET-DIRECTED THERAPY

PET with [^{18}F]2-fluorodeoxy-D-glucose scanning is emerging as an important tool to investigate response to therapy. Several studies in esophagogastric tumors have demonstrated that the degree of response detected by PET after preoperative chemo-radiation[32,33] or chemotherapy[34,35] is highly correlated with pathologic response at surgery and with patient survival.

The German MUNICON trial (the Metabolic response evalUatioN for Individualisa-tion of neoadjuvant Chemotherapy in oesOphageal and oesophagogastric adeNocar-cinoma) evaluated the strategy of taking patients with locally advanced GEJ adenocarcinomas with a suboptimal response to 2 weeks of induction chemotherapy with 5-FU/cisplatin—as determined by serial PET scans—directly to surgery, instead of continuing with presumably ineffective chemotherapy. Patients with a metabolic response by PET (defined as ≥35% reduction in the standard uptake value between baseline and repeat PET scan) continued with an additional 12 weeks of chemo-therapy before surgery.[36] This trial revealed a significantly improved R0 resection rate (96% vs 74%; P = .002), major pathologic response rate (58% vs 0%; P = .001), median event-free survival (29.7 vs 14.1 months; P = .002), and median OS (median not reached vs 25.8 months; P = .015) for PET responders versus PET nonresponders. The outcome for PET nonresponders referred for immediate surgery was similar to the outcome of such patients in an earlier trial who completed 3 months of preoperative chemotherapy,[34] indicating that nonresponding patients were not compromised by referral to immediate surgery. These results, therefore, support the early discontinuation of inactive preoperative chemotherapy in PET nonresponder patients.

Building on the results of the MUNICON trial, the MUNICON-2 trial attempted to improve outcome in the PET nonresponders to the same regimen of preoperative 5-FU/cisplatin by treating them with "salvage" chemoradiation with cisplatin before surgery.[37] When compared with the PET responders who completed 3 months of 5-FU/cisplatin before surgery, the PET nonresponders had inferior 2-year PFS (64% vs 33%; P = .035) and a trend toward inferior 2-year OS (71% vs 42%; P = .10). These results likely speak to the underlying unfavorable biology of the tumors of PET nonre-sponders but do not rule out the possibility that such patients can receive effective salvage therapy. In this trial, the chemotherapy administered with radiation (cisplatin) had already been assessed to be associated with suboptimal outcomes by PET when administered as induction therapy.

As such, another possible strategy would be to use PET assessment after induction chemotherapy to dictate subsequent chemotherapy during concurrent radiation. Responding patients can continue with the same chemotherapy regimen during con-current radiation while nonresponding patients can be switched to alternative, non–cross-resistant chemotherapy during radiation. Our group has reported long-term DFS in patients who progressed on induction chemotherapy but were changed to alternative chemotherapy during subsequent chemoradiation.[38]

Based on this concept, the CALGB has completed accrual to the 80,803 trial (NCT01333033), which is enrolling patients with esophageal/GEJ adenocarcinomas. Participants are randomized to receive induction chemotherapy with either carbopla-tin/paclitaxel or a modification of the FOLFOX6 regimen (infusional 5-FU/leucovorin/oxaliplatin). Responses to induction chemotherapy are then adjudicated with an early PET scan performed after induction chemotherapy. Whereas PET responders continue with the same regimen during concurrent radiation, PET nonresponders are changed to the alternative regimen with radiation before surgery. The primary endpoint is to improve the pCR rate in PET nonresponder patients by changing chemotherapy during combined chemoradiation.

We have also since retrospectively reviewed our experience of changing to alternative chemotherapy during radiation for some PET nonresponders to induction chemotherapy in 201 patients with esophageal/GEJ adenocarcinomas.[39] Our data suggest that improvements in pCR rate and PFS are possible and that there is also a trend toward improved OS. The results of the CALGB 80803 study are, therefore, eagerly awaited.

POSTOPERATIVE CHEMORADIATION

In the United States, a standard of care is postoperative chemoradiation for GEJ and gastric cancers undergoing upfront resection, based primarily on the results of the Intergroup 116 trial.[40] This trial randomized 556 patients (20% of whom had tumors that involved the GEJ) to adjuvant chemotherapy and chemoradiation with bolus 5-FU/leucovorin versus observation alone after surgery. Patients who received adjuvant chemoradiation had an improvement in relapse-free survival (3-year relapse-free survival of 48% vs 31%; $P<.001$) and 3-year (OS of 51% vs 40%; $P = .005$). Despite these positive results, this trial is frequently criticized because of the relatively inadequate surgical resections that were performed—54% of patients had less than a D1 or D2 resection, which is less than an optimal resection of the involved lymph nodes. It has been argued that radiation in this setting potentially compensated for inadequate surgery because the greatest impact of adjuvant chemoradiation was a reduction in local recurrence of cancer. Such benefits may not be seen for radiotherapy if a more complete D1 or D2 surgical resection is undertaken.

Based on the results of the Intergroup trial, the CALGB launched and completed the 80101 trial. Five hundred forty-six gastric cancer patients (30% of whom had tumors involving the GEJ and proximal stomach) were enrolled. The standard arm consisted of systemic bolus 5-FU/leucovorin preceding and after chemoradiation with infusional 5-FU, whereas the experimental arm intensified the systemic chemotherapy by replacing the bolus 5-FU/leucovorin with the ECF regimen. Results have been presented in abstract form and reveal no improvement in 3-year DFS (47% vs 46%) or OS (52% vs 50%) with the addition of an anthracycline and platinum compound to 5-FU.[41] These results are also virtually identical to the outcomes in the adjuvant chemoradiation arm of the Intergroup 116 trial. These results indicate that 5-FU monotherapy, combined with radiation, remains a standard of care and that adding cisplatin and epirubicin to adjuvant chemotherapy failed to improve survival. ECF should not be used as an adjuvant chemotherapy regimen, although preoperative and postoperative ECF without radiation therapy remains a care standard.

The Dutch CRITICS study evaluated an alternative to the perioperative ECF approach by randomizing patients (38% of whom had GEJ or proximal gastric adenocarcinomas) to perioperative ECX or EOX (epirubicin/oxaliplatin/capecitabine) chemotherapy (the control arm) versus preoperative ECX/EOX and adjuvant chemoradiation with capecitabine plus cisplatin. The results were presented recently and revealed no difference in PFS and OS for either treatment arm.[42] Although subgroup analyses are planned, the nearly superimposable Kaplan-Meier survival curves confirm, for now at least, that patients who have received preoperative chemotherapy should not receive adjuvant chemoradiation in a standard fashion. These results are summarized in Table 3.

POSTOPERATIVE CHEMOTHERAPY

In comparison with chemoradiation, trials in East Asia of resectable gastric cancer have frequently focused on postoperative chemotherapy alone. To date, 2 large phase

Table 3
Results of phase III postoperative chemoradiation trials in gastroesophageal junction and gastric adenocarcinoma

Treatment	No. of Patients	Disease-Free Survival Median (mo)	Overall	Overall Survival Median (mo)	Overall	Local Failure (%)[a]	Reference
Surgery	275	19	3-y 31%	27	3-y 41%	29	Macdonald
Postoperative 5FU/LV → 5FU/RT → 5FU/LV	281	**30**	3-y **48%**	**36**	3-y **50%**	19	et al,[40] 2001
Postoperative 5FU/LV → 5FU/RT → 5FU/LV	280	30	3-y 46%	36.6	3-y 50% 5-y 41%	NS	Fuchs et al,[41] 2011
Postoperative ECF → 5FU/RT → ECF	266	28	3-y 47%	37.8	3-y 52% 5-y 44%	NS	
ECX/EOX → Surgery → ECX/EOX	393	27.6	5-y 38.5%	42	5-y 40.8%	NS	Verheij et al,[42]
ECX/EOX → Surgery → chemoRT	395	30	5-y 39.5%	39.6	5-y 40.9%	NS	2016

Numbers in **bold** indicate statistically significant differences.
Abbreviations: Adeno, adenocarcinoma; ECF, epirubicin/cisplatin/infusional 5-fluorouracil; ECX, epirubicin/cisplatin/capecitabine; EOX, epirubicin/oxaliplatin/capecitabine LV, leucovorin; N/A, not applicable; NS, not stated; RT, radiotherapy.
[a] Local failure with or without distant recurrence.

III trials have demonstrated a benefit for this approach. These data support the use of adjuvant fluoropyrimidines as monotherapy and combination chemotherapy with a fluoropyrimidine plus a platinum agent. The results are summarized in Table 4, but should be interpreted with caution because these trials have exclusively enrolled patients with gastric adenocarcinoma. In East Asia, fewer than 10% of tumors occur in the proximal stomach/GEJ, making it unclear if they are applicable to the patient population discussed in this review article.

The ACTS-GC (Adjuvant Chemotherapy Trial of TS-1 for Gastric Cancer) study was performed in Japan. In this study of 1059 patients with stage II/III gastric cancer who had undergone D2 resections, patients were randomized to 1 year of adjuvant S-1 versus observation.[8] The 5-year outcomes for this trial were updated recently, confirming that adjuvant S-1 is associated with significant improvements in 5-year relapse-free survival (65.4% vs 53.1%; HR, 0.65; 95% CI, 0.54–0.79) and OS (71.7% vs 61.1%; HR, 0.67; 95% CI, 0.54–0.83) compared with observation alone.[43] Subgroup analyses revealed benefit for all groups, including by stage and histologic type.

The second of these trials is the CLASSIC trial (Capecitabine and Oxaliplatin Adjuvant Study in Stomach Cancer), which was performed in 1035 East Asian patients who had undergone a D2 resection of stage II to IIIB gastric cancer.[9] Patients were randomized to 6 months of adjuvant capecitabine/oxaliplatin versus observation. Updated survival data confirm improved 5-year OS for patients who received chemotherapy (78% vs 69%; HR, 0.66; *P* = .0015); 5-year DFS was also improved (68% vs 53%; HR, 0.58; *P*<.0001).[44]

In comparison, postoperative chemotherapy for resected esophageal SCC has not clearly been shown to be beneficial. This approach was studied in 2 Japanese

Table 4
Results of phase III postoperative chemotherapy trials in esophageal and gastric cancer

| Treatment | Histology | No. of Patients | Survival | | Local Failure (%) | Reference |
			Median	Overall		
Surgery	Adeno	530	NR	5-y **61%**	2.8	Sakuramoto et al,[8]
Surgery + S-1	(gastric)	529	NR	5-y **72%**	1.3	2007; Sasako et al,[43] 2011
Surgery	Adeno	515	NR[a]	5-y **78%**	44	Bang et al,[9] 2012;
Surgery + Capeox	(gastric)	520	NR[a]	5-y **69%**	21	Bang et al,[44] 2014
Surgery	SCC	100	NS	5-y 45%	30	Ando et al,[45] 1997
Surgery + cisplatin/ vindesine		105	NS	5-y 48%	30	
Surgery	SCC	122	NS	5-y 52%	**46**	Ando et al,[46] 2003
Surgery + 5-FU/ cisplatin		120	NS	5-y 61%	**8**	
5-FU/ cisplatin + surgery	SCC	164	NS	**5-y 55%**	NS	Ando et al,[47] 2012
Surgery + 5-FU/ cisplatin		166	NS	**5-y 43%**	NS	

Numbers in **bold** indicate statistically significant differences.
Abbreviations: Capeox, capecitabine/oxaliplatin; CR, complete response; NR, not reached; NS, not stated; UFT, tegafur/uracil.
[a] Disease-free survival.

randomized trials, where patients with SCC histology were randomized to receive 2 cycles of chemotherapy with cisplatin/vindesine[45] or 5-FU/cisplatin,[46] respectively. Although the trial with cisplatin/vindesine did not show any survival benefit, an unplanned subset analysis of the trial with 5-FU/cisplatin revealed a survival benefit for patients with lymph node involvement (5-year DFS of 52% vs 38%).

The possible benefit of postoperative therapy suggested by the trial as discussed led to a subsequent Japanese trial that randomized 330 patients with SCC histology to surgery and either 2 cycles of preoperative versus postoperative 5-FU/cisplatin.[47] The results showed improved 5-year OS for the preoperative chemotherapy group (55% vs 43%; $P = .04$), further raising questions about the value of adjuvant chemotherapy for these patients. However, interpretation of these results is confounded by the fact that only 96 of the 166 patients randomized to postoperative chemotherapy received any treatment; 38 patients who had pN0 disease were not treated per protocol because of the prior observation that adjuvant chemotherapy only benefited patients with lymph node involvement. Furthermore, this study observed that a survival benefit for preoperative chemotherapy was seen only in N0 patients, which contrasted with the prior postoperative adjuvant study that claimed a benefit only in N1 patients.

SUMMARY

Esophageal cancer remains a significant worldwide health problem, with adenocarcinoma of the esophagus an emerging epidemic in Western countries. Completed phase III studies now show clear improvements in outcomes in patients who present with locally advanced disease who receive additional treatment compared with surgery alone. For patients who are medically unresectable, definitive chemoradiation has been the standard of care since the 1990s. Studies now show that preoperative chemoradiation for esophageal/GEJ tumors is superior to surgery alone and that definitive chemoradiation is an option for patients with SCC who achieve a clinical CR. GEJ adenocarcinomas may also be treated with perioperative chemotherapy and surgery, although recent studies reveal R0 resection rates of only 70% with this approach. For patients with GEJ adenocarcinomas who undergo surgery upfront, adjuvant chemoradiation is a validated approach. Adjuvant chemotherapy alone is of proven benefit in East Asian studies that enrolled patients mostly with distal gastric cancer, so it is uncertain if such an approach can be extrapolated to GEJ tumors. A similar benefit for adjuvant chemotherapy for resected SCC has not been demonstrated.

REFERENCES

1. Siegel RL, Miller KD, Jemal A. Cancer statistics, 2016. CA Cancer J Clin 2016; 66(1):7–30.
2. Ferlay J, Shin HR, Bray F, et al. Estimates of worldwide burden of cancer in 2008: GLOBOCAN 2008. Int J Cancer 2010;127:2893–917.
3. Crew KD, Neugut AI. Epidemiology of upper gastrointestinal malignancies. Semin Oncol 2004;31:450–64.
4. Devesa SS, Fraumeni JF Jr. The rising incidence of gastric cardia cancer. J Natl Cancer Inst 1999;91:747–9.
5. Cunningham D, Allum WH, Stenning SP, et al. Perioperative chemotherapy versus surgery alone for resectable gastroesophageal cancer. N Engl J Med 2006;355: 11–20.
6. Ychou M, Boige V, Pignon JP, et al. Perioperative chemotherapy compared with surgery alone for resectable gastroesophageal adenocarcinoma: an FNCLCC and FFCD multicenter phase III trial. J Clin Oncol 2011;29:1715–21.
7. Alderson D, Langley R, Nankivell M, et al. Neoadjuvant chemotherapy for resectable oesophageal and junctional adenocarcinoma: results from the UK Medical Research Council randomised OEO5 trial (ISRCTN 01852072) [abstract]. J Clin Oncol 2015;33(4002):2015.
8. Sakuramoto S, Sasako M, Yamaguchi T, et al. Adjuvant chemotherapy for gastric cancer with S-1, an oral fluoropyrimidine. N Engl J Med 2007;357:1810–20.
9. Bang YJ, Kim YW, Yang HK, et al. Adjuvant capecitabine and oxaliplatin for gastric cancer after D2 gastrectomy (CLASSIC): a phase 3 open-label, randomised controlled trial. Lancet 2012;379:315–21.
10. van Hagen P, Hulshof MC, van Lanschot JJ, et al. Preoperative chemoradiotherapy for esophageal or junctional cancer. N Engl J Med 2012;366:2074–84.
11. Shapiro J, van Lanschot JJ, Hulshof MC, et al. Neoadjuvant chemoradiotherapy plus surgery versus surgery alone for oesophageal or junctional cancer (CROSS): long-term results of a randomised controlled trial. Lancet Oncol 2015;16:1090–8.
12. Kelsen DP, Ginsberg R, Pajak TF, et al. Chemotherapy followed by surgery compared with surgery alone for localized esophageal cancer. N Engl J Med 1998;339:1979–84.
13. Allum WH, Stenning SP, Bancewicz J, et al. Long-term results of a randomized trial of surgery with or without preoperative chemotherapy in esophageal cancer. J Clin Oncol 2009;27:5062–7.
14. Schuhmacher C, Gretschel S, Lordick F, et al. Neoadjuvant chemotherapy compared with surgery alone for locally advanced cancer of the stomach and

cardia: European Organisation for Research and Treatment of Cancer randomized trial 40954. J Clin Oncol 2010;28:5210–8.

15. Sjoquist KM, Burmeister BH, Smithers BM, et al. Survival after neoadjuvant chemotherapy or chemoradiotherapy for resectable oesophageal carcinoma: an updated meta-analysis. Lancet Oncol 2011;12:681–92.

16. Herskovic A, Martz K, al-Sarraf M, et al. Combined chemotherapy and radiotherapy compared with radiotherapy alone in patients with cancer of the esophagus. N Engl J Med 1992;326:1593–8.

17. Cooper JS, Guo MD, Herskovic A, et al. Chemoradiotherapy of locally advanced esophageal cancer: long-term follow-up of a prospective randomized trial (RTOG 85-01). Radiation Therapy Oncology Group. JAMA 1999;281:1623–7.

18. Bosset JF, Gignoux M, Triboulet JP, et al. Chemoradiotherapy followed by surgery compared with surgery alone in squamous-cell cancer of the esophagus. N Engl J Med 1997;337:161–7.

19. Burmeister BH, Smithers BM, Gebski V, et al. Surgery alone versus chemoradiotherapy followed by surgery for resectable cancer of the oesophagus: a randomised controlled phase III trial. Lancet Oncol 2005;6:659–68.

20. Urba SG, Orringer MB, Turrisi A, et al. Randomized trial of preoperative chemoradiation versus surgery alone in patients with locoregional esophageal carcinoma. J Clin Oncol 2001;19:305–13.

21. Walsh TN, Noonan N, Hollywood D, et al. A comparison of multimodal therapy and surgery for esophageal adenocarcinoma. N Engl J Med 1996;335:462–7.

22. Tepper J, Krasna MJ, Niedzwiecki D, et al. Phase III trial of trimodality therapy with cisplatin, fluorouracil, radiotherapy, and surgery compared with surgery alone for esophageal cancer: CALGB 9781. J Clin Oncol 2008;26:1086–92.

23. Mariette C, Dahan L, Mornex F, et al. surgery alone versus chemoradiotherapy followed by surgery for stage I and II esophageal cancer: final analysis of randomized controlled phase III Trial FFCD 9901. J Clin Oncol 2014;32:2416–22.

24. Stahl M, Walz MK, Stuschke M, et al. Phase III comparison of preoperative chemotherapy compared with chemoradiotherapy in patients with locally advanced adenocarcinoma of the esophagogastric junction. J Clin Oncol 2009;27:851–6.

25. Stahl M, Stuschke M, Lehmann N, et al. Chemoradiation with and without surgery in patients with locally advanced squamous cell carcinoma of the esophagus. J Clin Oncol 2005;23:2310–7.

26. Bedenne L, Michel P, Bouche O, et al. Chemoradiation followed by surgery compared with chemoradiation alone in squamous cancer of the esophagus: FFCD 9102. J Clin Oncol 2007;25:1160–8.

27. Conroy T, Galais MP, Raoul JL, et al. Definitive chemoradiotherapy with FOLFOX versus fluorouracil and cisplatin in patients with oesophageal cancer (PRODIGE5/ACCORD17): final results of a randomised, phase 2/3 trial. Lancet Oncol 2014;15:305–14.

28. Vincent J, Mariette C, Pezet D, et al. Early surgery for failure after chemoradiation in operable thoracic oesophageal cancer. Analysis of the non-randomised patients in FFCD 9102 phase III trial: chemoradiation followed by surgery versus chemoradiation alone. Eur J Cancer 2015;51:1683–93.

29. Marks JL, Hofstetter W, Correa AM, et al. Salvage esophagectomy after failed definitive chemoradiation for esophageal adenocarcinoma. Ann Thorac Surg 2012;94:1126–32 [discussion: 1132–3].

30. Markar S, Gronnier C, Duhamel A, et al. Salvage surgery after chemoradiotherapy in the management of esophageal cancer: is it a viable therapeutic option? J Clin Oncol 2015;33:3866–73.
31. Swisher SG, Winter KA, Komaki RU, et al. A phase II study of a paclitaxel-based chemoradiation regimen with selective surgical salvage for resectable locoregionally advanced esophageal cancer: initial reporting of RTOG 0246. Int J Radiat Oncol Biol Phys 2012;82:1967–72.
32. Downey RJ, Akhurst T, Ilson D, et al. Whole body 18FDG-PET and the response of esophageal cancer to induction therapy: results of a prospective trial. J Clin Oncol 2003;21:428–32.
33. Flamen P, Van Cutsem E, Lerut A, et al. Positron emission tomography for assessment of the response to induction radiochemotherapy in locally advanced oesophageal cancer. Ann Oncol 2002;13:361–8.
34. Ott K, Weber WA, Lordick F, et al. Metabolic imaging predicts response, survival, and recurrence in adenocarcinomas of the esophagogastric junction. J Clin Oncol 2006;24:4692–8.
35. Weber WA, Ott K, Becker K, et al. Prediction of response to preoperative chemotherapy in adenocarcinomas of the esophagogastric junction by metabolic imaging. J Clin Oncol 2001;19:3058–65.
36. Lordick F, Ott K, Krause BJ, et al. PET to assess early metabolic response and to guide treatment of adenocarcinoma of the oesophagogastric junction: the MUNICON phase II trial. Lancet Oncol 2007;8:797–805.
37. zum Buschenfelde CM, Herrmann K, Schuster T, et al. (18)F-FDG PET-guided salvage neoadjuvant radiochemotherapy of adenocarcinoma of the esophagogastric junction: the MUNICON II trial. J Nucl Med 2011;52:1189–96.
38. Ilson DH, Bains M, Kelsen DP, et al. Phase I trial of escalating-dose irinotecan given weekly with cisplatin and concurrent radiotherapy in locally advanced esophageal cancer. J Clin Oncol 2003;21:2926–32.
39. Ku GY, Kriplani A, Janjigian YY, et al. Change in chemotherapy during concurrent radiation followed by surgery after a suboptimal positron emission tomography response to induction chemotherapy improves outcomes for locally advanced esophageal adenocarcinoma. Cancer 2016;122:2083–90.
40. Macdonald JS, Smalley SR, Benedetti J, et al. Chemoradiotherapy after surgery compared with surgery alone for adenocarcinoma of the stomach or gastroesophageal junction. N Engl J Med 2001;345:725–30.
41. Fuchs C, Tepper J, Niedzwiecki D, et al. Postoperative adjuvant chemoradiation for gastric or gastroesophageal junction (GEJ) adenocarcinoma using epirubicin, cisplatin, and infusional (CI) 5-FU (ECF) before and after CI 5-FU and radiotherapy (CRT) compared with bolus 5-FU/LV before and after CRT: Intergroup trial CALGB 80101 [abstract]. J Clin Oncol 2011;29:4003.
42. Verheij M, Jansen E, Cats A, et al. A multicenter randomized phase III trial of neoadjuvant chemotherapy followed by surgery and chemotherapy or by surgery and chemoradiotherapy in resectable gastric cancer: first results from the CRITICS study [abstract]. J Clin Oncol 2016;34:4000.
43. Sasako M, Sakuramoto S, Katai H, et al. Five-year outcomes of a randomized phase III trial comparing adjuvant chemotherapy with S-1 versus surgery alone in stage II or III gastric cancer. J Clin Oncol 2011;29:4387–93.
44. Noh SH, Park SR, Yang HK, et al. Adjuvant capecitabine plus oxaliplatin for gastric cancer after D2 gastrectomy (CLASSIC): 5-year follow-up of an open-label, randomised phase 3 trial. Lancet Oncol 2014;15:1389–96.

45. Ando N, Iizuka T, Kakegawa T, et al. A randomized trial of surgery with and without chemotherapy for localized squamous carcinoma of the thoracic esophagus: the Japan Clinical Oncology Group Study. J Thorac Cardiovasc Surg 1997; 114:205–9.

46. Ando N, Iizuka T, Ide H, et al. Surgery plus chemotherapy compared with surgery alone for localized squamous cell carcinoma of the thoracic esophagus: a Japan Clinical Oncology Group Study–JCOG9204. J Clin Oncol 2003;21:4592–6.

47. Ando N, Kato H, Igaki H, et al. A randomized trial comparing postoperative adjuvant chemotherapy with cisplatin and 5-fluorouracil versus preoperative chemotherapy for localized advanced squamous cell carcinoma of the thoracic esophagus (JCOG9907). Ann Surg Oncol 2012;19:68–74.

48. Medical Research Council Oesophageal Cancer Working Group. Surgical resection with or without preoperative chemotherapy in oesophageal cancer: a randomised controlled trial. Lancet 2002;359:1727–33.

Radiation Therapy for Locally Advanced Esophageal Cancer

Stephen G. Chun, MD*, Heath D. Skinner, MD, PhD,
Bruce D. Minsky, MD

KEYWORDS

- Esophageal cancer • Radiation • Chemotherapy • IMRT • Dose-escalation

KEY POINTS

- General guidelines for treatment of locally advanced esophageal cancer include both pre-operative and nonoperative approaches, predicated upon resectability, histology, and location.
- In patients with resectable disease who are medically fit for this procedure, pre-operative chemoradiation to 50.4 Gy, with consideration of a lower dose (41.4 Gy) based on the CROSS trial, is recommended.
- In non-operative patients, definitive chemoradiation to 50.4 Gy is standard; however, enrollment of these patients on dose-escalation or other protocols is encouraged.
- Clinicians should make use of all available imaging and diagnostic modalities to delineate tumor and involved lymphadenopathy.

OVERVIEW

Locally-advanced esophageal cancer (LAEC) is broadly defined as American Joint Commission on Cancer, version 7, clinical stage III or IVA (T3-4 and/or N+) disease. Therapeutic approaches commonly include preoperative concurrent chemotherapy plus radiation (chemoradiation) or definitive chemoradiation alone. There is controversy regarding the ideal therapeutic approach to this disease. The US Patterns of Care Study offers a historical perspective. A total of 414 patients (51%: adenocarcinoma and 49%: squamous cell carcinoma [SCC]) received radiation therapy as part of definitive or adjuvant management at 59 institutions from 1996 to 1999.[1,2] Overall, patients who received chemoradiation followed by surgery had a significant decrease in locoregional recurrence (hazard ratio [HR], 0.40, P<.0001) and survival improvement

Disclosure Statement: The authors have nothing to disclose.
Division of Radiation Oncology, The University of Texas, M.D. Anderson Cancer Center, 1515 Holcombe Boulevard, Houston, TX 77030, USA
* Corresponding author.
E-mail address: sgchun@mdanderson.org

Surg Oncol Clin N Am 26 (2017) 257–276
http://dx.doi.org/10.1016/j.soc.2016.10.006
surgonc.theclinics.com

(HR, 0.32, $P<.001$) compared with those who did not undergo surgery. A similar significant decrease in locoregional recurrence (HR, 1.36, $P = .01$) and survival (HR 1.32, $P<.03$) was seen in those patients who received their care at large radiation oncology centers (treating ≥500 new patients with cancer per year) compared with small centers (treating <500 new patients with cancer per year).

In the current review, the authors discuss the management of inoperable esophageal cancer and review neoadjuvant chemoradiation, perioperative chemotherapy, and radiotherapy techniques.

DEFINITIVE THERAPY IN UNRESECTABLE LOCALLY ADVANCED ESOPHAGEAL CANCER
Radiation Monotherapy

In LAEC, radiation therapy alone should be reserved for palliation or for patients who are medically unfit to receive concurrent chemotherapy. The 5-year survival rate for patients treated with conventional doses of radiation therapy alone is suboptimal.[3–5] In the landmark Radiation Therapy Oncology Group (RTOG) 85-01 trial in which patients were randomized to receive either 64 Gy at 2 Gy/d or chemoradiation, all patients who received radiation alone were all dead of disease by 3 years.[6,7] Shi and colleagues[8] reported a 33% 5-year survival rate with the use of late course accelerated fractionation to a total dose of 68.4 Gy.

Primary radiation is more successful in patients with cT1N0 disease. Sai and colleagues[9] from Kyoto University treated 34 patients who were either medically inoperable or refused surgery with either external beam alone (64 Gy) or external beam (52 Gy) plus 8 to 12 Gy with brachytherapy. The 5-year results included 59% overall survival, 68% local relapse-free survival, and 80% cause-specific survival. Yamada and colleagues[10] reported the results in a similar group of 63 patients treated with chemoradiation plus brachytherapy. The 5-year results included 66% overall survival, 64% disease-free survival, and 76% cause-specific survival.

Brachytherapy Boost

Brachytherapy can be delivered by low- or high-dose rates and has previously been used as a boost following external beam radiation therapy or chemoradiation.[11–16] This technique is limited by the effective treatment distance. The primary isotope is Iridium 192 (Ir-192), which is usually prescribed to treat to a distance of 1 cm from the source. Therefore, as confirmed by pathologic analysis of treated specimens, any portion of the tumor that is greater than 1 cm from the source will receive a suboptimal radiation dose.[17]

There does not appear to be an advantage of adding brachytherapy to external beam radiation. One series reported a local failure rate of 57% and a 5-year actuarial survival of 28% in 46 patients with stage T2-3N0-1M0 disease.[18] Even in patients with earlier stage disease (clinical T1-2), brachytherapy likely does not offer an advantage. Yorozu and colleagues[19] reported a local failure rate of 44% and a 5-year survival of 26%, and Pasquier and associates[20] reported local failure of 23% and the 5-year survival of 36%. However, in an updated series by Ishikawa and colleagues,[21] 59 patients with submucosal esophageal cancer received external beam followed by brachytherapy in a subset of 36 patients with either low-dose-rate Caesium 137 (17 patients) or high-dose-rate Ir-192 (19 patients). Patients selected to receive a brachytherapy boost had a significantly higher 5-year cause-specific survival (86% vs 62%, $P = .04$).

Chemoradiation plus brachytherapy was tested prospectively by the RTOG Trial 9207. A total of 75 patients with cancers of the thoracic esophagus (92% squamous cell, 8% adenocarcinoma) received the RTOG 8501 50-Gy chemoradiation regimen followed by a boost during cycle 3 of chemotherapy with either low-dose-rate or high-dose-rate intraluminal brachytherapy.[22] Because of low accrual, the low-dose-rate option was discontinued, and the analysis was limited to patients who received the high-dose-rate treatment. High-dose-rate brachytherapy was delivered in weekly fractions of 5 Gy during weeks 8, 9, and 10. Several patients developed fistulas, and the fraction delivered at week 10 was discontinued. The complete response rate was 73%. With a median follow-up of only 11 months, local failure as the first site of failure was 27%. Acute toxicities were high. These acute toxicities included 58% grade 3, 26% grade 4, and 8% grade 5 (treatment-related death). The cumulative incidence of fistula was 18%/y and the crude incidence was 14%. Of the 6 treatment-related fistulas, 3 were fatal. Significant toxicity, combined with the lack of dramatic efficacy and the labor-intensive nature of brachytherapy, has resulted in limited interest in developing this technique further in esophageal cancer.

If brachytherapy is to be used, guidelines for esophageal brachytherapy published by the American Brachytherapy Society are available.[23] For patients treated in the curative setting, brachytherapy should be limited to tumors 10 cm or less with no evidence of distant metastasis. Contraindications include tracheal or bronchial involvement, cervical esophagus location, or stenosis that cannot be bypassed. The applicator should have an external diameter of 6 to 10 cm. If chemoradiation is used (defined as 5-fluorouracil [5-FU]–based chemotherapy plus 45–50 Gy), the recommended doses of brachytherapy are 10 Gy in 2 weekly fractions of 5 Gy each for high-dose rate and 20 Gy in a single fraction at 4 to 10 Gy/h for low-dose rate. The doses should be prescribed to 1 cm from the source. Last, brachytherapy should be delivered after the completion of external beam and not concurrently with chemotherapy.

Definitive Chemoradiation

Although there are 6 randomized trials comparing definitive radiation therapy alone with chemoradiation, the only trial designed to deliver adequate doses of systemic chemotherapy with concurrent radiation therapy was the RTOG 85-01 trial reported by Herskovic and colleagues.[24–26] As was common in the 1980s, most patients had SCC. Treatment included 4 cycles of 5-FU (1000 mg/m^2/24 h × 4 days) and cisplatin (CDDP; 75 mg/m^2, day 1). Radiation therapy (50 Gy at 2 Gy/d) was given concurrently with the first day of cycle 1 of chemotherapy. Cycles 3 and 4 of chemotherapy were delivered every 3 weeks rather than every 4 weeks. Only 50% of the patients finished all 4 cycles of the chemotherapy. The control arm was radiation therapy alone, albeit a higher dose (64 Gy) than the chemoradiation arm.

Patients treated with chemoradiation had a significant improvement in both median (14 months vs 9 months) and 5-year survival (27% vs 0%, $P<.0001$).[25] The 8-year survival was 22%.[26] Histology did not significantly influence the results. The 5-year survival was 21% for the 107 patients with SCC versus 13% of the 23 patients with adenocarcinoma, P = NS. Local failure (defined as local persistence plus recurrence) was also lower in the chemoradiation arm (47% vs 65%). Although African Americans had larger primary tumors of which all were SCC, there was no difference in survival compared with Caucasians.[27]

Dose Escalation—2-Dimensional and 3-Dimensional Techniques

These promising results led to Intergroup 0122, a phase II trial of dose-escalated chemoradiation to 64.8 Gy delivered concurrently with CDDP and 5-FU.[28] This regimen appeared to have acceptable toxicity and formed the experimental arm of INT 0123 (RTOG 9405).[29] In this trial, patients selected for a nonsurgical approach were randomized to a slightly modified RTOG 85-01 chemoradiation regimen with 50.4 Gy versus the same chemotherapy with 64.8 Gy, based on INT 0122. As with RTOG 85-01, most patients (85%) had SCC.

There were several modifications to the original RTOG 85-01 chemoradiation arm. These modifications included using 1.8-Gy fractions to 50.4 Gy rather than 2-Gy fractions to 50 Gy, treating with 5 cm proximal and distal margins for 50.4 Gy rather than treating the whole esophagus for the first 30 Gy followed by a cone down with 5-cm margins to 50 Gy; cycle 3 of 5-FU/CDDP did not begin until 4 weeks following the completion of radiation therapy rather than 3 weeks, and last, cycles 3 and 4 of chemotherapy were delivered every 4 weeks rather than every 3 weeks. The trial opened in late 1994 and was closed in 1999 when an interim analysis revealed that it was unlikely that the high-dose arm would achieve a superior survival compared with the standard dose arm.

For the 218 eligible patients, there was no significant difference in median survival (13.0 months vs 18.1 months), 2-year survival (31% vs 40%), or local/regional failure and/or local/regional persistence of disease (56% vs 52%) between the high-dose and standard-dose arms. Although 11 treatment-related deaths occurred in the high-dose arm compared with 2 in the standard-dose arm, 7 of the 11 occurred in patients who had received 50.4 Gy or less.

An alternative approach to dose escalation is altered fractionation; this has been investigated in LAEC with modest results. Zaho and colleagues[30] treated 201 patients with squamous cell cancer using 41.4 Gy followed by late-course accelerated hyperfractionation to 68.4 Gy. The results were similar to RTOG 85-01 (38% local failure and 26% 5-year survival). Choi and colleagues[31] treated 46 patients with 5-FU/CDDP and twice-a-day radiation using a concurrent boost technique and reported a 37% 5-year survival. In addition, Lee and colleagues[32] reported a trial of 102 patients with LAEC, limited to SCC, randomized to surgery alone versus preoperative therapy with 45.6 Gy (1.2 Gy twice a day) plus 5-FU/CDDP. There was no difference in median survival (28 vs 27 months). Thus, although these approaches may appear to be reasonable, there appears to be a significant increase in acute toxicity without any clear therapeutic benefit.

Dose Escalation—Intensity-Modulated Radiation Therapy and Protons

A criticism of many dose escalation trials in the definitive management of LAEC is the use of conventional 2-dimensional (2D) and 3-dimensional (3D) radiation techniques. Trials using newer techniques such as intensity-modulated radiation therapy (IMRT) may be able to deliver higher doses of radiation with a more tolerable toxicity profile. Multiple dosimetric studies comparing standard 3-D conformal radiotherapy (3D-CRT) and IMRT generally have found improved sparing of the heart, lung, or both using either static field or arc-based IMRT.[33–44] The dosimetric advantages of IMRT has led multiple clinical centers to begin the routine use of IMRT in this disease. Retrospective analysis of these data does not suggest inferior outcome and may provide decreased toxicity versus non-IMRT treatment techniques.[45–47] Investigators at MD Anderson Cancer Center reported the results of 676 patients with LAEC treated with either IMRT (263) or 3D-CRT (413).[45] On multivariate analysis, IMRT was associated with improved survival ($P = .004$), but not cancer-specific survival ($P = .86$). The survival difference between 3D-CRT and IMRT was thought to be due to a higher level of cardiac ($P = .05$) and unexplained deaths ($P = .003$) in the 3D-CRT patients, suggesting that decreased cardiac dose may have a direct impact on patient outcome. Although this and other comparisons between 3D-CRT and IMRT in LAEC are retrospective, a randomized trial is unlikely; thus, the available data may represent the best comparison.

Another theoretic advantage of IMRT is the possibility of dose escalation. With the use of IMRT, a simultaneous integrated boost may be performed while maintaining commonly used lung and heart dosimetric constraints. Retrospective data from Zhang and colleagues[48] suggest a positive correlation between radiation dose and locoregional control. This positive correlation has led to a phase I studying examining this approach in LAEC at MD Anderson Cancer Center. However, at this point, based on results of the INT 0123 trial, the standard dose of external beam radiation remains 50.4 Gy.

The use of proton therapy remains investigational.

Perioperative and Induction Chemotherapy

For locally advanced lower esophageal and gastroesophageal (GE) junction cancers, perioperative chemotherapy may be considered as a therapeutic option, although such an approach has not been validated for midthoracic or upper esophageal cancers.[49] The UK Medical Research Council Adjuvant Gastric Infusional Chemotherapy (MAGIC) trial that showed perioperative epirubicin, CDDP, and 5-FU chemotherapy provides a 10% survival advantage when given in addition to definitive surgery. However, lower esophageal and GE junction cancers represented less than 25% of patients enrolled in the MAGIC trial with the vast majority of patients having gastric cancer, creating challenges for interpreting these data in esophageal cancer. Pathologic complete response rate, not reported in this trial, is generally relatively low with chemotherapy alone.

The ideal approach for lower esophageal cancer with either perioperative chemotherapy or trimodality therapy has been debated.[50] Interpretation of the data is also challenging because these trials have primarily enrolled gastric cancer with only small numbers of lower esophageal cancer. Given the limited number of esophageal cancers limited to the lower esophagus in these perioperative chemotherapy trials, caution should be exercised in interpreting these data.

A potential advantage of neoadjuvant chemotherapy is the early identification of those patients who may or may not respond to the chemotherapeutic regimen being delivered concurrently with chemoradiation. Lordick and colleagues[51] demonstrated that patients without a response to preoperative chemotherapy on fluorodeoxyglucose (FDG)-PET scan did not benefit from continuing this therapy and could be sent to immediate surgery without compromising survival. Ilson and colleagues[52] have shown that the change in standardized uptake value (SUV) on FDG-PET scan during induction chemotherapy was able to predict which patients showed a response to subsequent chemoradiotherapy. Wieder and associates[53] reported similar findings in 38 patients with squamous cell cancers. Although this approach is investigational, if the nonresponders can be identified early, changing the chemotherapeutic regimen may be helpful. However, in the context of induction chemotherapy before definitive chemoradiation, the data do not support its routine use. For example, Ruhstaller and colleagues[54] report the outcomes from a phase II trial using CDDP/docetaxel followed by chemoradiation in unresectable LAEC. In this study, median survival was 16 months, with 29% of patients surviving long term, suggesting no benefit over chemoradiation alone. Recently, the Cancer and Acute Leukemia Group B (CALGB)/Alliance completed a randomized phase II trial using PET scan response to guide selection of chemotherapy to use during preoperative chemoradiotherapy, and results are expected in 2017.

In summary, either perioperative chemotherapy or neoadjuvant chemoradiotherapy can be considered for lower and GE junction cancers. However, for patients who have positive margins or progress after induction chemotherapy, chemoradiotherapy should be considered. For patients with LAEC above the low esophagus and GE junction, neoadjuvant chemoradiotherapy remains the standard of care (Table 1).

Table 1
Randomized trials of neoadjuvant chemoradiation in locally advanced esophageal cancer

Trial	N	Patients	Comparison	Concurrent Chemotherapy	Outcome	Comments
Urba et al,[55] 1993	100	Adenocarcinoma: 75% SCC: 25%	Arm 1: Surgery Arm 2: 45 Gy/1.5 Gy BID → Surgery	CDDP, 5-FU, and vinblastine	MS: 17.6 mo Arm 2 vs 16.9 mo Arm 1 (NS) LRF: 19% Arm 2 vs 42% Arm 1 ($P = .02$)	Small study, required a >1 y improvement in MS to be significant
Walsh et al,[56] 2012	113	Adenocarcinoma: 100%	Arm 1: Surgery Arm 2: 40 Gy/2.67 Gy QD → Surgery	CDDP and 5-FU	MS: 16 mo Arm 2 vs 11 mo Arm 1 ($P = .01$)	Low survival rate in Arm 1 compared with other trials
FFCD 8805/EORTC 40881[57]	282	SCC: 100%	Arm 1: Surgery Arm 2: 18.5 Gy/3.7 QD→ 2 wk break → 18.5 Gy/3.7 QD →Surgery	CDDP	MS: 18.6 for both arms (NS) DFS: 40% Arm 2 vs 28% Arm 1 ($P = .003$)	Unconventional radiotherapy
TTROG/AGITG[58]	128	Adenocarcinoma: 63% SCC: 35%	Arm 1: Surgery Arm 2: 30 Gy/3 Gy QD → Surgery	CDDP and 5-FU	MS: 22.2 mo Arm 2 vs 19.3 mo Arm 1 (NS)	R0 80% in Arm 2 vs 59% Arm 1
Lee et al,[32] 2004	101	SCC: 100%	Arm 1: Surgery Arm 2: 45.6 Gy/1.2 Gy BID → Surgery	CDDP and 5-FU	MS: 28.2 mo Arm 2 vs 27.3 mo Arm 1 (NS)	31% of patients in Arm 2 did not have a surgical resection
CALGB 9781[59]	56	Adenocarcinoma: 75% SCC: 25%	Arm 1: Surgery Arm 2: 50.4 Gy/1.8 Gy QD → Surgery	CDDP and 5-FU	MS: 53.8 mo Arm 2 vs 21.5 mo Arm 1 ($P = .002$)	Closed early due to poor accrual
CROSS[60]	366	Adenocarcinoma: 75% SCC: 23%	Arm 1: Surgery Arm 2: 41.4 Gy/1.8 Gy QD → Surgery	Carboplatin and paclitaxel	MS: 49.4 mo Arm 2 vs 24 mo Arm 1 ($P = .003$)	R0: 93% in Arm 2 vs 69% in Arm 1

Abbreviations: BID, twice daily; MS, median survival; NS, not significant; QD, daily.

Tracheoesophageal Fistula

A malignant tracheoesophageal (TE) fistula is an unfavorable prognostic feature, and its management deserves special attention. Although the survival of such patients is low, occasionally they may have long-term survival. Historically, the use of radiation therapy was contraindicated due to the concern of exacerbating the fistula as the tumor responded. However, some data suggest that this is not the case. At the Mayo Clinic, 10 patients with a malignant TE fistula received 30 to 66 Gy and their median survival was 5 months.[55] None of the patients experienced an enlarging or more debilitating fistula following radiation. Rueth and colleagues[56] showed improved survival with a palliative course of radiation compared with stent placement alone (3.3 vs 1 month) and no significant difference in complications. Finally, in a series of 24 patients with TE fistulae, Muto and colleagues[57] found a 71% TE fistula closure rate following chemoradiation, with a median survival time of 6.7 months. The data, albeit limited, suggest that radiation does not necessarily increase the severity of a malignant TE fistula, and it is not a contraindication to its use. However, given the overall poor prognosis of this subset of patients, the impact on outcome is not clear.

TRIMODALITY THERAPY

Preoperative Chemoradiation

There are 7 randomized trials comparing preoperative combined modality therapy with surgery alone in patients with clinically resectable disease, the most recent being the Chemoradiotherapy for Oesophageal Cancer followed by Surgery Study (CROSS).[32,58–63]

The CROSS trial randomized 366 patients with LAEC (75% adenocarcinoma, 23% SCC) to receive either neoadjuvant chemoradiation with 41.4 Gy and carboplatin/paclitaxel followed by surgical resection versus surgical resection alone.[63] In this trial, median survival was effectively doubled by the addition of chemoradiation (49.4 vs 24 months, $P = .003$). Improved survival was seen in both adenocarcinoma and SCC, although the magnitude was slightly greater in SCC. The R0 resection was 93% in the chemoradiation arm, compared with 69% in the surgery alone arm ($P<.001$). Despite concerns that a lower radiation dose combined with carboplatin and paclitaxel may not be as effective, the pathologic complete response (pCR) rate was 29%. The pCR rate and survival in the CROSS trial is comparable to most previous trials and retrospective reviews.[64] In addition, no significant difference in perioperative complications was seen between treatment arms.

Before the publication of the CROSS trial, the role of preoperative chemoradiation was controversial. The first 6 trials (Urba,[58] Walsh,[59] EORTC,[60] Australasian,[61] Korea,[32] and CALGB 9781[62]) had limited patient numbers and heterogeneous treatment regimens, and in some, the dose of radiation was insufficient based on a dose response analysis by Geh and colleagues.[65] Despite all of these limitations, a meta-analysis did suggest a survival benefit.[66] However, with the publication of the CROSS trial, the standard of care for patients with locally advanced but medically resectable adenocarcinoma of the esophagus is now preoperative chemoradiation.

Necessity for Surgery Following Chemoradiation

Because of the known response of LAEC to chemoradiation as well as the significant morbidity of an esophagectomy, questions arise as to the necessity of this procedure. Two randomized trials examine whether surgery is necessary after chemoradiation. In the Federation Francaise de Cancerologie Digestive (FFCD) 9102 trial, 445 patients with clinically resectable T3-4N0-1M0 SCC or adenocarcinoma of the esophagus received initial chemoradiation.[67] The vast majority of patients (90%) in this trial had squamous cancers. Patients initially received 2 cycles of 5-FU, CDDP, and concurrent radiation (either 46 Gy at 2 Gy/d or split course 15 Gy weeks 1 and 3). The 259 patients who had at least some evidence of clinical response were then randomized to surgery versus additional chemoradiation, which included 3 cycles of 5-FU, CDDP, and concurrent radiation (either 20 Gy at 2 Gy/d or split course 15 Gy). There was no significant difference in 2-year survival (34% vs 40%, $P = .56$) or median survival (18 months vs 19 months) in patients who underwent surgery versus additional chemoradiation. These data suggest that for patients who initially respond to chemoradiation, they should complete chemoradiation rather than stop and undergo surgery. Using the Spitzer index, there was no difference in global quality of life; however, a significantly greater decrease in quality of life was observed in the surgery arm during the postoperative period (7.52 vs 8.45, $P<.01$, respectively).[68] In a separate trial that compared with split course radiation, patients who received standard course radiation had improved 2-year local relapse-free survival rates (77% vs 57%, $P = .002$), but no significant difference in overall survival (37% vs 31%).[69]

The German Oesophageal Cancer Study Group compared preoperative chemoradiation followed by surgery versus chemoradiation alone.[70] In this trial, 172 eligible patients less than 70 years old with uT3-4N0-1M0 SCC were randomized to preoperative therapy (3 cycles of 5-FU, leucovorin, etoposide, and CDDP, followed by concurrent etoposide, CDDP, plus 40 Gy) followed by surgery versus chemoradiation alone (the same chemotherapy but the radiation dose was increased to 60–65 Gy ± brachytherapy). The pCR rate was 33%. Although there was a decrease in 2-year local failure (36% vs 58%, $P = .003$), there was no significant difference in 3-year survival (31% vs 24%) for those who were randomized to preoperative chemoradiation followed by surgery versus chemoradiation alone.

Despite the above data, the current standard of care is to perform esophagectomy following chemoradiation in patients who can tolerate this approach. However, it is known that a subset of patients will have a complete response to chemoradiation. Furthermore, it is known that patients with pCR have improved survival. Data from both Berger and colleagues[71] and Rohatgi and colleagues[72] suggest that patients who achieve a pCR had an improvement in survival compared with those who do not (5 year: 48% vs 15%, and median: 133 months vs 34 months, respectively). In these patients, surgical resection may not be necessary and has led to the concept of "selective" surgery after preoperative chemoradiation.

Swisher and colleagues[73] have also reported a retrospective analysis of patients who underwent a salvage compared with a planned esophagectomy. The operative mortality was higher in those who underwent salvage versus planned surgery (15% vs 6%), but there was no difference in survival (25%). However, only 13 patients were identified who had salvage, limiting the broad interpretation of these findings. However, a recent phase II trial, RTOG 0246, prospectively examined the approach of preoperative paclitaxel/CDDP and 50.4 Gy followed by selective surgery in patients with either residual disease or recurrent disease in the absence of distant metastasis. In this trial of 43 patients with LAEC, 21 patients required surgical resection after chemoradiation due to residual (17 patients) or recurrent (3 patients) disease.[74] This approach led to a 1-year overall survival of 71%, lower than the predetermined survival rate (77.5%).

For patients with adenocarcinoma, there is substantial evidence that esophagectomy is critically important for oncologic outcomes. Although definitive chemoradiotherapy with CDDP and 5-FU in RTOG 8501 had an overall survival of 26%, nearly all of these survivors had squamous histology and only 1 of 23 patients with adenocarcinoma was alive at 5 years.[26] The importance of definitive surgical management for adenocarcinoma is further corroborated by findings in the CROSS trial showing that there was a pCR rate of only 23% for adenocarcinoma compared with 49% for SCC. Thus, for patients who receive concurrent chemoradiotherapy either with carboplatin and paclitaxel or with CDDP and 5-FU, there is no clear evidence that esophagectomy can be omitted for adenocarcinoma.

Evaluation of Response to Chemoradiation

To further pursue the selective surgical approach as a treatment modality, it will be critical to establish the definition of an adequate response. However, the ability to predict a pCR before surgery is variable. A multivariate analysis by Gaca and colleagues[75] reported that posttreatment nodal status ($P = .03$) but not the degree of primary tumor response predicted disease-free survival.

Current available imaging modalities and/or postchemoradiation biopsies are also of limited value in predicting a pCR. Bates and colleagues[76] noted a 41% false-negative rate with preoperative endoscopy and biopsy. Jones and colleagues[77] reported that computed tomography (CT) had a sensitivity of 65%, a specificity of 33%, a positive predictive value of 58%, and a negative predictive value of 41% in evaluating pathologic response after preoperative chemoradiation. Many studies show that endoscopic ultrasound (EUS) performed after chemoradiation is a suboptimal predictor of complete response because of the inability to distinguish postirradiation fibrosis and inflammation from residual tumor. Reported accuracy is generally at or less than 50%.[78] For example, Sarkaria and colleagues[79] found that in 165 patients a negative endoscopic biopsy was not a useful predictor of a pCR after chemoradiation (31% negative predictive value), final nodal status, or overall survival.

The value of FDG-PET for staging after chemoradiation is unclear. Several studies of patients with esophageal cancer show that an early decrease in FDG uptake after chemotherapy can predict clinical response.[80,81] In addition, multiple studies have evaluated the ability of FDG-PET to predict a pCR following chemoradiation.[82–87] Flamen and colleagues[83] evaluated the predictive value of PET after chemoradiation in patients receiving preoperative treatment. The sensitivity and positive predictive value of PET for identifying a pCR were 67% and 50%, respectively. Both false-positive PET findings (residual FDG activity in an area of intense inflammatory activity on histopathologic analysis) and false-negative findings occurred at the primary tumor site. Vallbohmer and colleagues[82] treated 119 patients with preoperative chemoradiation and reported a nonsignificant association between major responders and FDG-PET results ($P = .056$). There was no clear SUV threshold that predicted response. The inflammatory effect of chemoradiation as well as a lack of standardization of FDG-PET protocols and techniques and definitions of a pathologic response may be responsible for the variation in results.[88] Thus, although most studies investigating the role of posttreatment FDG-PET in evaluating pCR found some correlation between the 2, a wide array of SUV threshold values and a lack of specificity preclude its use as a surrogate marker of pCR.

Biomarkers of Response

Because of the marginal results of using clinical variables to predict and assess pCR following chemoradiation, attention has been shown to the use of pathologic or molecular markers to this end. Studies have linked tumor lymphocytic infiltration as well as apoptotic index with response to chemoradiation.[89] Additional studies have linked a large number of proteins and genes involved in a wide array of signaling cascades with response to chemoradiation. Examples include alterations in diverse signaling cascades involving PI3 kinase, p53, EGFR, and HIF-1α.[90-99] Unfortunately, the vast majority of these studies lack validation and the specificity required to be used clinically. One recent study generated a micro-RNA signature to predict pCR from LAEC tumors in 52 patients treated uniformly with chemoradiation.[100] This signature was then validated in a separate cohort of 72 patients treated similarly. When combined with clinical stage, the area under the curve for pCR was 0.77 (p = 2 $\times$ 10^{-41}). These validated data argue for further investigation, possibly within the context of a clinical trial.

The human epidermal growth factor receptor 2 (Her2) is expressed in 20% to 30% of patients, where it is thought to contribute to tumor progression and therapeutic resistance.[101] Initially, Her2-directed therapy was used in metastatic esophageal cancer in the Trastuzumab for Gastric Cancer trial for Her2 overexpressing tumors where traztuzumab provided a modest, but significant survival benefit. However, the utility of Her2 as a predictive biomarker for chemoradiotherapy in esophageal cancer is under investigation. The current NSABP, RTOG, GOG (NRG) Oncology/RTOG 1010 trial evaluated neoadjuvant concurrent carboplatin and paclitaxel $\pm$ traztuzumab (concurrent and maintenance) followed by surgical resection for Her2 overexpressing LAEC. The study is completed and the results are pending. Given the known cardiac toxicity of traztuzumab and potential synergistic toxicity with thoracic radiation therapy, it is not recommended to offer concurrent traztuzumab with cytotoxic chemotherapy and radiation off-protocol until results of NRG/RTOG 1010 are available.

Palliative Radiation Therapy

Despite advances in oncologic treatments for LAEC, the vast majority of patients will develop locoregional recurrence and/or metastatic disease. For patients with incurable esophageal cancer, systemic chemotherapy is the mainstay of therapy. However, locally advanced esophageal primary tumors can produce symptoms including dysphagia, chest pain, and bleeding. For such situations, radiation is a potent and effective palliative therapy. Most patients treated with radiation therapy will experience subjective relief of dysphagia from radiation therapy. Gastrointestinal bleeding is also effectively palliated by radiation therapy that may facilitate systemic therapy by reducing transfusion requirements. Although hypofractionated palliative radiation regimens have been used for other sites, hypofractionation can produce acute nausea and esophagitis. In the palliative setting, regimens, such as 30 Gy in 10 fractions or 37.5 Gy in 15 fractions, improve symptoms without excess toxicity.

TECHNIQUES OF RADIATION THERAPY
Radiation Dose and Fractionation

Historically, the standard radiation dose, based on INT 0123, for patients selected for chemoradiation is 50.4 Gy at 1.8 Gy per fraction.[29] However, recent data from the CROSS trial suggest that 41.4 Gy in the same fractionation may be sufficient to treat in the preoperative setting.[63] As previously described, some investigators have performed dose escalation; however, based on INT 0113, dose escalation greater than 50.4 Gy should not be performed off-protocol. In addition, radiation should be delivered without treatment breaks, as randomized data from France reveal a higher local control (57% vs 29%) and 2-year survival rate (37% vs 23%) with continuous course compared with split course radiation.[102]

There is considerable debate regarding the appropriate radiation fields for LAEC. Typically, in the major prospective trials for LAEC, radiation field has included the primary tumor with 5 cm superior and inferior margins and 2 cm lateral margins. The primary local/regional lymph nodes should receive the same dose. For cervical (proximal) primary tumors (defined as at or proximal to the carina), the treatment volume includes the bilateral supraclavicular nodes, and for GE junction (distal) primaries, the celiac axis nodes should be included. However, with modern imaging, the necessity for large elective coverage has been questioned.

Treatment Modality

At many centers, the standard of care in radiotherapy for LAEC is 3D-CRT using a beam arrangement optimized via CT-based planning. However, as mentioned previously, many clinicians have used IMRT with a possible benefit in regards to toxicity and no apparent compromise in oncologic outcome.[45] A comparison of 3 techniques is shown in Fig. 1. If IMRT is to be used, careful attention should be given to target delineation. In addition, particularly in the case of distal/GE junction tumors, 4-dimensional CT or other forms of motion management should be considered.

For patients treated with IMRT, plan optimization should be centered on maximizing conformity of the high- and intermediate-radiation dose volumes to the PTV. Although retrospective studies have correlated the V5 with respiratory outcomes in LAEC treated with IMRT, the significance of this finding is unclear and should not be used as a reason to optimize plans by the V5. An important hallmark of IMRT is its ability to reduce the volume of the high- and intermediate-dose regions, which are likely to have an even bigger impact on lung toxicity than the V5. There is little radiobiologic

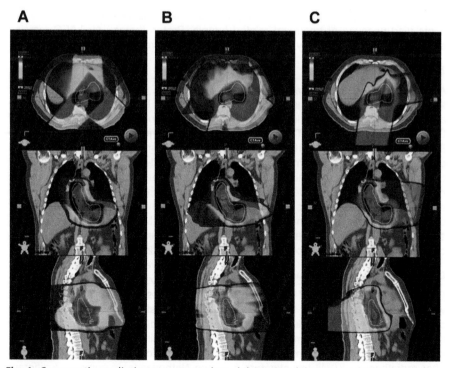

Fig. 1. Comparative radiation treatment plans. (*A*) 3D-CRT, (*B*) IMRT, and (*C*) proton beam comparison between treatment modalities. In this case, both IMRT and protons provide improved lung and cardiac sparing compared with 3D-CRT. Proton beam decreases liver dose compared with other modalities.

evidence to suggest that the V5 is the causative factor for lung toxicity. Rather, it is entirely possible that in these retrospective analyses, the V5 was a surrogate indicator for truly causative factors for pneumonitis such as the lung V20. Conformity of the high- and intermediate-dose regions are the most critical objectives for reducing likelihood of radiation-induced side effects. Because the evidence for the importance of the low-dose bath is weak, IMRT plan optimization by the V5 is discouraged because it will inevitably reduce conformity.

Recently, proton radiotherapy has become more available as a treatment modality. By virtue of its physical characteristics, proton radiotherapy can potentially reduce cardiac doses as well as reduce the low-dose "bath" often seen with IMRT. Emerging evidence suggests that cardiac doses are important predictors of survival for thoracic cancers. The potential dosimetric advantages of protons compared with IMRT for dose reduction to the lung and heart are compared in Fig. 1.[103] Several studies have examined patient outcome after treating with proton radiotherapy. Sugahara and colleagues[104] examined outcomes in 46 patients with SCC treated with protons with or without photons to a median total dose of 76 Gy. The 5-year local control rate was T1: 83%, T2-4: 29% and survival T1: 55% and T2-4: 13%. Koyama and Tsujii[105] reported mean actuarial survival rates of 60% for patients with superficial and 39% for those with advanced disease treated to mean total doses of 78 to 81 Gy. The incidence of esophageal ulcer was 67%. In the United States, Lin and colleagues[106] retrospectively reviewed 62 patients treated with proton radiotherapy for LAEC at the MD Anderson Cancer Center. Overall, 47% were treated with surgical resection following chemoradiation, with a pCR rate in these patients of 28%. In this series, 2 patients (3.2%) developed symptomatic pneumonitis and an additional 2 patients died because of treatment-related factors. Proton therapy for LAEC remains experimental and is currently being evaluated in a randomized trial.

Target Delineation

Although CT can identify adjacent organs and structures, it may be limited in defining the extent of the primary tumor. Leong and colleagues[107] have demonstrated that the addition of PET/CT information for treatment planning improved the identification of the gross tumor volume (GTV). The GTV based on CT information alone excluded PET-avid disease in 11 of 16 patients (69%), 5 of whom would have resulted in a geographic miss of gross tumor. Thus, in many centers, it is customary to obtain pretreatment FDG-PET scans, not only to identify patients with occult metastatic disease but also to assist in target delineation. Conversely, MRI has also been suggested to delineate esophageal tumors, although initial studies showed limited benefit in tumor or positive lymph node delineation.[108] Thus, the use of MRI in this context remains experimental. Thus, the current recommendation for target delineation includes using contrasted CT and esophagogastroduodenoscopy/EUS findings as well as FDG-PET.

Limiting Toxicity of Chemoradiation

Depending on the location of the primary tumor, there are several sensitive organs that will be in the radiation field. Specifically, the most well-studied organs at risk in the context of treating LAEC include the lungs and heart. Radiation pneumonitis is clearly linked to the dose and volume of lung treated. Various single dosimetric parameters have been proposed to estimate the probability of developing radiation pneumonitis after radiotherapy.[109–115] Investigators from the Netherlands[113] compared different normal tissue complication probability models to predict radiation pneumonitis. Using the observed incidence of radiation pneumonitis among patients with breast cancer, malignant lymphoma, and inoperable non–small cell lung cancer, they found that the underlying local dose-effect relation for radiation pneumonitis was linear. Willner and colleagues[110] performed an analysis of pneumonitis risk from dose-volume histogram (DVH) parameters among patients treated with 3D-CRT. Their data indicated that it is reasonable to disperse the dose outside the target volume over large areas in order to reduce the volumes of lung receiving greater than 40 Gy (lung V40). They found that reducing the high-dose volume reduces the pneumonitis rate more than a corresponding reduction in the low-dose regions of the DVH. In addition, Konski and colleagues[116] were able to correlate cardiac toxicity to dosimetric and patient factors. Specifically, they recommended a threshold of V20, V30, and V40 less than 70%, 65%, and 60%, respectively, to decrease symptomatic cardiac toxicity. In general practice, an MLD less than 20 Gy is standard. Cardiac dose constraints are not as clearly defined, but at the authors' institution, a V30 less than 35% is thought to be reasonable.

SUMMARY

The management of esophageal cancer continues to evolve. General guidelines for treatment of LAEC include both preoperative and nonoperative approaches, predicated on resectability, histology, and location. In patients with resectable disease, who are medically fit for this procedure, the authors recommend preoperative chemoradiation to 50.4 Gy, with consideration of a lower dose (41.4 Gy) based on the CROSS trial. One possible exception to this recommendation is SCC of the cervical esophagus, for which definitive chemoradiation should be considered. In addition, in nonoperative patients, definitive chemoradiation to 50.4 Gy is standard; however, enrollment of these patients on dose-escalation or other protocols is encouraged. Clinicians should make use of all available imaging modalities to delineate tumor and involved lymphadenopathy. Motion management should be considered, particularly if the tumor is distal and IMRT is the preferred treatment modality. Reasonable goal dose constraints for treatment planning include an MLD less than 20 Gy and heart V30 less than 45%. Future directions include evaluation of tumor biomarkers of response to chemoradiation with a goal of possibly omitting surgery in favorable patients, while targeting nonresponders for protocol-based chemosensitizers and radiosensitizers.

REFERENCES

1. Kenjo M, Uno T, Murakami Y, et al. Radiation therapy for esophageal cancer in Japan: results of the patterns of care study 1999-2001. Int J Radiat Oncol Biol Phys 2009;75:357–63.
2. Suntharalingam M, Moughhan J, Coia LR, et al. Outcome results of the 1996-1999 patterns of care survey of the national practice for patients receiving radiation therapy for carcinoma of the esophagus. J Clin Oncol 2005;23:2325–31.
3. De-Ren S. Ten-year follow-up of esophageal cancer treated by radical radiation therapy: analysis of 869 patients. Int J Radiat Oncol Biol Phys 1989;16:329–34.
4. Newaishy GA, Read GA, Duncan W, et al. Results of radical radiotherapy of squamous cell carcinoma of the esophagus. Clin Radiol 1982;33:347–52.
5. Okawa T, Kita M, Tanaka M, et al. Results of radiotherapy for inoperable locally advanced esophageal cancer. Int J Radiat Oncol Biol Phys 1989;17:49–54.
6. Smyth E, Schoder H, Strong VE, et al. A prospective evaluation of the utility of 2-deoxy-2-18F Fluoro-D-glucose positron emission tomography and computed tomography in staging locally advanced gastric cancer. Cancer 2012;118:5481–8.

7. Kozak KR, Moody JS. The survival impact of the Intergroup 0116 trial on patients with gastric cancer. Int J Radiat Oncol Biol Phys 2008;72:517–21.

8. Shi X, Yao W, Liu T. Late course accelerated fractionation in radiotherapy of esophageal carcinoma. Radiother Oncol 1999;51:21–6.

9. Sai H, Mitsumori M, Arai K, et al. Long-term results of definitive radiotherapy for stage I esophageal cancer. Int J Radiat Oncol Biol Phys 2005;62:1339–44.

10. Yamada K, Murakami M, Okamoto Y, et al. Treatment results of chemoradiotherapy for clinical stage I (T1N0M0) esophageal carcinoma. Int J Radiat Oncol Biol Phys 2006;64:1106–11.

11. Moni J, Armstrong JG, Minsky BD, et al. High dose rate intraluminal brachytherapy for carcinoma of the esophagus. Dis Esophagus 1996;9:123–7.

12. Calais G, Dorval E, Louisot P, et al. Radiotherapy with high dose rate brachytherapy boost and concomitant chemotherapy for stages IIB and III esophageal carcinoma: results of a pilot study. Int J Radiat Oncol Biol Phys 1997;38:769–75.

13. Schraube P, Fritz P, Wannenmacher MF. Combined endoluminal and external irradiation of inoperable oesophageal carcinoma. Radiother Oncol 1997;44:45–51.

14. Akagi Y, Hirokawa Y, Kagemoto M, et al. Optimum fractionation for high-dose-rate endoesophageal brachytherapy following external irradiation of early stage esophageal cancer. Int J Radiat Oncol Biol Phys 1999;43:525–30.

15. Okawa T, Dokiya T, Nishio M, et al. Multi-institutional randomized trial of external radiotherapy with and without intraluminal brachytherapy for esophageal cancer in Japan. Int J Radiat Oncol Biol Phys 1999;45:623–8.

16. Caspers RJL, Zwinderman AH, Griffioen G, et al. Combined external beam and low dose rate intraluminal radiotherapy in oesophageal cancer. Radiother Oncol 1993;27:7–12.

17. Sur M, Sur R, Cooper K, et al. Morphologic alterations in esophageal squamous cell carcinoma after preoperative high dose rate intraluminal brachytherapy. Cancer 1996;77:2200–5.

18. Yorozu A, Toya K, Dokiya T. Long-term results of concurrent chemoradiotherapy followed by high dose rate brachytherapy for T2-3N0-1M0 esophageal cancer. Esophagus 2006;3:1–5.

19. Yorozu A, Dokiya T, Oki Y, et al. Curative radiotherapy with high-dose-rate brachytherapy boost for localized esophageal carcinoma: dose-effect relationship of brachytherapy with the balloon type applicator system. Radiother Oncol 1999;51:133–9.

20. Pasquier D, Mirabel X, Adenis A, et al. External beam radiation therapy followed by high-dose-rate brachytherapy for inoperable superficial esophageal carcinoma. Int J Radiat Oncol Biol Phys 2006;65:1456–61.

21. Ishikawa H, Nonaka T, Sakurai H, et al. Usefulness of intraluminal brachytherapy combined with external beam radiation therapy for submucosal esophageal cancer: long-term follow-up results. Int J Radiat Oncol Biol Phys 2010;76:452–9.

22. Gaspar LE, Qian C, Kocha WI, et al. A phase I/II study of external beam radiation, brachytherapy, and concurrent chemotherapy in localized cancer of the esophagus (RTOG 9207): Preliminary toxicity report. Int J Radiat Oncol Biol Phys 1995;32:160.

23. Gaspar LE, Nag S, Herskovic A, et al. American Brachytherapy Society (ABS) consensus guidelines for brachytherapy of esophageal cancer. Int J Radiat Oncol Biol Phys 1997;38:127–32.

24. Herskovic A, Martz LK, Al-Sarraf M, et al. Combined chemotherapy and radio-therapy compared with radiotherapy alone in patients with cancer of the esophagus. N Engl J Med 1992;326:1593–8.

25. Al-Sarraf M, Martz K, Herskovic A, et al. Progress report of combined chemoradiotherapy versus radiotherapy alone in patients with esophageal cancer: an intergroup study. J Clin Oncol 1997;15:277–84.

26. Cooper JS, Guo MD, Herskovic A, et al. Chemoradiotherapy of locally advanced esophageal cancer: long-term follow-up of a prospective randomized trial (RTOG 85-01). Radiation Therapy Oncology Group. JAMA 1999;281(17): 1623–7.

27. Streeter OE, Martz KL, Gaspar LE, et al. Does race influence survival for esophageal cancer patients treated on the radiation and chemotherapy arm of RTOG # 85-01? Int J Radiat Oncol Biol Phys 1999;44:1047–52.

28. Minsky BD, Neuberg D, Kelsen DP, et al. Final report of intergroup trial 0122 (ECOG PE-289, RTOG 90-12): phase II trial of neoadjuvant chemotherapy plus concurrent chemotherapy and high-dose radiation for squamous cell carcinoma of the esophagus. Int J Radiat Oncol Biol Phys 1999;43:517–23.

29. Minsky BD, Pajak T, Ginsberg RJ, et al. INT 0123 (RTOG 94-05) phase III trial of combined modality therapy for esophageal cancer: high dose (64.8 Gy) vs. standard dose (50.4 Gy) radiation therapy. J Clin Oncol 2002;20:1167–74.

30. Zaho KL, Shi XH, Jiang GL, et al. Late course accelerated hyperfractionated radiotherapy for localized esophageal carcinoma. Int J Radiat Oncol Biol Phys 2004;60:123–9.

31. Choi N, Park SD, Lynch T, et al. Twice-daily radiotherapy as concurrent boost technique during chemotherapy cycles in neoadjuvant chemoradiotherapy for resectable esophageal carcinoma: mature results of a phase II study. Int J Radiat Oncol Biol Phys 2004;60:111–22.

32. Lee JL, Kim SB, Jung HY, et al. A single institutional phase III trial of preoperative chemotherapy with hyperfractionation radiotherapy plus surgery versus surgery alone for resectable esophageal squamous cell carcinoma. Ann Oncol 2004;15:947–54.

33. Wu VWC, Sham JST, Kwong DLW. Inverse planning in three-dimensional conformal and intensity-modulated radiotherapy of mid-thoracic oesophageal cancer. Br J Radiol 2004;77(919):568–72.

34. Woudstra E, Heijmen BJM, Storchi PRM. Automated selection of beam orientations and segmented intensity-modulated radiotherapy (IMRT) for treatment of oesophagus tumors. Radiother Oncol 2005;77(3):254–61.

35. Chandra A, Guerrero TM, Liu HH, et al. Feasibility of using intensity-modulated radiotherapy to improve lung sparing in treatment planning for distal esophageal cancer. Radiother Oncol 2005;77:247–53.

36. Fenkell L, Kaminsky I, Breen S, et al. Dosimetric comparison of IMRT vs. 3D conformal radiotherapy in the treatment of cancer of the cervical esophagus. Radiother Oncol 2008;89(3):287–91.

37. Kole TP, Aghayere O, Kwah J, et al. Comparison of heart and coronary artery doses associated with intensity-modulated radiotherapy versus three-dimensional conformal radiotherapy for distal esophageal cancer. Int J Radiat Oncol Biol Phys 2012;83(5):1580–6.

38. Yin L, Wu H, Gong J, et al. Volumetric-modulated arc therapy vs. c-IMRT in esophageal cancer: a treatment planning comparison. World J Gastroenterol 2012;18(37):5266–75.

39. Nicolini G, Ghosh-Laskar S, Shrivastava SK, et al. Volumetric modulation arc radiotherapy with flattening filter-free beams compared with static gantry IMRT and 3D conformal radiotherapy for advanced esophageal cancer: a feasibility study. Int J Radiat Oncol Biol Phys 2012;84(2):553–60.

40. Martin S, Chen JZ, Rashid Dar A, et al. Dosimetric comparison of helical tomotherapy, RapidArc, and a novel IMRT & Arc technique for esophageal carcinoma. Radiother Oncol 2011;101(3):431–7.

41. Vivekanandan N, Sriram P, Kumar SAS, et al. Volumetric modulated arc radiotherapy for esophageal cancer. Med Dosim 2012;37(1):108–13.

42. Yin Y, Chen J, Xing L, et al. Applications of IMAT in cervical esophageal cancer radiotherapy: a comparison with fixed-field IMRT in dosimetry and implementation. J Appl Clin Med Phys 2011;12(2):3343.

43. Van Benthuysen L, Hales L, Podgorsak MB. Volumetric modulated arc therapy vs. IMRT for the treatment of distal esophageal cancer. Med Dosim 2011; 36(4):404–9.

44. Gong Y, Wang S, Zhou L, et al. Dosimetric comparison using different multileaf collimeters in intensity-modulated radiotherapy for upper thoracic esophageal cancer. Radiat Oncol 2010;5:65.

45. Lin SH, Wang L, Myles B, et al. Propensity score-based comparison of long-term outcomes with 3-dimensional conformal radiotherapy vs intensity-modulated radiotherapy for esophageal cancer. Int J Radiat Oncol Biol Phys 2012;84(5): 1078–85.

46. Wang S-L, Liao Z, Liu H, et al. Intensity-modulated radiation therapy with concurrent chemotherapy for locally advanced cervical and upper thoracic esophageal cancer. World J Gastroenterol 2006;12(34):5501–8.

47. La TH, Minn AY, Su Z, et al. Multimodality treatment with intensity modulated radiation therapy for esophageal cancer. Dis Esophagus 2010;23(4):300–8.

48. Zhang Z, Liao Z, Jin J, et al. Dose response relationship in locoregional control for patients with stage II-III esophageal cancer treated with concurrent chemotherapy and radiotherapy. Int J Radiat Oncol Biol Phys 2005;61:656–64.

49. Cunningham D, Allum WH, Stenning SP, et al. Perioperative chemotherapy versus surgery alone for resectable gastroesophageal cancer. N Engl J Med 2006;355(1):11–20.

50. Goodman KA. Refining the role for adjuvant radiotherapy in gastric cancer: risk stratification is key. J Clin Oncol 2015;33(28):3082–4.

51. Lordick F, Ott K, Krause B-J, et al. PET to assess early metabolic response and to guide treatment of adenocarcinoma of the oesophagogastric junction: the MUNICON phase II trial. Lancet Oncol 2007;8(9):797–805.

52. Ilson DH, Minsky BD, Ku GY, et al. Phase 2 trial of induction and concurrent chemoradiotherapy with weekly irinotecan and cisplatin followed by surgery for esophageal cancer. Cancer 2012;118(11):2820–7.

53. Wieder HA, Brucher BLDM, Zimmermann F, et al. Time course of tumor metabolic activity during chemoradiotherapy of esophageal squamous cell carcinoma and response to treatment. J Clin Oncol 2004;22:900–8.

54. Ruhstaller T, Templeton A, Ribi K, et al. Intense therapy in patients with locally advanced esophageal cancer beyond hope for surgical cure: a prospective, multicenter phase II trial of the Swiss Group for Clinical Cancer Research (SAKK 76/02). Onkologie 2010;33(5):222–8.

55. Gschossmann JM, Bonner JA, Foote RL, et al. Malignant tracheoesophageal fistula in patients with esophageal cancer. Cancer 1993;72:1513–21.

56. Rueth NM, Shaw D, D'Cunha J, et al. Esophageal stenting and radiotherapy: a multimodal approach for the palliation of symptomatic malignant dysphagia. Ann Surg Oncol 2012;19:4223–8.
57. Muto M, Ohtsu A, Miyamoto S, et al. Concurrent chemoradiotherapy for esophageal carcinoma patients with malignant fistulae. Cancer 1999;86:1406–13.
58. Urba SG, Orringer MB, Turrisi A, et al. Randomized trial of preoperative chemoradiation versus surgery alone in patients with locoregional esophageal carcinoma. J Clin Oncol 2001;19:305–13.
59. Walsh TN, Noonan N, Hollywood D, et al. A comparison of multimodal therapy and surgery for esophageal adenocarcinoma. N Engl J Med 1996;335:462–7.
60. Bosset JF, Gignoux M, Triboulet JP, et al. Chemoradiotherapy followed by surgery compared with surgery alone in squamous cell cancer of the esophagus. N Engl J Med 1997;337:161–7.
61. Burmeister BH, Smithers BM, Fitzgerald L, et al. Surgery alone versus chemoradiotherapy followed by surgery for resectable cancer of the oesophagus: a randomised controlled phase III trial. Lancet Oncol 2005;6:659–68.
62. Tepper JE, Krasna MJ, Niedzwieki D, et al. Phase III trial of trimodality therapy with cisplatin, fluorouracil, radiotherapy, and surgery compared with surgery alone for esophageal cancer: CALGB 9781. J Clin Oncol 2008;26:1086–92.
63. van Hagen P, Hulshof MCCM, van Lanschot JJB, et al. Preoperative chemoradiotherapy for esophageal or junctional cancer. N Engl J Med 2012;366(22): 2074–84.
64. Scheer RV, Fakiris AJ, Johnstone PAS. Quantifying the benefit of a pathologic complete response after neoadjuvant chemoradiotherapy in the treatment of esophageal cancer. Int J Radiat Oncol Biol Phys 2011;80(4):996–1001.
65. Geh JI, Bond SJ, Bentzen SM, et al. Systematic overview of preoperative (neoadjuvant) chemoradiotherapy trials in oesophageal cancer: evidence of a radiation and chemotherapy dose response. Radiother Oncol 2006;78:236–44.
66. Urschel JD, Vasan H. A meta-analysis of randomized controlled clinical trials that compared neoadjuvant chemoradiation and surgery to surgery alone for resectable esophageal cancer. Am J Surg 2002;185:538–43.
67. Bedenne L, Michel P, Bouche O, et al. Chemoradiation followed by surgery compared with chemoradiation alone in squamous cell cancer of the esophagus: FFCD 9102. J Clin Oncol 2007;25:1160–8.
68. Bonnetain F, Bouche O, Michel P, et al. A comparative longitudinal quality of life study using the Spitzer quality of life index in a randomized multicenter phase III trial (FFCD 9102): chemoradiation followed by surgery compared with chemoradiation alone in locally advanced squamous resectable thoracic esophageal cancer. Ann Oncol 2006;17:827–34.
69. Crehange G, Maingon P, Peignaux K, et al. Phase III trial of protracted compared with split-course chemoradiation for esophageal cancer: Federation Francophone de Cancerologie Digestive 9102. J Clin Oncol 2007;25:4895–901.
70. Stahl M, Stuschke M, Lehmann N, et al. Chemoradiation with and without surgery in patients with locally advanced squamous cell carcinoma of the esophagus. J Clin Oncol 2005;23:2310–7.
71. Berger AC, Farma J, Scott WJ, et al. Complete response to neoadjuvant chemoradiotherapy in esophageal carcinoma is associated with significantly improved survival. J Clin Oncol 2005;23(19):4330–7.
72. Rohatgi P, Swisher S, Correa AM, et al. Characterization of pathologic complete response after preoperative chemoradiotherapy in carcinoma of the esophagus and outcome after pathologic response. Cancer 2005;104:2365–72.

73. Swisher SG, Hofsetter W, Wu TT, et al. Proposed revision of the esophageal cancer staging system to accommodate pathologic response (pP) following preoperative chemoradiation (CRT). Ann Surg 2005;241:810–20.

74. Swisher SG, Winter KA, Komaki RU, et al. A phase II study of a paclitaxel-based chemoradiation regimen with selective surgical salvage for resectable locoregionally advanced esophageal cancer: initial reporting of RTOG 0246. Int J Radiat Oncol Biol Phys 2012;82:1967–72.

75. Gaca JG, Petersen RP, Peterson BL, et al. Pathologic nodal status predicts disease-free survival after neoadjuvant chemoradiation for gastroesophageal junction carcinoma. Ann Surg Oncol 2006;13:340–6.

76. Bates BA, Detterbeck FC, Bernard SA, et al. Concurrent radiation therapy and chemotherapy followed by esophagectomy for localized esophageal carcinoma. J Clin Oncol 1996;14:156–63.

77. Jones DR, Parker LA, Detterbeck FC, et al. Inadequacy of computed tomography in assessing patients with esophageal carcinoma after induction chemoradiotherapy. Cancer 1999;85:1026–32.

78. Lightdale CJ, Kulkarni KG. Role of endoscopic ultrasonography in the staging and follow-up of esophageal cancer. J Clin Oncol 2005;23(20):4483–9.

79. Sarkaria IS, Rizk NP, Bains MS, et al. Post-treatment endoscopic biopsy is a poor-predictor of pathologic response in patients undergoing chemoradiation therapy for esophageal cancer. Ann Surg 2009;249:764–7.

80. Wieder HA, Ott K, Lordick F, et al. Prediction of tumor response by FDG-PET: comparison of the accuracy of single and sequential studies in patients with adenocarcinomas of the esophagogastric junction. Eur J Nucl Med Mol Imaging 2007;34(12):1925–32.

81. Ott K, Weber WA, Lordick F, et al. Metabolic imaging predicts response, survival, and recurrence in adenocarcinomas of the esophagogastric junction. J Clin Oncol 2006;24(29):4692–8.

82. Vallbohmer D, Holscher AH, Dietlein M, et al. [18F] fluorodeoxyglucose-positron emission tomography for the assessment of histologic response and prognosis after completion of neoadjuvant chemoradiation in esophageal cancer. Ann Surg 2009;250:888–94.

83. Flamen P, van Cutsem E, Lerut T, et al. Positron emission tomography for assessment of the response to induction radiochemotherapy in locally advanced oesophageal cancer. Ann Oncol 2002;13:361–8.

84. Klayton T, Li T, Yu JQ, et al. The role of qualitative and quantitative analysis of F18-FDG positron emission tomography in predicting pathologic response following chemoradiotherapy in patients with esophageal carcinoma. J Gastrointest Cancer 2012;43(4):612–8.

85. Swisher SG, Erasmus J, Maish M, et al. 2-Fluoro-2-deoxy-D-glucose positron emission tomography imaging is predictive of pathologic response and survival after preoperative chemoradiation in patients with esophageal carcinoma. Cancer 2004;101(8):1776–85.

86. Monjazeb AM, Riedlinger G, Aklilu M, et al. Outcomes of patients with esophageal cancer staged with [18F] fluorodeoxyglucose positron emission tomography (FDG-PET): can postradiochemotherapy FDG-PED predict the utility of resection? J Clin Oncol 2010;28:4714–21.

87. Eng CW, Fuqua JL 3rd, Grewal R, et al. Evaluation of response to induction chemotherapy in esophageal cancer: is barium esophagography or PET-CT useful? Clin Imaging 2013;37(3):468–74.

88. Erasmus JJ, Munden RF, Truong MT, et al. Preoperative chemo-radiation-induced ulceration in patients with esophageal cancer: a confounding factor in tumor response assessment in integrated computed tomographic-positron emission tomographic imaging. J Thorac Oncol 2006;1(5):478–86.

89. Morita M, Kuwano H, Araki K, et al. Prognostic significance of lymphocytic infiltration following preoperative chemoradiotherapy and hyperthermia for esophageal cancer. Int J Radiat Oncol Biol Phys 2001;49:1259–66.

90. Alexander BM, Wang XZ, Niemierko A, et al. DNA repair biomarkers predict response to neoadjuvant chemoradiotherapy in esophageal cancer. Int J Radiat Oncol Biol Phys 2012;83(1):164–71.

91. Kuwahara A, Yamamori M, Fujita M, et al. TNFRSF1B A1466G genotype is predictive of clinical efficacy after treatment with a definitive 5-fluorouracil/cisplatin-based chemoradiotherapy in Japanese patients with esophageal squamous cell carcinoma. J Exp Clin Cancer Res 2010;29:100.

92. Yi Y, Li B, Sun H, et al. Predictors of sensitivity to chemoradiotherapy of esophageal squamous cell carcinoma. Tumour Biol 2010;31(4):333–40.

93. Gotoh M, Takiuchi H, Kawabe S, et al. Epidermal growth factor receptor is a possible predictor of sensitivity to chemoradiotherapy in the primary lesion of esophageal squamous cell carcinoma. Jpn J Clin Oncol 2007;37(9):652–7.

94. Luthra R, Luthra MG, Izzo J, et al. Biomarkers of response to preoperative chemoradiation in esophageal cancers. Semin Oncol 2006;33(6 Suppl 11):S2–5.

95. Izzo JG, Correa AM, Wu T-T, et al. Pretherapy nuclear factor-kappaB status, chemoradiation resistance, and metastatic progression in esophageal carcinoma. Mol Cancer Ther 2006;5(11):2844–50.

96. Wu X, Gu J, Wu T-T, et al. Genetic variations in radiation and chemotherapy drug action pathways predict clinical outcomes in esophageal cancer. J Clin Oncol 2006;24(23):3789–98.

97. Okumura H, Natsugoe S, Matsumoto M, et al. The predictive value of p53, p53R2, and p21 for the effect of chemoradiation therapy on oesophageal squamous cell carcinoma. Br J Cancer 2005;92(2):284–9.

98. Sohda M, Ishikawa H, Masuda N, et al. Pretreatment evaluation of combined HIF-1alpha, p53 and p21 expression is a useful and sensitive indicator of response to radiation and chemotherapy in esophageal cancer. Int J Cancer 2004;110(6):838–44.

99. Harpole DHJ, Moore MB, Herndon JE 2nd, et al. The prognostic value of molecular marker analysis in patients treated with trimodality therapy for esophageal cancer. Clin Cancer Res 2001;7(3):562–9.

100. Skinner HD, Xu E, Lee JH, et al. A validated miRNA expression profile for response to neoadjuvant therapy in esophageal cancer. J Clin Oncol 2013;31 [Internet] [suppl; abstract 4078]. Available at: http://meetinglibrary.asco.org/content/82991. Accessed June 26, 2013.

101. Lloyd S, Chang BW. Current strategies in chemoradiation for esophageal cancer. J Gastrointest Oncol 2014;5(3):156–65.

102. Jacob JH, Seitz JF, Langlois C, et al. Definitive concurrent chemo-radiation therapy (CRT) in squamous cell carcinoma of the esophagus (SCCE): preliminary results of a French randomized trial comparing standard vs. split course irradiation (FNCLCC-FFCD 9305). Proc ASCO 1999;18:270a.

103. Zhang X, Zhao K, Guerrero TM, et al. Four-dimensional computed tomography-based treatment planning for intensity-modulated radiation therapy and proton therapy for distal esophageal cancer. Int J Radiat Oncol Biol Phys 2008;72(1):278–87.

104. Sugahara S, Tokuuye K, Okumura T, et al. Clinical results of proton beam therapy for cancer of the esophagus. Int J Radiat Oncol Biol Phys 2005;61:76–84.
105. Koyama S, Tsujii H. Proton beam therapy with high-dose irradiation for superficial and advanced esophageal carcinomas. Clin Cancer Res 2003;9(10 Pt 1): 3571–7.
106. Lin SH, Komaki R, Liao Z, et al. Proton beam therapy and concurrent chemotherapy for esophageal cancer. Int J Radiat Oncol Biol Phys 2012;83(3): e345–51.
107. Leong T, Everitt C, Yuen K, et al. A prospective study to evaluate the impact of FDG-PET on CT-based radiotherapy treatment planning for oesophageal cancer. Radiother Oncol 2006;78:254–61.
108. Sakurada A, Takahara T, Kwee TC, et al. Diagnostic performance of diffusion-weighted magnetic resonance imaging in esophageal cancer. Eur Radiol 2009;19(6):1461–9.
109. Seppenwoolde Y, Lebesque JV, de Jaeger K, et al. Comparing different NTCP models that predict the incidence of radiation pneumonitis. Normal tissue complication probability. Int J Radiat Oncol Biol Phys 2003;55:724–35.
110. Willner J, Jost A, Baier K, et al. A little to a lot or a lot to a little? An analysis of pneumonitis risk from dose-volume histogram parameters of the lung in patients with lung cancer treated with 3-D conformal radiotherapy. Strahlenther Onkol 2003;179:548–56.
111. Yorke ED, Jackson A, Rosenzweig KE, et al. Dose-volume factors contributing to the incidence of radiation pneumonitis in non-small-cell lung cancer patients treated with three-dimensional conformal radiation therapy. Int J Radiat Oncol Biol Phys 2002;54:329–39.
112. Kwa SL, Lebesque JV, Theuws JC, et al. Radiation pneumonitis as a function of mean lung dose: an analysis of pooled data of 540 patients. Int J Radiat Oncol Biol Phys 1998;42:1–9.
113. Schallenkamp J, Miller R, Brinkmann D, et al. Incidence of radiation pneumonitis after thoracic irradiation: dose-volume correlates. Int J Radiat Oncol Biol Phys 2007;67:410–6.
114. Wang S, Liao Z, Wej X, et al. Analysis of clinical and dosimetric factors associated with treatment-related pneumonitis (TRP) in patients with non-small-cell lung cancer (NSCLC) treated with concurrent chemotherapy and three-dimensional conformal radiotherapy (3D-CRT). Int J Radiat Oncol Biol Phys 2006;66:1399–407.
115. Kong F-M, Hayman JA, Griffith KA, et al. Final toxicity results of a radiation-dose escalation study in patients with non-small-cell lung cancer (NSCLC): predictors for radiation pneumonitis and fibrosis. Int J Radiat Oncol Biol Phys 2006;65(4): 1075–86.
116. Konski A, Li T, Christensen M, et al. Symptomatic cardiac toxicity is predicted by dosimetric and patient factors rather than changes in 18F-FDG PET determination of myocardial activity after chemoradiotherapy for esophageal cancer. Radiother Oncol 2012;104:72–7.

The Current Status of Immunotherapies in Esophagogastric Cancer

Geoffrey Y. Ku, MD

KEYWORDS

- Adenocarcinoma • Squamous cell carcinoma • Gastric • Esophageal
- Immunotherapy • Immune checkpoint • PD-1 • PD-L1

KEY POINTS

- Immune checkpoint inhibitors that target cytotoxic T lymphocyte antigen-4 or the programmed death-1/programmed death–ligand 1 axis have transformed the treatment of many solid tumors.
- Initial phase I/II studies in esophagogastric cancer suggest significant activity for these drugs.
- Ongoing phase III studies will determine if there is a role for these drugs in the next several years.
- Correlative analyses are ongoing to identify the group of patients most likely to benefit from these therapies.

INTRODUCTION

Outcomes for patients with advanced esophagogastric cancer (EGC) are poor.[1] Approximately 50% of patients with EGC present with overt metastatic disease, and chemotherapy is the mainstay of palliation in this setting. With the high likelihood that patients with initial locoregional disease will eventually have metastatic disease, palliative chemotherapy will ultimately be used in most patients. In recent years, the incorporation of targeted agents—trastuzumab with first-line chemotherapy for Her2-positive disease[2] and ramucirumab as monotherapy[3] or with paclitaxel chemotherapy[4] in the second-line setting—has incrementally improved outcomes, but median overall survival (OS) remains at best only 1 year.

In this gloomy context, excitement is growing among oncologists and patients alike for the use of immunotherapy or, more specifically, immune checkpoint inhibitors. Since the landmark approval by the US Food and Drug Administration (FDA) of

Disclosure: Dr G.Y. Ku received research support from Merck and AstraZeneca/Medimmune.
Gastrointestinal Oncology Service, Department of Medicine, Memorial Sloan Kettering Cancer Center, 300 East 66th Street, Room 1035, New York, NY 10065, USA
E-mail address: kug@mskcc.org

Surg Oncol Clin N Am 26 (2017) 277–292
http://dx.doi.org/10.1016/j.soc.2016.10.012
1055-3207/17/© 2016 Elsevier Inc. All rights reserved.

surgonc.theclinics.com

the anti–cytotoxic T-lymphocyte antigen-4 (CTLA-4) antibody ipilimumab in advanced melanoma,[5,6] these and other antibodies (namely, antagonists of the programmed death [PD]-1/PD-ligand 1 pathway) that de-repress the immune system have undergone extensive evaluation in multiple other solid tumors, including EGC. These studies have led to the FDA approval of additional immune checkpoint inhibitors in several solid tumor malignancies and, in EGC, have culminated in ongoing phase III studies.

This review focuses on the role of the immune system in cancer, a brief history of immunotherapy, the role of immune checkpoint molecules in normal immune homeostasis and, the rapidly accumulating data in EGC.

THE IMMUNE SYSTEM

The immune system protects us from external threats (infectious diseases) and also from internal ones (cancers) while not attacking healthy tissue (which would lead to the development of autoimmune diseases). To fulfill these critical and synchronous roles, it must recognize self from non–self-antigens with unerring accuracy.

The immune system consists of an innate and an adaptive component.[7] The innate immune system involves rapid immune responses, which are mediated by macrophages, neutrophils, dendritic cells, and natural killer cells. These cells are hard wired to recognize non–self-antigens, such as those from infectious organisms, but have (1) relatively low potency, (2) limited specificity for the specific microorganism, and (3) no memory (ie, no ability to generate an enhanced response if re-exposed to the same microorganism).

If a microbe or cancer cell is not rapidly eliminated by innate immune mechanisms, adaptive immune responses are then engendered. These responses are produced by B cells (the humoral arm, which produces antibodies that typically target extracellular antigens) and T cells (the cellular arm, which destroys infected cells that harbor intracellular organisms or malignant cells). In contrast to innate immunity, adaptive immunity develops over days to weeks and is (1) much more potent, (2) highly specific for a specific antigen, and (3) leads to a memory response (which results in a much more rapid and potent response upon re-exposure).

Despite these coordinated mechanisms, the development of cancer necessarily implies a failure of immunosurveillance of incipient malignant cells. Dunn and colleagues[8] proposed the concept of immunoediting to explain this phenomenon. They envisaged that this process comprises 3 phases that are collectively denoted as the 3 Es of cancer immunoediting: elimination, equilibrium, and escape. The first E refers to the fact that most cancer cells are indeed recognized and successfully killed by the immune system, leading to the second E, where the surviving cancer cells acquire multiple mechanisms that allow them to exist alongside increasingly ineffective immune responses (eg, down-regulating immunogenic molecules on the tumor cell surface or recruiting immunosuppressive mechanisms in the tumor microenvironment). This second E lasts the longest and may occur over many years. Finally, the balance of forces shifts decidedly in the favor of the cancer cells, allowing them to escape from immune control.

COLEY'S TOXINS

The idea of harnessing the immune system to attack cancer is an intuitively appealing concept but not a new one. The attractiveness of such a proposed treatment stems from the belief that recruitment of the immune system to attack cancer cells potentially offers more durable benefit and less toxicity than conventional therapies (akin to fighting off a virulent influenza infection) and, in some fashion, is more natural than the harsh chemicals and x-rays that comprise modern anticancer therapy.

The earliest proof of the potential of the immune system to directly combat malignant tumors stems from a series of observations and experiments by William Coley, a surgeon at the New York Cancer Hospital (the precursor to Memorial Sloan Kettering Cancer Center).[9] He noted the regression of a soft tissue sarcoma in a patient who had erysipelas, an infection caused by *Streptococcus pyogenes*. He then inoculated the tumors of 10 patients directly with a culture of the bacterium and noted durable curative responses in some patients. The immune basis of these observations is not known with certainty but is presumed to involve the nonspecific recruitment to the tumor site and activation of immune cells by the bacterial products.[10]

Although Coley's concoction of toxins fell out of favor, other approaches to stimulate the immune system continued to be investigated in the 20th century. Most of these methods focused on vaccinating patients against preidentified antigens that are expressed preferentially or exclusively on tumor cells.[11] Uniformly, despite laboratory evidence of cellular immune responses to these vaccines, few clinically relevant responses were noted.

The sole exception is sipuleucel-T, a recombinant human protein consisting of prostatic acid phosphatase linked to granulocyte-macrophage colony-stimulating factor, which has to be introduced into autologous peripheral blood mononuclear cells obtained from patients by leukopheresis. It was approved in 2010 for the treatment of castrate-resistant prostate cancer based on a phase III study, which found an improvement in OS in the absence of an improvement in time to progression.[12]

The low effectiveness of most cancer vaccines is likely because of their lack of antigenicity and the failure to provide adequate costimulation (to be discussed later), which results in inactivation of T cells against the tumor.[13]

IMMUNE CHECKPOINTS

The generation of an effective cellular immune response by T cells against a cancer cell requires a primary signal and cosignals.[14] As shown in Fig. 1, the primary signal comes from recognition of a cancer-associated antigen by a T-cell receptor with high specificity for the antigen, presented in the context of a class I/II major histocompatibility complex molecule, which is expressed on so-called antigen-present cells (APCs), such as dendritic cells or on the tumor cell itself. In addition to this primary signal, a secondary signal is required, in the absence of which the T cell may be rendered anergic or nonfunctional.

As noted in Fig. 1, it is now well established that the interactions between multiple molecules at the interface between the T cell and tumor cell create multiple secondary signals, some of which are costimulatory and some of which are inhibitory. The ultimate activation or quiescence of the immune response depends on the complex interplay and net signal—positive or negative—of these diverse interactions, which occur at different times in the process of successful T-cell engagement and activation.

Under normal physiologic conditions, immune checkpoints are crucial for the maintenance of self-tolerance (and the avoidance of autoimmunity) and also to protect tissues from excessive damage if the immune system were to respond too exuberantly to an infection. However, many of these molecules have become co-opted by cancer cells (in the process of achieving equilibrium and escape from the immune system). Their identification and targeting with neutralizing (or agonist) antibodies now forms the basis of modern-era immunotherapy.

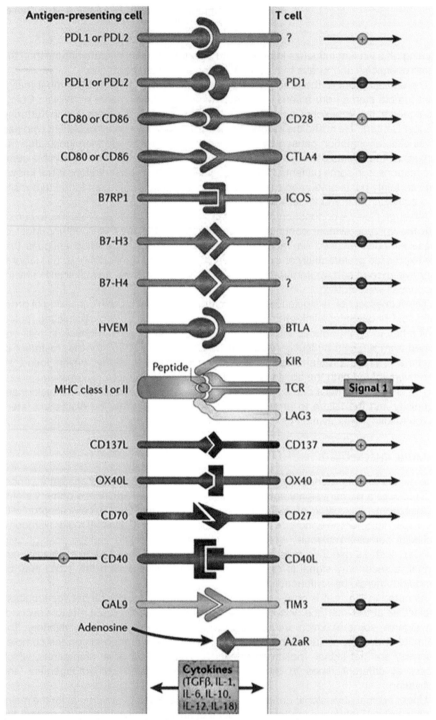

Fig. 1. Immune checkpoint molecules at the T cell–tumor interface. A2aR, adenosine A2a receptor; B7RP1, B7-related protein 1; BTLA, B and T lymphocyte attenuator; GAL9, galectin 9; HVEM, herpesvirus entry mediator; ICOS, inducible T-cell costimulator; IL, interleukin; KIR, killer cell immunoglobulinlike receptor; LAG3, lymphocyte activation gene 3; PD1, programmed cell death protein 1; PDL, PD1 ligand; TGFβ, transforming growth factor-β; TIM3, T cell membrane protein 3. (*From* Pardoll DM. The blockade of immune checkpoints in cancer immunotherapy. Nat Rev Cancer 2012;12:252; with permission.)

Cytotoxic T-Lymphocyte Antigen-4 and the Programmed Death-1/Programmed Death–ligand 1/2 Pathway

In 1995, James Allison and colleagues[15] were 1 of 2 groups that simultaneously characterized the function of CTLA-4, a protein that has high homology with CD28, which was already known to be a costimulatory molecule expressed on T cells necessary to provide the secondary signal for T-cell activation. Just like CD28, CTLA-4 also binds their cognate ligands, the B7 molecules (which are found on APCs), but with much higher affinity. However, unlike CD28, CTLA-4 expression is induced only when a T cell becomes activated. It then competes with CD28 for binding to the B7 molecules but leads to down-regulation and eventual abrogation of the immune response.

Subsequently, PD-1 was also identified as another negative immune checkpoint molecule.[16] PD-1 has 2 ligands, PD-L1 and PD-L2. PD-L2 is mostly expressed on APCs, whereas PD-L1 is expressed on numerous tissues, including immune and tumor cells. In the tumor microenvironment, PD-L1 expressed on tumor cells binds to PD-1 on activated T cells reaching the tumor. This delivers an inhibitory signal to those T cells, preventing them from killing target cancer cells and protecting the tumor from immune elimination.[17] Unlike CTLA-4, which is thought to be necessary for T-cell activation, the PD-1/PD-L1/2 pathway is thought to protect cells from T-cell attack.[18]

Anti–Cytotoxic T-Lymphocyte Antigen-4 Antibodies

The 2 anti–CTLA-4 antibodies that have been evaluated in EGC are ipilimumab and tremelimumab. In the first-line phase III study of ipilimumab in advanced melanoma, immune-related adverse events (irAEs) resulted from nonspecific immune activation and included diarrhea (33% all grade, 4% grade 3), pruritus (27% all grade, 2% grade 3), rash (22% all grade, 1.2% grade 3), and elevation in liver enzymes (about 29% all grade, 15% grade 3/4).[6] No treatment-related deaths were reported. Since that time, the growing clinical experience with ipilimumab and other immune checkpoint inhibitors has also led to well-established algorithms for treating irAEs with the use of steroids and other immunosuppressants, which do not appear to reduce the benefit from ipilimumab in melanoma patients.[19]

Historically, the first immune checkpoint inhibitor to be studied in EGC was tremelimumab. In a phase II study, Ralph and colleagues[20] evaluated tremelimumab, 15 mg/kg every 90 days, in 18 patients with advanced esophageal, gastroesophageal junction (GEJ), or gastric adenocarcinoma; 15 received prior first-line chemotherapy, and 3 received prior second-line treatment. One patient achieved a partial response (PR, 6%) by standard Response Evaluation Criteria in Solid Tumors (RECIST) criteria that was ongoing at 33 months of follow-up, whereas 4 other patients achieved stable disease (SD, 22%). Although median time to progression and OS were disappointing (2.83 and 4.83 months respectively), one-third of patients were alive at 12 months. Grade ≥ 3 toxicities included rash and diarrhea in 2 and 3 patients, respectively, consistent with the known toxicities of these drugs. Correlative analyses included evaluating T-cell proliferative responses to carcinoembryonic antigen; the 5 patients with a posttreatment response had improved OS compared with the 8 assayed patients without a carcinoembryonic antigen response (17.1 vs 4.7 months; $P = .004$).

The dose of tremelimumab in this study is now considered subtherapeutic. In an ongoing study of tremelimumab (with or without the anti–PD-L1 antibody, durvalumab), the dose of tremelimumab monotherapy is 10 mg/kg every 4 weeks.

Data for ipilimumab were recently reported in abstract form.[21] This was for a randomized phase II study in which 114 patients with either a PR or SD to first-line fluoropyrimidine/platinum chemotherapy were randomly assigned to best supportive care

(BSC, which mostly consisted of continuation of the fluoropyrimidine) versus ipilimumab. The primary endpoint was immune-related progression-free survival (PFS), which used a modification of the modified World Health Organization criteria, in which the appearance of new lesions does not automatically constitute progressive disease. Unfortunately, the immune-related PFS was only 2.9 months in patients who received ipilimumab versus 4.9 months for patients who continued on fluoropyrimidine maintenance chemotherapy. The median OS was similar in both groups (12.7 vs 12.1 months). Toxicities were also higher in the ipilimumab versus BSC arm (72% vs 56%) and included pruritus (32%), diarrhea (25%), fatigue (23%), and rash (18%).

These 2 studies contain the only data for anti–CTLA-4 antibody monotherapy in EGC (Table 1). They suggest modest activity for these drugs at best, and toxicity profiles comparable with the known irAEs of ipilimumab in other cancers.

Anti–Programmed Death-1 and Programmed Death–Ligand 1 Antibodies

Several anti–PD-1 and anti–PD-L1 antibodies are now approved for the treatment of various cancers. Pembrolizumab, an antibody against PD-1, was initially approved in 2014 for the treatment of advanced melanoma.[22] Since then, it has also obtained approval in non–small cell lung cancer in 2015. In general, toxicities associated with pembrolizumab (and other anti–PD-1 inhibitors) seem to be less than with ipilimumab, as was noted in a phase III study in melanoma that compared 2 doses of pembrolizumab with ipilimumab and found lower rates of grade $\geq$3 toxicities for pembrolizumab (10%–13% vs 20%).[23] The rates of treatment discontinuation were also lower in the pembrolizumab arms than in the ipilimumab arm (4%–6.9% vs 9.4%). Individual grade $\geq$3 toxicities with pembrolizumab were less than 5% and include colitis, hepatitis, and pneumonitis.

Another anti–PD-1 antibody, nivolumab, is also now FDA approved for several malignancies, including melanoma, non–small cell lung cancer, renal cell carcinoma, and Hodgkin lymphoma. Toxicities of nivolumab are qualitatively and quantitatively similar to those of pembrolizumab.[24]

Nivolumab's labeling indication was expanded in 2016 to permit for combination with ipilimumab as first-line therapy for advanced melanoma. This approval was based on a phase III study, which showed improvement in PFS for the combination versus ipilimumab or nivolumab alone.[25] However, this increased efficacy is at the expense of significantly added toxicity (grade $\geq$3 toxicity rate of 55.0% vs 16.3% for the nivolumab arm and 27.3% for the ipilimumab arm).

An interesting observation is that, in patients whose tumors were PD-L1 negative, the addition of ipilimumab to nivolumab improved outcomes compared with nivolumab only (PFS 11.2 vs 5.3 months), whereas the addition of ipilimumab did not

Table 1
Results of anticytotoxic T lymphocyte antigen-4 antibody studies in esophagogastric cancer

Treatment	Location/ Histology	No. of Patients	Response Rate, %	PFS Median	PFS Overall	OS Median	OS Overall	Reference
Tremelimumab	E/GEJ/G adenoCA	18	6	2.83	NS	4.83	33% 1-y	Ralph et al,[20] 2010
Ipilimumab	GEJ/G adenoCA	57	NS	2.9 mo	NS	12.7	NS	Moehler et al,[21] 2016
BSC (including chemo)		57	NS	4.9 mo	NS	12.1	NS	

Abbreviations: adenoCA, adenocarcinoma; BSC, best supportive care; E, esophageal; G, gastric; NS, not stated.

improve outcomes in patients with PD-L1–positive tumors (PFS, 14.0 months in both groups). This finding gives rise to the intriguing theory that PD-L1 may be upregulated by a tumor as a defense mechanism to dampen the immune system after it has been infiltrated and recognized by T cells. Therefore, in such an inflamed tumor microenvironment, PD-1 blockade alone may be sufficient to exert a significant effect. On the other hand, the absence of PD-L1 inhibition suggests a noninflamed tumor, which requires CTLA-4 blockade to drive T cells into the tumor to facilitate tumor recognition to benefit from blockade of the PD-1/PD-L1 axis.[18]

Finally, an anti–PD-L1 antibody, atezolizumab, was recently approved to treat advanced urothelial carcinoma, based on a single-arm phase II study that treated 310 patients.[26] Toxicities seem to be qualitatively similar to those of the anti–PD-1 antibodies and less than ipilimumab; 5% of patients had a grade ≥3 irAE, which included colitis, pneumonitis, and elevation of liver enzymes in 1% of patients each.

Although many of these anti–PD-1 and anti–PD-L1 antibodies have been evaluated in EGC (results are summarized in **Table 2**), only 1 study has been published.[27] The KEYNOTE-012 study is a phase Ib dose-expansion study that evaluated 39 patients with GEJ/gastric adenocarcinomas, whose tumors were found to be PD-L1 positive using an experimental immunohistochemistry (IHC) assay that used the Merck 22C3 antibody. Based on the cutoff for positivity of ≥1% membrane staining of tumor or peritumoral mononuclear inflammatory cells, 40% of tumors were noted to be PD-L1 positive.

Nineteen patients were from Asia, and the remainder was from the rest of the world. Patients were heavily pretreated and two-thirds received ≥2 prior therapies. The confirmed response rate was 22% for all patients; 4 of these 8 patients had ongoing responses at the time of data analysis, and the median duration of response was 40 weeks. Median PFS was 1.9 months, and median OS was 11.4 months; the 6- and 12-month OS rates were 66% and 42%, respectively. Toxicities seemed to be in line with the known side effects of pembrolizumab and included grade ≥3 pneumonitis, pemphigoid, peripheral neuropathy, and hypothyroidism in 1 patient (3%) each.

In the similarly designed KEYNOTE-028 study, 23 patients with PD-L1–positive esophageal cancer were treated, 17 had squamous cell cancer (SCC) and 5 had adenocarcinoma.[28,29] The PD-L1 positivity rate in the screened patients was 41%, virtually identical to the rate in GEJ/gastric adenocarcinoma. This was, again, a heavily pretreated group, with 87% of patients receiving ≥2 prior therapies. Seven of 23 patients (30%) had a PR, with 5 of the PRs ongoing at the time of data analysis. The median duration of response was 40.0 weeks. Six- and 12-month PFS rates were 30.4% and 21.7%, respectively.

Nivolumab has also shown promising activity in EGC. Recently, data presented in abstract form suggest similar activity to that of pembrolizumab.[30] Fifty-nine patients with unselected GEJ/gastric adenocarcinoma were treated in a phase I/II study. Eighty-three percent of patients received ≥2 prior therapies. The relative risk was 14%, with a median time to response of 1.6 months and duration of response of 7.1 months in the responders. Median OS was 6.8 months for the entire group, and the 12-month survival rate was 36%. PD-L1 positivity was assessed using a cutoff of ≥1% for IHC positivity. The relative response rates in patients with PD-L1–positive and PD-L1–negative tumors were 27% and 12%, respectively.

Similar activity was also noted for nivolumab in a Japanese study of 64 patients with esophageal SCC who received a median of 3 prior therapies.[31] PD-L1 positivity was not required nor was it reported in the presented data. The response rate was 17.2%, including a complete response in 1 patient. Median PFS was 1.5 months and median OS was 10.8 months.

In addition, anti–PD-L1 antibodies also seem to be active. Avelumab produced a response rate of 15% in 20 patients who received it as second-line therapy (although

Table 2
Results of antiprogrammed death or anti-PD-ligand 1 antibody studies in esophagogastric cancer

Treatment	Location/Histology	No. of Patients	Response Rate, %	PFS		OS		Reference
				Median	Overall	Median	Overall	
Pembrolizumab (anti–PD-1)	GEJ/G adenoCA (PD-L1 +ve only)	39	22	1.9 mo	NS	11.4 mo	6-mo 66% 12-mo 42%	KEYNOTE-012, Muro et al,[27] 2016
	E adenoCA	23	30	NS	6-mo 30% 12-mo 22%	NS	NS	KEYNOTE-028, Doi et al,[28] 2015; Doi et al,[29] 2016
	adenoCA	5	40					
	SCC (PD-L1 +ve only)	17	27					
Nivolumab (anti–PD-1)	E/GEJ/G adenoCA	59	14	NS	NS	5.0 mo	6-mo 49% 12-mo 36%	Checkmate-032, Le et al,[30] 2016
	PD-L1 +ve		27					
	PD-L1 −ve		12					
	E SCC	64	17.2	1.51 mo	NS	10.8 mo	NS	Kojima et al,[31] 2016
Nivolumab 3 mg/kg q3 wk + Ipilimumab 1 mg/kg q3 wk	GEJ/G adenoCA	52	10	1.58 mo	6-mo 9% 12-mo N/A	4.8 mo	6-mo 43% 12-mo N/A	Checkmate-032, Janjigian et al,[35] 2016
	PD-L1 +ve		27					
	PD-L1 −ve		0					
Nivolumab 1 mg/kg q3 wk + Ipilimumab 3 mg/kg q3 wk	GEJ/G adenoCA	49	26	1.45 mo	6-mo 24% 12-mo 18%	6.9 mo	6-mo 54% 12-mo 34%	
	PD-L1 +ve		44					
	PD-L1 −ve		21					

Drug	Phenotype	n		PFS	OS			Reference
Avelumab (anti-PD-L1)	GEJ/G adenoCA (2nd-line)	20	15	11.6 wk	3-mo 39%, 6-mo 19%	NS	NS	JAVELIN, Chung et al,[32] 2016
	PD-L1 +ve		20	36 wk	3-mo 60%			
	PD-L1 −ve		0	11.6 wk	3-mo 29%			
	GEJ/G adenoCA (Maintenance)	55	7	14.1 wk	3-mo 54%, 6-mo 34%	NS	NS	
	PD-L1 +ve		6.7	17.6 wk	3-mo 59%			
	PD-L1 −ve		3.6	11.6 wk	3-mo 44%			
Durvalumab (MEDI4736) (anti-PD-L1)	GEJ/G adenoCA	16	25	NS	NS	NS	NS	Segal et al,[33] 2014
Atezolizumab (MPDL3280A) (anti-PD-L1)	G adenoCA	1	100	NS	NS	NS	NS	Herbst et al,[34] 2013

Abbreviations: adenoCA, adenocarcinoma; E, esophageal; G, gastric; NS, not stated.

20% of patients had actually received ≥2 prior therapies).[32] The disease control rate (PR and SD rate) was 50%. Forty-two percent of the 12 tumors in this group that were tested were PD-L1 positive by IHC, using a cutoff of ≥1%. The response rate was 20% versus 0% in the PD-L1–positive versus PD-L1–negative tumors. The median PFS was 36.0 weeks versus 11.6 weeks for PD-L1–positive versus PD-L1–negative tumors.

This study also treated another 55 patients with maintenance avelumab after they achieved a PR/SD on first-line chemotherapy. Four responses were seen (7%), including 1 complete response. Of the 43 patients who had tumor for PD-L1 testing, the response rates were 6.7% versus 3.6% for PD-L1–positive and PD-L1–negative tumors, respectively. Median PFS for the PD-L1–positive versus PD-L1–negative tumors was 17.6 versus 11.6 weeks, respectively.

Finally, abstract presentations also show responses for the PD-L1 antibody MEDI4736 (now called *durvalumab*) in 16 patients with EGC, in which 4 patients had a PR.[33] A PR in 1 gastric cancer patient treated with the anti–PD-L1 antibody, MPDL3280A (now called *atezolizumab*), has also been reported.[34]

The only data for combination immune checkpoint blockade in EGC comes from the Checkmate-032 study, which was recently presented in abstract form.[35] In addition to the 59 patients treated with nivolumab alone (and discussed above), an additional 2 cohorts received different doses of nivolumab together with ipilimumab. Baseline characteristics in these other 2 groups were similar to the nivolumab-only arm. The highest response rate was reported for patients who received nivolumab 3 mg/kg and ipilimumab 1 mg/kg every 3 weeks for 4 cycles (followed by nivolumab 3 mg/kg every 2 weeks), although survival data in these small groups of patients seemed comparable. Grade ≥3 toxicities were also highest in this group (35% vs 5% in the nivolumab arm and 15% in the other arm of ipilimumab 1 mg/kg and nivolumab 3 mg/kg). Nevertheless, this dose has been selected as the basis for a proposed phase III study (see later discussion).

FUTURE DIRECTIONS

Based on the results above, numerous phase III studies are ongoing or planned, as noted in Table 3. Many of these studies are testing similar concepts in the first-, second- and third-line settings for advanced EGC.

Of note, the KEYNOTE-059 study, which has completed accrual, included a first-line arm in which patients received pembrolizumab in combination with 5-fluorouracil/cisplatin. Although efficacy data have not been presented, data presented in abstract form suggested an acceptable toxicity profile for this combination.[36] This combination is being further tested in the phase III first-line KEYNOTE-062 study. The results of both of these studies will therefore determine if there is a benefit for combination immune checkpoint blockade and chemotherapy in EGC.

Also of interest is the Checkmate-577 study, which is evaluating the benefit of adjuvant nivolumab versus placebo in patients with locally advanced esophageal/GEJ tumors (both adenocarcinomas and SCC), who have undergone chemoradiation and surgery but are found to have persistent disease (ypT1-4Nany or ypTanyN+ tumor).

Finally, a phase Ib/II study is evaluating combination immune checkpoint blockade, this time with a PD-L1 inhibitor (durvalumab) and an anti–CTLA-4 antibody (tremelimumab).

These studies represent only a small fraction of ongoing or planned phase I/II studies that will combine immune checkpoint inhibitors with other immunotherapy drugs, chemotherapy, targeted therapies, or locoregional approaches (such as radiation or ablative procedures). Many of these studies are specifically enrolling EGC patients but also include studies that are enrolling EGC patients in dose-expansion cohorts.

Table 3
Ongoing phase II/III studies of immune checkpoint inhibitors in esophagogastric cancer

Drug	Treatment	Setting	Status	Study Id
Pembrolizumab	Pembrolizumab + 5-FU/cisplatin Pembrolizumab Pembrolizumab	1st-line, PD-L1 +ve, Her2 −ve GEJ/G adenoCA ≥3rd-line, PD-L1 +ve or −ve, Her2 +ve allowed if prior trastuzumab GEJ/G adenoCA	Completed	KEYNOTE-059 (NCT02335411)
	Pembrolizumab vs paclitaxel	2nd-line, PD-L1 +ve, Her2 +ve allowed if prior trastuzumab GEJ/G adenoCA	Recruiting	KEYNOTE-061 (NCT02370498)
	Pembrolizumab vs 5-FU/cisplatin vs pembrolizumab/5-FU/cisplatin	1st-line, Her2 −ve, PD-L1 +ve GEJ/G adenoCA	Recruiting	KEYNOTE-062 (NCT02494583)
	Pembrolizumab vs irinotecan or taxane	2nd-line, PD-L1 not assessed, E/GEJ SCC or adenoCA	Recruiting	KEYNOTE-181 (NCT02564263)
	Pembrolizumab	3rd-line, PD-L1 not assessed, E/GEJ SCC or adenoCA	Recruiting	KEYNOTE-182 (NCT02559687)
Nivolumab	Ipilimumab 3 mg/kg/nivolumab 1 mg/kg vs chemotherapy	1st-line, PD-L1 not assessed, Her2 −ve, GEJ/G adenoCA	Planned	Checkmate-649 (NCT02872116)
	Nivolumab vs taxane	2nd-line, PD-L1 not assessed, E/GEJ adenoCA or SCC	Ongoing	NCT02569242
	Nivolumab vs placebo	Adjuvant, PD-L1 not assessed, R0 resection, $ypT_{any}N_{any}$ tumor E/GEJ adenoCA or SCC	Recruiting	Checkmate-577 (NCT02743494)
Avelumab	Avelumab vs fluoropyrimidine/oxaliplatin	1st-line, maintenance, PD-L1 not assessed, GEJ/G adenoCA	Recruiting	JAVELIN-100 (NCT02625610)
	Avelumab vs BSC (includes paclitaxel or irinotecan)	3rd-line, PD-L1 not assessed, GEJ/G adenoCA	Recruiting	JAVELIN-300 (NCT02625623)
Durvalumab (MEDI4736)	Durvalumab vs tremelimumab vs durvalumab/tremelimumab Durvalumab/tremelimumab	2nd-line, PD-L1 not assessed, Her2 −ve, GEJ/G adenoCA 3rd-line, PD-L1 not assessed, Her2 −ve, GEJ/G adenoCA	Recruiting	(NCT02340975)

Abbreviations: 5-FU, 5-fluorouracil; adenoCA, adenocarcinoma; BSC, best supportive care; E, esophageal; G, gastric; N/A, not available.

BIOMARKERS OF RESPONSE

The results of the studies discussed above uniformly suggest that less than 25% of patients who receive immune checkpoint inhibitors derive significant benefit. Most studies report a median PFS of less than 2 months, even in the setting of encouraging OS, suggesting that most patients are rapidly progressing on these treatments and that most of the OS benefit may be experienced by the small group who do respond or have disease stabilization. Therefore, the identification of biomarkers to select patients most likely to benefit from these expensive and potentially toxic agents is a priority.

At this time, PD-L1 status by IHC is a leading contender as a biomarker. Although PD-L1–positive tumors seem more likely to respond to treatment with anti–PD-1 and anti–PD-L1 antibodies, many of the studies above suggest the possibility of response and disease control even for patients with PD-L1 negative tumors. Therefore, many ongoing and phase III studies are enrolling patients irrespective of the tumor PD-L1 status.

The situation is further complicated by the fact that there are currently several antibodies available for PD-L1 testing. These antibodies have not been compared against each other to determine if PD-L1 positivity by one test is comparable to the results of another. In fact, there can be issues with reproducibility even using experimental and clinical versions of the same assay[27] and intratumoral and intertumoral heterogeneity and dynamic temporal variability.

Therefore, another possibility is to identify a genetic signature within the tumor and peritumoral tissue that may correlate with an increased chance of benefit from immune checkpoint inhibitors. In the KEYNOTE-012 study with pembrolizumab, a 6-gene signature of interferon-γ genes (CXCL9, CXCL10, IDO1, IFNG, HLA-DRA, and STAT1) was assessed using gene expression profiling of RNA isolated from tumor samples to generate a composite score, which was the average of the normalized values of the 6 genes.[27] There was a trend between a higher interferon-γ signature score and response, but it did not achieve statistical significance ($P = .070$), possibly a reflection of the small numbers involved (only 30 tumor samples could be tested). One benefit of this gene signature is that it may be more reproducible and robust than PD-L1 testing, and efforts continue to evaluate it in EGC and other cancers.

Finally, there are also ongoing efforts to correlate response and benefit on these studies with the 4 subtypes of gastric cancer, identified by the Cancer Genome Atlas (TCGA) as Epstein-Barr virus (EBV) positive, microsatellite unstable (MSI), genomically stable, and chromosomal instability.[37] Of these subtypes, both the EBV and MSI groups may be more responsive to immune checkpoint inhibition. The EBV subtype accounted for 9% of the tumors in the TCGA analysis and are associated with CD274 and PDCD1LG2 amplifications, which encode for the PD-L1 and PD-L2 proteins.

The MSI subgroup accounts for 22% of gastric cancer patients. It is characterized by MLH1 promoter hypermethylation, which is associated with an elevated mutation rate. A seminal report by Alexandrov and colleagues[38] showed that the prevalence of somatic mutations varies widely among different cancers (Fig. 2). The mutation rate is highest in cancers that respond strongly to immune checkpoint inhibition (such as melanoma or bladder cancer), whereas EGC has mutation rates that are less than these cancers but still significantly higher than many other malignancies. Proof-of-principle for this concept comes from activity of pembrolizumab only in MSI-high colorectal cancer.[39] Recent data also suggest significant activity in other mismatch repair-deficient gastrointestinal cancers, including gastric cancer.[40]

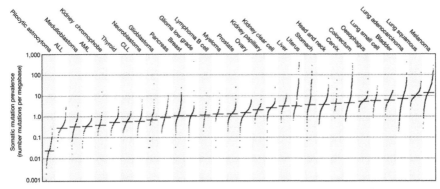

Fig. 2. The prevalence of somatic mutations across human cancer types. Every dot represents a sample, whereas the red horizontal lines are the median numbers of mutations in the respective cancer types. The vertical axis (log scaled) shows the number of mutations per megabase, whereas the different cancer types are ordered on the horizontal axis based on their median numbers of somatic mutations. (*From* Alexandrov LB, Nik-Zainal S, Wedge DC, et al. Signatures of mutational processes in human cancer. Nature 2013;500:415; with permission.)

Recapitulation of the TCGA subtypes in a clinical context will be difficult, given that the TCGA analyses were multiplex research tests that required fresh-frozen tissue. However, next-generation sequencing platforms that are now performed semiroutinely in standard clinical care and the IHC characterization of DNA mismatch repair protein status of tumor tissue may permit for the proactive identification of patients more likely to respond to immune checkpoint blockade or to correlate responses with these genetic profiles.

SUMMARY

The evaluation of immune checkpoint inhibitors in solid tumors in general but also in EGC has occurred at a breathtaking pace. The phase Ib studies that generated significant interest a little more than a year ago have now been overtaken by nearly completed phase III studies.

The results of these phase III studies are, of course, awaited with eager anticipation, and it is hoped that they will establish a new treatment paradigm in EGC, just as these drugs have transformed the treatment of several other cancers. If there is proven benefit for an immune checkpoint inhibitor in EGC, ongoing correlative efforts and the next generation of studies will better delineate the small but significant subpopulation that is most likely to benefit. These efforts will also try to further increase the proportion of patients who will derive benefit by evaluating combinatorial strategies.

In this regard, the many other potential targets noted in Fig. 1 for antagonist or agonist strategies (many of which are already in phase I/II testing), which can be combined with the current stable of immune checkpoint inhibitors, are a source of promise and a reminder of the significant work that remains to improve outcomes in this difficult disease.

REFERENCES

1. Ku GY, Ilson DH. Management of gastric cancer. Curr Opin Gastroenterol 2014; 30:596–602.
2. Bang YJ, Van Cutsem E, Feyereislova A, et al. Trastuzumab in combination with chemotherapy versus chemotherapy alone for treatment of HER2-positive

advanced gastric or gastro-oesophageal junction cancer (ToGA): a phase 3, open-label, randomised controlled trial. Lancet 2010;376:687–97.

3. Fuchs CS, Tomasek J, Yong CJ, et al. Ramucirumab monotherapy for previously treated advanced gastric or gastro-oesophageal junction adenocarcinoma (RE-GARD): an international, randomised, multicentre, placebo-controlled, phase 3 trial. Lancet 2014;383:31–9.

4. Wilke H, Muro K, Van Cutsem E, et al. Ramucirumab plus paclitaxel versus placebo plus paclitaxel in patients with previously treated advanced gastric or gastro-oesophageal junction adenocarcinoma (RAINBOW): a double-blind, randomised phase 3 trial. Lancet Oncol 2014;15:1224–35.

5. Hodi FS, O'Day SJ, McDermott DF, et al. Improved survival with ipilimumab in patients with metastatic melanoma. N Engl J Med 2010;363:711–23.

6. Robert C, Thomas L, Bondarenko I, et al. Ipilimumab plus dacarbazine for previously untreated metastatic melanoma. N Engl J Med 2011;364:2517–26.

7. Kuby J. Overview of the immune system. In: Kuby J, editor. Immunology. New York: W.H. Freeman; 1992. p. 1–17.

8. Dunn GP, Old LJ, Schreiber RD. The three Es of cancer immunoediting. Annu Rev Immunol 2004;22:329–60.

9. WB C. The treatment of malignant tumors by repeated inoculations of erysipelas: with a report of ten original cases. Am J Med Sci 1893;105:487–510.

10. Karbach J, Neumann A, Brand K, et al. Phase I clinical trial of mixed bacterial vaccine (Coley's toxins) in patients with NY-ESO-1 expressing cancers: immunological effects and clinical activity. Clin Cancer Res 2012;18:5449–59.

11. Old LJ. Cancer vaccines 2003: opening address. Cancer Immun 2003;3(Suppl 2):1.

12. Kantoff PW, Higano CS, Shore ND, et al. Sipuleucel-T immunotherapy for castration-resistant prostate cancer. N Engl J Med 2010;363:411–22.

13. Melero I, Gaudernack G, Gerritsen W, et al. Therapeutic vaccines for cancer: an overview of clinical trials. Nat Rev Clin Oncol 2014;11:509–24.

14. Pardoll DM. The blockade of immune checkpoints in cancer immunotherapy. Nat Rev Cancer 2012;12:252–64.

15. Krummel MF, Allison JP. CD28 and CTLA-4 have opposing effects on the response of T cells to stimulation. J Exp Med 1995;182:459–65.

16. Freeman GJ, Long AJ, Iwai Y, et al. Engagement of the PD-1 immunoinhibitory receptor by a novel B7 family member leads to negative regulation of lymphocyte activation. J Exp Med 2000;192:1027–34.

17. Zou W, Chen L. Inhibitory B7-family molecules in the tumour microenvironment. Nat Rev Immunol 2008;8:467–77.

18. Sharma P, Allison JP. The future of immune checkpoint therapy. Science 2015; 348:56–61.

19. Horvat TZ, Adel NG, Dang TO, et al. Immune-related adverse events, need for systemic immunosuppression, and effects on survival and time to treatment failure in patients with melanoma treated with ipilimumab at Memorial Sloan Kettering Cancer Center. J Clin Oncol 2015;33:3193–8.

20. Ralph C, Elkord E, Burt DJ, et al. Modulation of lymphocyte regulation for cancer therapy: a phase II trial of tremelimumab in advanced gastric and esophageal adenocarcinoma. Clin Cancer Res 2010;16:1662–72.

21. Moehler M, Cho J, Kim Y, et al. A randomized, open-label, two-arm phase II trial comparing the efficacy of sequential ipilimumab (ipi) versus best supportive care (BSC) following first-line (1L) chemotherapy in patients with unresectable, locally

advanced/metastatic (A/M) gastric or gastro-esophageal junction (G/GEJ) cancer [abstract]. J Clin Oncol 2016;34:4011.

22. Ribas A, Puzanov I, Dummer R, et al. Pembrolizumab versus investigator-choice chemotherapy for ipilimumab-refractory melanoma (KEYNOTE-002): a randomised, controlled, phase 2 trial. Lancet Oncol 2015;16:908–18.

23. Robert C, Schachter J, Long GV, et al. Pembrolizumab versus Ipilimumab in Advanced Melanoma. N Engl J Med 2015;372:2521–32.

24. Robert C, Long GV, Brady B, et al. Nivolumab in previously untreated melanoma without BRAF mutation. N Engl J Med 2015;372:320–30.

25. Larkin J, Chiarion-Sileni V, Gonzalez R, et al. Combined Nivolumab and Ipilimumab or Monotherapy in Untreated Melanoma. N Engl J Med 2015;373:23–34.

26. Rosenberg JE, Hoffman-Censits J, Powles T, et al. Atezolizumab in patients with locally advanced and metastatic urothelial carcinoma who have progressed following treatment with platinum-based chemotherapy: a single-arm, multicentre, phase 2 trial. Lancet 2016;387:1909–20.

27. Muro K, Chung HC, Shankaran V, et al. Pembrolizumab for patients with PD-L1-positive advanced gastric cancer (KEYNOTE-012): a multicentre, open-label, phase 1b trial. Lancet Oncol 2016;17:717–26.

28. Doi T, Piha-Paul S, Jalal S, et al. Pembrolizumab (MK-3475) for patients (pts) with advanced esophageal carcinoma: Preliminary results from KEYNOTE-028 [abstract]. J Clin Oncol 2015;33:4010.

29. Doi T, Piha-Paul S, Jalal S, et al. Updated results for the advanced esophageal carcinoma cohort of the phase Ib KEYNOTE-028 study of pembrolizumab (MK-3475) [abstract]. J Clin Oncol 2016;34:7.

30. Le D, Bendell J, Calvo E, et al. Safety and activity of nivolumab monotherapy in advanced and metastatic (A/M) gastric or gastroesophageal junction cancer (GC/GEC): results from the CheckMate-032 study [abstract]. J Clin Oncol 2016;34:6.

31. Kojima T, Hara H, Yamaguchi K, et al. Phase II study of nivolumab (ONO-4538/BMS-936558) in patients with esophageal cancer: preliminary report of overall survival [abstract]. J Clin Oncol 2016;34:TPS175.

32. Chung H, Arkenau H-T, Wyrwicz L, et al. Safety, PD-L1 expression, and clinical activity of avelumab (MSB0010718C), an anti-PD-L1 antibody, in patients with advanced gastric or gastroesophageal junction cancer [abstract]. J Clin Oncol 2016;34:167.

33. Segal N, Hamid O, Hwu W, et al. 1058PD - A phase I multi-arm dose-expansion study of the anti-programmed cell death-ligand-1 (PD-L1) antibody MEDI4736: preliminary data, ESMO [abstract]. Ann Oncol 2014;25:iv361–72.

34. Herbst R, Gordon M, Fine G, et al. A study of MPDL3280A, an engineered PD-L1 antibody in patients with locally advanced or metastatic tumors [abstract]. J Clin Oncol 2013;31:3000.

35. Janjigian Y, Bendell J, Calvo E, et al. CheckMate-032: phase I/II, open-label study of safety and activity of nivolumab (nivo) alone or with ipilimumab (ipi) in advanced and metastatic (A/M) gastric cancer (GC) [abstract]. J Clin Oncol 2016;34:4010.

36. Fuchs C, Ohtsu A, Tabernero J, et al. Pembrolizumab (MK-3475) plus 5-fluorouracil (5-FU) and cisplatin for first-line treatment of advanced gastric cancer: preliminary safety data from KEYNOTE-059 [abstract]. J Clin Oncol 2016;34:161.

37. Cancer Genome Atlas Research Network. Comprehensive molecular characterization of gastric adenocarcinoma. Nature 2014;513:202–9.

38. Alexandrov LB, Nik-Zainal S, Wedge DC, et al. Signatures of mutational processes in human cancer. Nature 2013;500(7463):415–21.
39. Le DT, Uram JN, Wang H, et al. PD-1 blockade in tumors with mismatch-repair deficiency. N Engl J Med 2015;372:2509–20.
40. Le D, Uram J, Wang H, et al. PD-1 blockade in mismatch repair deficient non-colorectal gastrointestinal cancers [abstract]. J Clin Oncol 2016;34:195.

Novel Targeted Therapies for Esophagogastric Cancer

Steven B. Maron, MD, Daniel V.T. Catenacci, MD*

KEYWORDS

- Gastric cancer • Esophagogastric junction cancer
- Gastroesophageal adenocarcinoma • HER2 • VEGFR2 • EGFR • MET • FGFR2

KEY POINTS

- Anti-human epidermal growth factor receptor 2 (HER2) trastuzumab therapy is standard for HER2 amplified/overexpressed gastroesophageal adenocarcinoma, whereas second/later lines of anti-HER2–directed therapy have not shown definitive benefit to date.
- Anti–vascular endothelial growth factor receptor 2 (VEGFR2) ramucirumab modestly improves survival as monotherapy and in combination with paclitaxel in second-line treatment of patients with gastroesophageal adenocarcinoma.
- Anti–epidermal growth factor receptor (EFGR) therapy has not shown benefit in unselected gastroesophageal patients in any line of therapy, although gene amplification/overexpression warrants further investigation.
- Anti-MET therapy has not shown benefit in overexpressing gastroesophageal patients in any line of therapy, although gene amplification/overexpression may merit further investigation.
- Other promising predictive biomarkers and targeted therapies, including fibroblast growth factor type 2 and claudin 18.2, require further investigation in larger trials to confirm therapeutic benefits for patients with gastroesophageal adenocarcinoma.

BACKGROUND

Distal gastric adenocarcinoma (GC) incidence ranks fifth globally and third for cancer-related mortality of all malignancies.[1–3] Approximately 25,000 new GC cases and 11,000 deaths occurred in the United States in 2015.[4] In contrast,

Disclosure: Dr D.V.T. Catenacci has received research funding from Genentech/Roche, Amgen, OncoplexDx/Nantomics and honoraria from Genentech/Roche, Amgen, Eli Lilly, Five Prime, OncoplexDx/Nantomics, Guardant Health, Foundation Medicine. Dr S.B. Maron has nothing to disclose.
Funding: NIH (CA178203-01A1).
Section of Hematology/Oncology, University of Chicago Comprehensive Cancer Center, 900 E 57th St, Suite 7128, Chicago, IL 60637, USA
* Corresponding author.
E-mail address: dcatenac@medicine.bsd.uchicago.edu

esophagogastric junction adenocarcinoma (EGJ), is increasing in incidence. For both (gastroesophageal cancer [GEC]), most patients present with metastatic disease, or locally advanced disease with a high risk of recurrence despite aggressive perioperative therapy. In the metastatic setting, median overall survival (OS) remains approximately 11 months with optimal palliative chemotherapy in *ERRB2*-nonamplified patients. Over the past decade, molecular subtyping of GEC has highlighted the interpatient heterogeneity of GEC and uncovered potentially actionable molecular pathways.[5] Routine next-generation sequencing identified that at least 37% of patients with GC harbor genetic alterations in receptor tyrosine kinases (RTKs), including *ERBB2, MET, EGFR, KRAS*, and *FGFR2*.[6–8] These genomic events, as well as recently derived key subsets of the disease, namely microsatellite instability-high (MSI-high), Epstein-Barr virus (EBV) associated, chromosomal instability (CIN), and genomically stable (GS), provide more molecularly targeted therapeutic possibilities.[9]

Erb-B2 Receptor Tyrosine Kinase 2

Erb-B2 receptor tyrosine kinase 2 (Erb-B2), or HER2, is a transmembrane RTK within the epidermal growth factor receptor (EGFR) family, encoded at chromosome 17q21. HER2 regulates proliferation, adhesion, differentiation, and migration via activation of the Ras and Mitogen-activated protein kinases (RAS-MAPK) and phosphatidylinositol-3-kinase and AKT (PI3K-AKT) pathways. HER2 lacks an exogenous ligand and is transactivated via heterodimerization with other HER family members, leading to downstream kinase activation. Significant and therapeutically relevant overexpression results predominantly from gene amplification. HER2 IHC expression localizes to the cell membrane in well-differentiated adenocarcinoma and to the cytoplasm in poorly differentiated adenocarcinomas, which may affect treatment response.[10] HER2-expressing tumors are more common with EGJ (15%–20%) compared with distal GC (10%–15%), and the prognostic impact of HER2 expression remains controversial.[11–16]

Effective targeting of HER2 in GEC was initially shown using trastuzumab, a humanized monoclonal anti-HER2 antibody against the HER2 ectodomain (Table 1). The phase III ToGA trial evaluated first-line fluoropyrimidine/cisplatin chemotherapy doublet with or without trastuzumab in patients with HER-2 over-expressing (any IHC 3+ or fluorescence in-situ hybridization [FISH] HER2/CEP17 ratio $\geq$2) unresectable or metastatic GEC. Patients receiving trastuzumab survived a median of 13.8 months versus 11.1 months with chemotherapy alone, and response rates were 47% and 35% respectively in the intention-to-treat (ITT) population. In a subset analysis, median survival was 16 versus 11.8 months in the combined IHC2+/FISH+ and IHC3+ groups, accounting for 77% of the patients. This trial therefore led to the approval of trastuzumab in HER2 overexpressing GEC for the IHC2+/FISH+ and IHC3+ subsets of the trial.[16,17]

Although HER-2 overexpression/*ERBB2* amplification predicts benefit from the anti-HER2 antibody trastuzumab in the first-line setting,[16] the definition of positivity and trial inclusion criteria within trials has evolved over time. Current clinical diagnostic testing requires evaluation by a combination of IHC (membranous reactivity in $\geq$10% of cancer cells in a surgical specimen or a cluster of at least 5 cells in a biopsy specimen), and FISH (with HER2/CEP17 ratio $\geq$2). IHC 0/1 is considered negative, and IHC3+ is considered positive, whereas IHC2+ requires reflex FISH assessment. Higher throughput assays, including mass spectrometry and next-generation sequencing, have emerged with potential to refine diagnostic accuracy as well as possessing multiplexing capability to assess for other relevant aberrations.[5,18,19] Assessment of ERBB2 amplification by cell-free DNA is also emerging as a potential noninvasive strategy for serial assessment of HER2 status that can monitor intrapatient tumoral evolution.[19–23]

Table 1
Phase III trials evaluating HER2-targeted therapies

Line	Trial	N	Treatment	Primary End Point (Met?)	mOS (mo)	HR	mPFS (mo)	HR	RR (%)
1L	Bang et al,[16] 2010 ToGA	584	Cis/FP + placebo Cis/FP + trastuzumab	OS (Yes)	11.1 13.8	0.74 P<.0046	5.5 6.7	0.71 P<.001	35 47
1L	Hecht et al,[24] 2016 LOGiC	545 (487)	Cis/FP + placebo Cis/FP + lapatinib	OS (No)	10.5 12.2	0.91 P = NS	5.4 6	0.82 P = .03	39 53
2L	Satoh et al,[29] 2014 TyTAN	261	Paclitaxel + placebo Paclitaxel + lapatinib	OS (No)	8.9 11	0.84 P = NS	4.4 5.5	0.84 P<.001	9 27
2L	Kang et al,[30] 2016 GATSBY	345 (1:2)	Paclitaxel (38%)/Doc (62%) T-DM1	OS (No)	8.6 7.9	1.15 P = NS	2.9 2.7	1.13 P = NS	20 21

Abbreviations: Cis, cisplatin; Doc, docetaxel; FP, fluoropyrimidine; HR, hazard ratio; mOS, mean overall survival; mPFS, mean progression-free survival; NS, not significant; RR, response rate; T-DM1, trastuzumab emtansine.

Lapatinib, a selective intracellular tyrosine kinase inhibitor (TKI) of ErbB1 and ErbB2, was also studied in first-line and second-line GEC (see Table 1). The phase III TRIO-013/LOGiC trial randomized 545 untreated patients with HER2-positive (HER2/CEP17 ratio ≥2 by FISH or IHC 3+ if FISH not available) GEC to receive capecitabine and oxaliplatin in addition to either lapatinib or placebo. Lapatinib increased objective response from 39% to 53%, and modestly increased median progression-free survival (PFS) from 5.4 to 6 months, but failed to confer an OS benefit in the ITT population.[24] Younger and Asian patients seemed to derive the most benefit in subset analyses. The absolute level of amplification positively correlated with outcome,[25] as previously described,[26,27] signifying heterogeneity of benefit within the current HER2-positive classification. Recently, the degree of amplification has been shown to correlate closely with absolute protein expression level, which is associated with clinical benefit.[18,28] Inter-trial variation in absolute amplification/expression as well as lack of antibody-dependent cell-mediated cytotoxicity (ADCC) with lapatinib compared with trastuzumab, serve as two of the many potential explanations when contrasting outcomes of ToGA and LOGiC. In the second line, the phase III Asian TyTAN trial enrolled patients with GEC regardless of HER2 expression (FISH ratios ≥2 were eligible), and 31% of patients enrolled were FISH+ and IHC 0/1+.[29] Patients received paclitaxel alone or in combination with lapatinib. Despite response rates of 27% versus 9%, no significant PFS or OS benefit was shown in the ITT population. Of note, when evaluating only those patients with 3+ HER2 expression by IHC, median survival improved from 7.6 to 14 months in this subgroup ($P = .0176$), and PFS 4.2 to 5.6 months ($P = .0101$). This finding highlights the need to improve patient selection for targeted therapies.

Trastuzumab emtansine (T-DM1), an antibody-drug conjugate that is approved in HER2-positive metastatic breast cancer, was studied in the second-line GATSBY trial (see Table 1), but failed to demonstrate a response or survival benefit versus paclitaxel monotherapy.[30] Possible explanations for this negative trial include intrapatient tumor heterogeneity, recognized to be more frequent in GEC than observed in breast cancer, with HER2-negative clones not controlled by targeted cytotoxic therapy. Another possible explanation is the recent appreciation of conversion of HER2 status after first-line therapy, making archived samples, as used in GATSBY (and TyTAN), inadequate for selecting appropriate HER2+ patients in the second line.[19,21–23]

In addition, although trastuzumab binds domain IV of HER2, pertuzumab binds domain II and thereby prevents dimerization. The CLEOPATRA trial revealed PFS and OS benefits with the addition of pertuzumab to trastuzumab and chemotherapy in breast cancer,[31] and initial results from the JACOB trial evaluating pertuzumab in combination with trastuzumab and chemotherapy are eagerly awaited.

Thus, to date, no standard anti-HER2–directed approaches are recognized in trastuzumab-refractory HER2+ GEC. However, standard chemotherapy with irinotecan-based or taxane-based regimens are recommended. Notably, although second-line ramucirumab trials, discussed later, included HER2-positive and trastuzumab-treated patients, this accounted for only ~6% of patients enrolled in RAINBOW and less than 1% of REGARD.[32,33] Other strategies under evaluation in the second and later lines include novel TKIs like apatinib,[34] trastuzumab beyond progression,[21,23] novel HER2 antibodies,[35] and combination therapy with immune checkpoint inhibitors (see Table 5).[36]

Vascular Endothelial Growth Factor

Vascular endothelial growth factor (VEGF) induces angiogenesis and neovascularization. Overexpression is found in up to 58% of patients with resected gastric cancer ,[37] and 7% of The Cancer Genome Atlas (TCGA) patients with gastric cancer have *VEGF-A* gene amplification.[9] Ramucirumab, a human immunoglobulin G1 (IgG1) monoclonal antibody that directly binds to VEGFR2 and inhibits VEGF ligand binding, was evaluated in the second-line setting in the phase III REGARD trial (Table 2).[33] Compared with supportive care, ramucirumab demonstrated an OS of 5.2 versus 3.8 months (*P* = .047), despite a response rate of only 3% (the same as the placebo control).[33] The phase III RAINBOW trial subsequently compared paclitaxel with or without ramucirumab in the second-line setting (see Table 2). Patients had a significant OS benefit of 9.6 versus 7.4 months (*P* = .017) as well as statistically significant PFS and objective response rate (ORR) benefits.[32] In the third-line setting, apatinib, a multi-TKI, including VEGF receptor (VEGFR) kinases, showed an absolute 0.8-month PFS advantage (2.6 vs 1.8 months) as well as a nearly 2-month OS benefit compared with placebo in a Chinese population.[38]

However, evaluation of antiangiogenesis in the first-line setting of GEC has been disappointing to date. The AVAGAST trial evaluated chemotherapy (cisplatin and capecitabine) with or without bevacizumab, a humanized IgG1 VEGF-A monoclonal antibody. Despite PFS (6.7 vs 5.3 months; *P* = .0037) and ORR (46% vs 37.4%; *P* = .0315) benefits, the improved median OS of 12.1 over 10.1 months observed in the control was not statistically significant.[39] An Asian trial, AVATAR, confirmed these negative findings.[40] A phase II trial of first-line ziv-aflibercept with FOLFOX recently did not meet its primary end point of 6-month PFS compared with FOLFOX alone.[41] In addition, a phase II trial in first-line GEC comparing FOLFOX with or without ramucirumab was negative.[42] Despite this, the phase III RAINFALL trial is currently evaluating first-line ramucirumab/placebo in combination with capecitabine and cisplatin in metastatic GEC, with results eagerly awaited (NCT02314117).

Predictive biomarkers of response to antiangiogenesis, to be incorporated into routine practice, have remained elusive.[43] The AVAGAST trial suggested that patients with high plasma VEGF-A levels had increased OS compared with those expressing low VEGF-A levels,[12] and hypertension as a biomarker has been noted.[41] Further biomarker development may help identify a subset of patients who derive the most benefit from targeting this axis. However, biomarkers of response may remain undefined, potentially because of a marginal benefit realized by most patients.

Epidermal Growth Factor Receptor

EGFR, or Erb-B1 is a transmembrane receptor and a well-recognized mediator of oncogenic phenotype that is overexpressed in approximately 30% of GEC.[44,45] EGFR-overexpressing tumors are associated with higher stage, more poorly differentiated histology, increased vascular invasion, and potentially shorter survival.[14,46] *EGFR* amplification is found in only ~5% of patients.[9,47,48]

EGFR-directed therapies evaluated in GEC include cetuximab and panitumumab, which are monoclonal antibodies that antagonize the extracellular binding domain. Preclinical data also suggested that cetuximab, a recombinant human-murine chimeric monoclonal antibody of a murine Fv region and a human IgG1 heavy and k light chain Fc region, induces ADCC.[49] Small-molecule TKIs, such as gefitinib, erlotinib, lapatinib, and afatinib, competitively bind intracellularly to the tyrosine kinase domain. Early phase II trials combining cetuximab, panitumumab, or erlotinib with cytotoxic chemotherapy in GEC reported first-line therapy response rates ranging from 41% to 65%.[50–53] Second-line phase II evaluation of gefitinib or erlotinib monotherapy led to more modest responses of ~9% to 11%, and responses seemed limited to proximal EGJ cancers rather than distal GC.[54,55]

Table 2
Phase II/III trials of vascular endothelial growth factor–targeted therapies in gastroesophageal cancer

Line	Trial	N	Treatment	Primary End Point (Met?)	mOS (mo)	HR	mPFS (mo)	HR	RR (%)
2L	Fuchs et al,[33] 2014 REGARD	335	Placebo / Ram	OS	3.5 / 5.2	0.78 P = .047	1.3 / 2.1	0.48	3 / 3
2L	Wilke et al,[32] 2014 RAINBOW	665	Paclitaxel + placebo / Paclitaxel + Ram	OS	7.4 / 9.6	0.8 P = .017	2.9 / 4.4	0.64	16 / 27
3L	Li et al,[38] 2016	267	Placebo / Apatinib	OS/PFS	4.7 / 6.5	0.71 P = .015	1.8 / 2.6	0.44	0 / 3
1L	Ohtsu et al,[39] 2011 AVAGAST	774	Cis/5FU + placebo / Cis/5FU + Bev	OS (No)	10.1 / 12.1	0.87 NS	5.3 / 6.7	0.8 P = .004	37.4 / 46
1L	Shen et al,[40] 2015 AVATAR	202	Cis/Cape + placebo / Cis/Cape + Bev	OS (No)	11.4 / 10.5	1.11 NS	6 / 6.3	0.89 NS	34 / 41
1L	Yoon et al,[42] 2014	168	FOLFOX + placebo / FOLFOX + Ram	PFS (No)	11.7 / 11.5	1.08 NS	6.7 / 6.4	0.98 NS	46 / 45
1L	Enzinger et al,[41] 2016	64 / 1:02	FOLFOX + placebo / FOLFOX + aflibercept	6m PFS (No)	18.7 / 13.7	0.7 NS	7.3 / 9.9	0.88 NS	75 / 61

Abbreviations: 5FU, 5-fluorouracil; Bev, bevacizumab; Cape, capecitabine; Ram, ramucirumab.

Subsequent phase III GEC trials targeting EGFR included EXPAND (cetuximab with capecitabine/cisplatin, first line), REAL-3 (panitumumab with epirubicin/oxaliplatin/capecitabine, first line), and COG (gefitinib, second line or higher) (**Table 3**).[56–58] Disappointingly, each trial was negative, and panitumumab resulted in worse survival compared with the control. Notably, each of these trials enrolled all-comers without biomarker selection of any kind.

Xenograft models evaluating anti-EGFR therapy for *EGFR*-amplified tumors have reported potential benefit.[59] In the phase II study combining FOLFOX with cetuximab, 22% of patients had greater than 4 *EGFR* copies, which correlated with increased OS.[60] Similarly, in TRANS-COG, the translational correlative study of COG, 15.6% of patients had increased gene copy number, including true *EGFR* amplification (~5%); this latter small subset of *EGFR*-amplified patients derived a statistically significant survival benefit with the addition of gefitinib (hazard ratio [HR], 0.19; $P = .007$). The EXPAND trial also showed survival benefit in the small subset with extremely high EGFR expression by IHC H-score (likely representing EGFR-amplified tumors, but yet to be confirmed).[61] With these recent promising subset analyses of *EGFR* amplification and consequent overexpression, future studies assessing the benefits of anti-EGFR therapy in these patients are being pursued.[62] Also, a phase III trial of second-line nimotuzumab with irinotecan (NCT01813253) is currently recruiting patients deemed to harbor EGFR-overexpressing (IHC 2/3+) tumors (see **Table 5**).

MET

The MET proto-oncogene encodes the c-MET receptor tyrosine kinase, which is involved in cell proliferation, angiogenesis, and migration. MET overexpression, as well as the subset with *MET* amplification, are each associated with worse survival in most reports.[46,47,63–71] Canonical MET activation occurs via binding of its ligand, hepatocyte growth factor (HGF), but MET activation can also occur in an HGF-independent manner through RTK crosstalk.[72,73] *MET* amplification leads to constitutive receptor activation independent of HGF ligand, and is reported in ~4% to 10% of GEC cases,[47,74–76] but overexpression ranges from 23.7% to 70% in GEC, depending on the cohort evaluated and method of analysis used.[66–68,77–79]

As a predictive biomarker, early-phase reports and trials initially suggested that patients with GEC with MET-expressing tumors may benefit from MET-directed therapy.[71,77] However, a subsequent phase II[80] and two phase III MET-directed trials in GEC have been reported with overall negative results (**Table 4**).[80,81] The METGastric study evaluated onartuzumab, a humanized IgG1 antibody against the extracellular domain of c-MET, in combination with mFOLFOX6, in patients with c-MET–expressing tumors (≥1+, ≥50% cells).[82] However, METGastric was terminated prematurely (70% of planned accrual) because of negative results (regardless of intensity of MET expression) in the prior/parallel YO28252 phase II biomarker evaluation trial of onartuzumab in unselected patients with GEC.[80] With this in mind, no benefit was seen in the ITT or in the MET IHC 2/3+ preplanned subgroup analysis of the phase III trial (~38% of enrolled patients; HR, 0.64; $P = .06$), which had less power to identify a true benefit because of early termination of the trial.[82] Similarly, RILOMET-1, which evaluated epirubicin, cisplatin, and capecitabine with or without the addition of rilotumumab, a fully human IgG2 antibody against HGF ligand, was terminated because of an increased risk of death from the study drug.[81]

One pitfall of these phase III trials was their loose definition of MET expression. In RILOMET-1, patient selection was defined as greater than or equal to 1+ MET expression by IHC in greater than or equal to 25% of tumor cells to be eligible, which amounted to 81% of all patients screened, and of all patients enrolled and treated

Table 3
Phase III trials evaluating endothelial growth factor receptor–targeted therapies

Line	Trial	N	Treatment	Primary End Point (Met?)	mOS (mo)	HR	mPFS (mo)	HR	RR (%)
1L	Lordick et al,[56] 2013 EXPAND	904	Cis/5FU + placebo Cis/5FU + Cetuximab	PFS (No)	10.7 9.4	1.00	5.6 4.4	1.09 P = .32	29 30
1L	Waddell et al,[57] 2013 REAL-3	553	Epi/Oxali/Cape + placebo Epi/Oxali/Cape + P	OS (No)	11.3 8.8	1.37 P = .013	7.4 6.0	1.22	42 46
2L	Dutton et al,[58] 2014 COG	450	Placebo Gefitinib	OS (No)	3.67 3.73	0.9	1.17 1.57	0.8	~1 ~4

Abbreviations: Cape, capecitabine; Epi, epirubicin; Oxali, oxaliplatin; P, panitumumab.

Table 4
Phase III trials evaluating MET-targeted therapies in gastroesophageal cancer

Line	Trial	N	Treatment	Primary End Point (Met?)	mOS (mo)	HR	mPFS (mo)	HR	RR (%)
1L	Cunningham,[82] 2015 RILOMET-1	609	Epi/Cis/5FU + placebo	OS (No)	11.5	1.37	5.7	1.3	39
			Epi/Cis/5FU + Rilo		9.6	$P = .016$	5.7		30
1L	Shah et al,[83] 2016 METGastric	562	FOLFOX + placebo	OS (No)	11.3	0.82	6.8	0.9	41
			FOLFOX + onartuzumab		11	$P = .24$	6.7		46

Abbreviation: Rilo, rilotumumab.

only 21% were in the very high MET expression group of IHC 2/3+ in greater than or equal to 50% of cells. Similarly, only 38% of METGastric patient samples were IHC 2/3+ in greater than or equal to 50% of cells, but, as discussed earlier, these patients showed a near-significant benefit in an underaccrued trial. Even with the large phase III MET inhibitor trials, it could be argued that the selection for MET-dependent cancers was too lenient and inadequate, and the highest expressing tumors under-represented.[47,74–76] Another negative trial in second line with the multi-TKI foretinib was observed, again without selecting patients by any biomarker.[83]

More promising results have been reported in smaller trials of MET inhibitors for *MET*-amplified patients (4%–5% of GEC),[47,67,74,76] with consequent overexpression.[74] AMG-337, a highly selective MET TKI, showed clinical responses in patients with *MET*-amplified advanced GEC (ORR, 50%), but the phase II study has been on hold after the expansion phase of the trial (results not publicly available).[84] Similarly, half of *MET*-amplified patients treated with crizotinib in a phase I expansion cohort experienced response,[47] and 75% of *MET*-amplified patients receiving ABT-700 monoclonal antibody monotherapy showed an objective response.[85] The challenge of molecular heterogeneity,[21,86] particularly in the CIN subset of GEC,[9] may account for general lack of durable response and rapidly acquired resistance to MET-directed monotherapy for *MET*-amplified GEC. Any future therapeutic attempts with MET inhibitors are likely to be directed toward the small subset of *MET*-amplified patients, likely with combination approaches with either chemotherapy, other targeted therapies, or immune checkpoint inhibition to address this complex biology (**Table 5**).[87]

Fibroblast Growth Factor Type 2

Fibroblast growth factor type 2 (*FGFR2*) encodes an RTK that regulates cell angiogenesis and proliferation, and, when highly expressed, portends a poor prognosis in both Western and Asian populations.[88] FGFR2 expression in GEC is primarily driven by gene copy number, with 4% to 10% of GEC patients harboring *FGFR2* amplification.[6,88,89] *FGFR2* amplification has been associated with diffuse-type GC but also CIN EGJ adenocarcinoma. Dovitinib, a TKI targeting FGFR1/2/3, VEGF1/2/3, PDGFR and c-KIT, exhibited activity in vitro.[6] The SHINE trial compared paclitaxel with AZD4547, another FGFR2 TKI, in advanced GC in Asia in previously treated patients, but the paclitaxel arm had superior survival, even in the *FGFR2*-amplified patient subset.[90] In contrast, another small phase IIa trial showed response in 3 out of 9 patients (33%) with promising durability in *FGFR2*-amplified patients, and also observed that higher and homogeneous gene amplification may better predict therapeutic benefit.[91] These early-phase trials suggest safety from this class of TKIs, with mainly hyperphosphatemia and ocular toxicities reported.[90] Phase II trials are ongoing in combination with cytotoxic therapies, which, similarly to HER2, may be a more promising approach than monotherapy. Recently, 2 out of 6 (33%) patients with FGFR2 overexpressing gastric cancer responded to FPA144, a novel humanized monoclonal IgG1 antibody against the FGFR2b isoform, in a chemotherapy-refractory phase I evaluation.[92] Another 3 out of 6 (50%) had stable disease, resulting in a 5 out of 6 (83%) disease control rate in this early assessment. Phase I expansion accrual remains ongoing in this patient population, with specific interest in patients with *FGFR2*-amplified GEC (see **Table 5**). FPA144 does not inhibit FGF23 signaling, which mitigates adverse hyperphosphatemia that has hindered FGF TKI development.

PI3K-AKT-mTOR

The PI3K-AKT-mammalian target of rapamycin (mTOR) pathway is commonly altered in GEC, leading to increased proliferation and apoptotic resistance. *PIK3CA* activating

Table 5
Additional targeted therapy trials in gastroesophageal cancer

Target	Line	Trial	Phase	Treatment	Primary End Point	Outcome
HER2	2L HER2+	NCT02689284	I/II	Margetuximab + pembrolizumab	MTD/ORR	Ongoing
HER2	1L	NCT01774786 JACOB	III	TP ± pertuzumab	OS	Ongoing
EGFR	1+, amplified	NCT02213289 PANGEA-IMBBP	I/II	Chemotherapy + ABT-806	OS	Ongoing
MET	2+L, MET-amplified	NCT02016534	II	AMG-337	ORR	Ongoing (HOLD)
EGFR	2, EGFR Exp 2/3+	NCT01813253	III	Irinotecan ± nimotuzumab	OS/PFS	Ongoing
FGFR2	3+L, amplified	NCT01719549	II	Dovitinib	RR/PFS	Ongoing
FGFR2	2+L, amplified	NCT01921673	I/II	Dovitinib + Doc	MTD/PFS	Ongoing
FGFR2	2L, polysomy/amplified	NCT01457846 SHINE[90]	II	AZD4547 vs paclitaxel	PFS	Negative (amplified mPFS 1.5 vs 2.3 mo)
FGFR2	Any	NCT02318329 [92]	I	FPA144	MTD/DLT	Ongoing
PI3K	2+L	NCT01576666	IB	LDE225 + BKM120	MTD/DLT	Ongoing
PI3K	2-4L, PIK3CA mutated/amplified or HER2+	NCT01613950	IB	BYL719 + AUY922	MTD/DLT	Ongoing
Akt	2L, PIK3CA mutated/amplified	NCT02451956	II	AZD5363 + paclitaxel	ORR	Ongoing
Akt/mTOR	2L	NCT02449655	II	Paclitaxel + AZD5363 or AZD2014	ORR	Ongoing
mTOR	2-3L	NCT00879333 GRANITE-1[94]	III	Everolimus vs placebo	OS	Negative (5.4 vs 4.3 mo, P = .124)
CLDN18.2	1L, CLDN18.2 expressing	NCT01630083 FAST[100]	II	EOX ± IMAB362	PFS	Positive – improved PFS, OS

Abbreviations: DLT, dose-limiting toxicity; Doc, docetaxel; Exp, expressing; HOLD, trial on hold; MTD, maximum tolerated dose.

mutations, loss of *PTEN*, *RICTOR* amplification, and *AKT* amplification have all been described.[5,9,48] *PIK3CA* activating mutation alone is observed in ~15% of GEC.

Attempted inhibition of mTOR with everolimus showed a median PFS of 2.7 months and OS of 10.1 months in an early study, but the subsequent phase III GRANITE-1 trial comparing everolimus with placebo in an unselected patient population of second-line or third-line therapy failed to show an OS benefit.[93,94] Results from a phase III trial of paclitaxel with or without everolimus are still awaited (NCT01248403). Numerous PI3K inhibitors have shown benefit in preclinical studies, including BEZ235 and BKM120 as monotherapy, or in combination with HSP90 or hedgehog inhibitors, suggesting a disconnect between preclinical models and GEC patients treated with these agents.[95,96] Second-line AKT inhibition trials are ongoing with AZD5363 in combination with paclitaxel (NCT02451956/NCT02449655), as well as the first-line JAGUAR trial combining FOLFOX with or without AKT inhibition using ipatasertib (NCT01896531). Strategies selecting for only those with tumors having a genomically activated PI3K-AKT-mTOR pathway may enrich for clinical benefit to these targeted therapies, but further investigation is required to support this notion (see Table 5).

CLDN18.2

Claudins are structural components of tight junctions that seal intercellular space, and are overexpressed in numerous cancers. *CLDN18* amplification is found in 3% of TCGA patients with gastric cancer and 3% of patients also harbor oncogenic gene fusions between *CLDN18* and *ARHGAP26*, a RHOA inhibitor.[97] These fusions impair cell-extracellular membrane adhesion, and in doing so promote migration. Claudiximab (IMAB362) is a chimeric IgG1 monoclonal antibody against CLDN18.2 that is intended to enhance T-cell infiltration and antibody-dependent cell-mediated toxicity (ADCC).[98] Claudiximab was developed from high-throughput screening of malignancy-specific cell surface molecules that identified gastric specificity of claudin 18 splice variant 2.[99] Phase II evaluation of claudiximab in combination with epirubicin/oxaliplatin/capecitabine (FAST trial) demonstrated a 39% ORR along with PFS and OS in patients expressing CLDN18.2 (defined as ≥2+ intensity) in at least 40% of cells. Benefit was more pronounced in patients with overexpression in over 70% of tumor cells (see Table 5).[100] Further evaluation is planned in a phase III study.

Programmed-death Ligand 1

Immune checkpoint inhibition using programmed-death 1 (PD-1) and programmed-death ligand 1 (PD-L1) inhibitors are under evaluation in many cancers, including GEC. PD-L1 normally binds to receptors on T lymphocytes, thereby inhibiting T-cell proliferation and inducing apoptosis, which impairs the cytotoxic immune response. EBV-associated GEC overexpresses PD-L1 and PD-L2 because of amplification of 9p24,[101] and MSI-high tumors are also associated with intense immune infiltration and overexpression of checkpoint inhibitor targets.[9,102] KEYNOTE-012 evaluated pembrolizumab, a PD-1 inhibitor, in PD-L1+ (~30%–40% of patients screened) advanced GC, and showed a 22% ORR.[103] Of note, although PD-L1 overexpression correlated with a higher response rate, PD-L1 expression remains a poor predictive biomarker; patients without PD-L1 expression can still respond, and most often those with expression do not derive benefit.[103] Similarly, in the CheckMate-032 trial, objective response to nivolumab, another PD-1 inhibitor, was 18% and 12% in PD-L1-positive and PD-L1-negative patients, respectively, in patients with chemorefractory GEC.[104] Second-line response rates, stratified by PD-L1 status, were similar in the Javelin GEC trial with avelumab, a PD-L1 antagonist (18.2% vs 9.1%), and less in subsequent lines (10% vs 3.1%).[105] RNA expression signatures reflecting interferon gamma activity and T-cell activity are are currently under development in order to improve patient selection.[106] Phase III evaluation of pembrolizumab (KEYNOTE-062, KEYNOTE-061) in the first-line and second-line metastatic settings respectively, and nivolumab (Check-Mate-577) in the adjuvant setting are ongoing, with various other approaches in all lines of therapy being assessed with multiple PD-1/PD-L1 inhibitors.[107]

Cytotoxic T Lymphocyte Antigen 4

Cytotoxic T lymphocyte antigen 4 (CTLA4) is constitutively expressed on the surface of T-regulatory cells and expression can be inducible on activated T lymphocytes and monocytes. Downregulation leads to interleukin (IL)-2 production and IL-2R expression, with subsequent priming of the T-cell response.[108] Mutations and copy number variation of CTLA4 occur rarely, in only 2.5% of TCGA patients with gastric cancer. Tremelimumab is a fully humanized IgG2 anti-CTLA4 monoclonal antibody that has undergone evaluation in numerous other malignancies. Of the 18 patients with metastatic GC enrolled in a second-line phase II trial, no objective responses were seen after cycle 1. However, 12-month survival was 33%, and 1 patient later derived a partial response after 25.4 months of therapy and was alive at 32.7 months at the time of publication.[109] Ipilimumab, another CTLA-4 antagonist, was evaluated as maintenance therapy after receiving a platinum fluoropyrimidine doublet, but failed to prolong PFS or OS.[110] Evaluation remains underway in combination with PD-1/PD-L1 antagonists as discussed earlier.[107]

SUMMARY

Despite dozens of trials evaluating targeted therapies for GEC, only trastuzumab and ramucirumab have shown benefit and been approved in the first-line and second-line settings, respectively. Subset analyses have successively identified patients with *MET*, *EGFR*, and *FGFR2* genomic aberrations that may benefit from matched targeted therapies, but designing traditional trials for such infrequent aberrations and interpatient heterogeneity remains extremely challenging. Tumor molecular heterogeneity within patients through space and over time/therapy are also obstacles to successful implementation of these targeted agents. Novel trial designs such as the PANGEA type II expansion platform may better identify and treat these uncommon actionable aberrations as a way forward by testing a treatment strategy.[21,62,111] Immune checkpoint inhibitors are being evaluated and hold promise, with investigations ongoing to determine subsets likely to derive benefit. Future directions should focus on improving diagnostic assays and validating predictive biomarkers for benefit from immuno-oncologic therapies.

REFERENCES

1. Torre LA, Bray F, Siegel RL, et al. Global cancer statistics, 2012. CA Cancer J Clin 2015;65(2):87–108.
2. Sehdev A, Catenacci DV. Gastroesophageal cancer: focus on epidemiology, classification, and staging. Discov Med 2013;16(87):103–11.
3. Sehdev A, Catenacci DV. Perioperative therapy for locally advanced gastro-esophageal cancer: current controversies and consensus of care. J Hematol Oncol 2013;6:66.
4. Siegel RL, Miller KD, Jemal A. Cancer statistics, 2015. CA Cancer J Clin 2015; 65(1):5–29.
5. Ali SM, Sanford EM, Klempner SJ, et al. Prospective comprehensive genomic profiling of advanced gastric carcinoma cases reveals frequent clinically

relevant genomic alterations and new routes for targeted therapies. Oncologist 2015;20(5):499–507.

6. Deng N, Goh LK, Wang H, et al. A comprehensive survey of genomic alterations in gastric cancer reveals systematic patterns of molecular exclusivity and co-occurrence among distinct therapeutic targets. Gut 2012;61(5):673–84.

7. Stachler MD, Taylor-Weiner A, Peng S, et al. Paired exome analysis of Barrett's esophagus and adenocarcinoma. Nat Genet 2015;47(9):1047–55.

8. Zang ZJ, Ong CK, Cutcutache I, et al. Genetic and structural variation in the gastric cancer kinome revealed through targeted deep sequencing. Cancer Res 2011;71(1):29–39.

9. Cancer Genome Atlas Research Network. Comprehensive molecular characterization of gastric adenocarcinoma. Nature 2014;513(7517):202–9.

10. Kameda T, Yasui W, Yoshida K, et al. Expression of ERBB2 in human gastric carcinomas: relationship between p185ERBB2 expression and the gene amplification. Cancer Res 1990;50(24):8002–9.

11. Okines AF, Thompson LC, Cunningham D, et al. Effect of HER2 on prognosis and benefit from peri-operative chemotherapy in early oesophago-gastric adenocarcinoma in the MAGIC trial. Ann Oncol 2013;24(5):1253–61.

12. Van Cutsem E, de Haas S, Kang YK, et al. Bevacizumab in combination with chemotherapy as first-line therapy in advanced gastric cancer: a biomarker evaluation from the AVAGAST randomized phase III trial. J Clin Oncol 2012; 30(17):2119–27.

13. Gordon MA, Gundacker HM, Benedetti J, et al. Assessment of HER2 gene amplification in adenocarcinomas of the stomach or gastroesophageal junction in the INT-0116/SWOG9008 clinical trial. Ann Oncol 2013;24(7):1754–61.

14. Terashima M, Kitada K, Ochiai A, et al. Impact of expression of human epidermal growth factor receptors EGFR and ERBB2 on survival in stage II/III gastric cancer. Clin Cancer Res 2012;18(21):5992–6000.

15. Kurokawa Y, Matsuura N, Kimura Y, et al. Multicenter large-scale study of prognostic impact of HER2 expression in patients with resectable gastric cancer. Gastric Cancer 2015;18(4):691–7.

16. Bang YJ, Van Cutsem E, Feyereislova A, et al. Trastuzumab in combination with chemotherapy versus chemotherapy alone for treatment of HER2-positive advanced gastric or gastro-oesophageal junction cancer (ToGA): a phase 3, open-label, randomised controlled trial. Lancet 2010;376(9742):687–97.

17. Hofmann M, Stoss O, Shi D, et al. Assessment of a HER2 scoring system for gastric cancer: results from a validation study. Histopathology 2008;52(7): 797–805.

18. Catenacci DV, Liao WL, Zhao L, et al. Mass-spectrometry-based quantitation of Her2 in gastroesophageal tumor tissue: comparison to IHC and FISH. Gastric Cancer 2016;19(4):1066–79.

19. Sellappan S, Blackler A, Liao WL, et al. Therapeutically induced changes in HER2, HER3, and EGFR protein expression for treatment guidance. J Natl Compr Canc Netw 2016;14(5):503–7.

20. Shoda K, Masuda K, Ichikawa D, et al. HER2 amplification detected in the circulating DNA of patients with gastric cancer: a retrospective pilot study. Gastric Cancer 2015;18(4):698–710.

21. Catenacci DV. Next-generation clinical trials: novel strategies to address the challenge of tumor molecular heterogeneity. Mol Oncol 2015;9(5):967–96.

22. Janjigian YY, Riches JC, Ku GY, et al. Loss of human epidermal growth factor receptor 2 (HER2) expression in HER2-overexpressing esophagogastric (EG)

tumors treated with trastuzumab. Paper presented at: ASCO Annual Meeting Proceedings. Chicago, 2015.

23. Denlinger CS, Alsina Maqueda M, Watkins DJ, et al. Randomized phase 2 study of paclitaxel (PTX), trastuzumab (T) with or without MM-111 in HER2 expressing gastroesophageal cancers (GEC). Paper presented at: ASCO Annual Meeting Proceedings. Chicago, 2016.

24. Hecht JR, Bang YJ, Qin SK, et al. Lapatinib in combination with capecitabine plus oxaliplatin in human epidermal growth factor receptor 2-positive advanced or metastatic gastric, esophageal, or gastroesophageal adenocarcinoma: TRIO-013/LOGiC–A randomized phase III trial. J Clin Oncol 2016;34(5):443–51.

25. Press MF, Ellis CE, Gagnon RC, et al. HER2 status in advanced or metastatic gastric, esophageal, or gastro-esophageal adenocarcinoma for entry to the TRIO-013/LOGiC trial of lapatinib. Mol Cancer Ther 2016. [Epub ahead of print].

26. Gomez-Martin C, Plaza JC, Pazo-Cid R, et al. Level of HER2 gene amplification predicts response and overall survival in HER2-positive advanced gastric cancer treated with trastuzumab. J Clin Oncol 2013;31(35):4445–52.

27. Ock CY, Lee KW, Kim JW, et al. Optimal patient selection for trastuzumab treatment in HER2-positive advanced gastric cancer. Clin Cancer Res 2015;21(11):2520–9.

28. An E, Ock CY, Kim TY, et al. Quantitative proteomic analysis of HER2 expression in the selection of gastric cancer patients for trastuzumab treatment. Ann Oncol 2016. [Epub ahead of print].

29. Satoh T, Xu RH, Chung HC, et al. Lapatinib plus paclitaxel versus paclitaxel alone in the second-line treatment of HER2-amplified advanced gastric cancer in Asian populations: TyTAN–a randomized, phase III study. J Clin Oncol 2014; 32(19):2039–49.

30. Kang YK, Shah MA, Ohtsu A, et al. A randomized, open-label, multicenter, adaptive phase 2/3 study of trastuzumab emtansine (T-DM1) versus a taxane (TAX) in patients (pts) with previously treated HER2-positive locally advanced or metastatic gastric/gastroesophageal junction adenocarcinoma (LA/MGC/GEJC). Paper presented at: ASCO Annual Meeting Proceedings. Chicago, 2016.

31. Swain SM, Kim SB, Cortes J, et al. Pertuzumab, trastuzumab, and docetaxel for HER2-positive metastatic breast cancer (CLEOPATRA study): overall survival results from a randomised, double-blind, placebo-controlled, phase 3 study. Lancet Oncol 2013;14(6):461–71.

32. Wilke H, Muro K, Van Cutsem E, et al. Ramucirumab plus paclitaxel versus placebo plus paclitaxel in patients with previously treated advanced gastric or gastro-oesophageal junction adenocarcinoma (RAINBOW): a double-blind, randomised phase 3 trial. Lancet Oncol 2014;15(11):1224–35.

33. Fuchs CS, Tomasek J, Yong CJ, et al. Ramucirumab monotherapy for previously treated advanced gastric or gastro-oesophageal junction adenocarcinoma (REGARD): an international, randomised, multicentre, placebo-controlled, phase 3 trial. Lancet 2014;383(9911):31–9.

34. Janjigian YY, Capanu M, Imtiaz T, et al. A phase II study of afatinib in patients (pts) with metastatic human epidermal growth factor receptor (HER2)-positive trastuzumab-refractory esophagogastric (EG) cancer. Paper presented at: ASCO Annual Meeting Proceedings. Chicago, 2014.

35. Rugo HS, Pegram MD, Gradishar WJ, et al. SOPHIA: A phase 3, randomized study of margetuximab (M) plus chemotherapy (CTX) vs trastuzumab (T) plus CTX in the treatment of patients with HER2+ metastatic breast cancer (MBC). ASCO Meeting Abstracts 2016;34(15 Suppl):TPS630. Available at: http:// meetinglibrary.asco.org/content/164475-176.

36. Combination margetuximab and pembrolizumab for advanced metastatic HER2(+) gastric or gastroesophageal junction cancer. Available at: https://ClinicalTrials.gov/show/NCT02689284. Accessed November 7, 2016.

37. Oh SY, Kwon HC, Kim SH, et al. Clinicopathologic significance of HIF-1alpha, p53, and VEGF expression and preoperative serum VEGF level in gastric cancer. BMC Cancer 2008;8:123.

38. Li J, Qin S, Xu J, et al. Randomized, double-blind, placebo-controlled phase III trial of apatinib in patients with chemotherapy-refractory advanced or metastatic adenocarcinoma of the stomach or gastroesophageal junction. J Clin Oncol 2016;34(13):1448–54.

39. Ohtsu A, Shah MA, Van Cutsem E, et al. Bevacizumab in combination with chemotherapy as first-line therapy in advanced gastric cancer: a randomized, double-blind, placebo-controlled phase III study. J Clin Oncol 2011;29(30):3968–76.

40. Shen L, Li J, Xu J, et al. Bevacizumab plus capecitabine and cisplatin in Chinese patients with inoperable locally advanced or metastatic gastric or gastroesophageal junction cancer: randomized, double-blind, phase III study (AVATAR study). Gastric Cancer 2015;18(1):168–76.

41. Enzinger PC, McCleary NJ, Zheng H, et al. Multicenter double-blind randomized phase II: FOLFOX + ziv-aflibercept/placebo for patients (pts) with chemo-naive metastatic esophagogastric adenocarcinoma (MEGA). Paper presented at: ASCO Annual Meeting Proceedings. Chicago, 2016.

42. Yoon HH, Bendell JC, Braiteh FS, et al. Ramucirumab (RAM) plus FOLFOX as front-line therapy (Rx) for advanced gastric or esophageal adenocarcinoma (GE-AC): randomized, double-blind, multicenter phase 2 trial. Paper presented at: ASCO Annual Meeting Proceedings. Chicago, 2014.

43. Murukesh N, Dive C, Jayson GC. Biomarkers of angiogenesis and their role in the development of VEGF inhibitors. Br J Cancer 2010;102(1):8–18.

44. Kim MA, Lee HS, Lee HE, et al. EGFR in gastric carcinomas: prognostic significance of protein overexpression and high gene copy number. Histopathology 2008;52(6):738–46.

45. Wang KL, Wu TT, Choi IS, et al. Expression of epidermal growth factor receptor in esophageal and esophagogastric junction adenocarcinomas: association with poor outcome. Cancer 2007;109(4):658–67.

46. Nagatsuma AK, Aizawa M, Kuwata T, et al. Expression profiles of HER2, EGFR, MET and FGFR2 in a large cohort of patients with gastric adenocarcinoma. Gastric Cancer 2015;18(2):227–38.

47. Lennerz JK, Kwak EL, Ackerman A, et al. MET amplification identifies a small and aggressive subgroup of esophagogastric adenocarcinoma with evidence of responsiveness to crizotinib. J Clin Oncol 2011;29(36):4803–10.

48. Dulak AM, Stojanov P, Peng S, et al. Exome and whole-genome sequencing of esophageal adenocarcinoma identifies recurrent driver events and mutational complexity. Nat Genet 2013;45(5):478–86.

49. Kimura H, Sakai K, Arao T, et al. Antibody-dependent cellular cytotoxicity of cetuximab against tumor cells with wild-type or mutant epidermal growth factor receptor. Cancer Sci 2007;98(8):1275–80.

50. Enzinger PC, Burtness BA, Niedzwiecki D, et al. CALGB 80403 (Alliance)/E1206: a randomized phase II study of three chemotherapy regimens plus cetuximab in metastatic esophageal and gastroesophageal junction cancers. J Clin Oncol 2016;34(23):2736–42.

51. Wainberg ZA, Lin LS, DiCarlo B, et al. Phase II trial of modified FOLFOX6 and erlotinib in patients with metastatic or advanced adenocarcinoma of the oesophagus and gastro-oesophageal junction. Br J Cancer 2011;105(6):760–5.

52. Lordick F, Luber B, Lorenzen S, et al. Cetuximab plus oxaliplatin/leucovorin/5-fluorouracil in first-line metastatic gastric cancer: a phase II study of the Arbeitsgemeinschaft Internistische Onkologie (AIO). Br J Cancer 2010;102(3):500–5.

53. Tebbutt NC, Price TJ, Ferraro DA, et al. Panitumumab added to docetaxel, cisplatin and fluoropyrimidine in oesophagogastric cancer: ATTAX3 phase II trial. Br J Cancer 2016;114(5):505–9.

54. Ferry DR, Anderson M, Beddard K, et al. A phase II study of gefitinib monotherapy in advanced esophageal adenocarcinoma: evidence of gene expression, cellular, and clinical response. Clin Cancer Res 2007;13(19):5869–75.

55. Dragovich T, McCoy S, Fenoglio-Preiser CM, et al. Phase II trial of erlotinib in gastroesophageal junction and gastric adenocarcinomas: SWOG 0127. J Clin Oncol 2006;24(30):4922–7.

56. Lordick F, Kang YK, Chung HC, et al. Capecitabine and cisplatin with or without cetuximab for patients with previously untreated advanced gastric cancer (EXPAND): a randomised, open-label phase 3 trial. Lancet Oncol 2013;14(6):490–9.

57. Waddell T, Chau I, Cunningham D, et al. Epirubicin, oxaliplatin, and capecitabine with or without panitumumab for patients with previously untreated advanced oesophagogastric cancer (REAL3): a randomised, open-label phase 3 trial. Lancet Oncol 2013;14(6):481–9.

58. Dutton SJ, Ferry DR, Blazeby JM, et al. Gefitinib for oesophageal cancer progressing after chemotherapy (COG): a phase 3, multicentre, double-blind, placebo-controlled randomised trial. Lancet Oncol 2014;15(8):894–904.

59. Zhang L, Yang J, Cai J, et al. A subset of gastric cancers with EGFR amplification and overexpression respond to cetuximab therapy. Sci Rep 2013;3:2992.

60. Luber B, Deplazes J, Keller G, et al. Biomarker analysis of cetuximab plus oxaliplatin/leucovorin/5-fluorouracil in first-line metastatic gastric and oesophago-gastric junction cancer: results from a phase II trial of the Arbeitsgemeinschaft Internistische Onkologie (AIO). BMC Cancer 2011;11:509.

61. Lordick F, Kang YK, Salman P, et al. Clinical outcome according to tumor HER2 status and EGFR expression in advanced gastric cancer patients from the EXPAND study. Paper presented at: ASCO Annual Meeting Proceedings. Chicago, 2013.

62. Catenacci DVT, Polite BN, Henderson L, et al. Toward personalized treatment for gastroesophageal adenocarcinoma (GEC): strategies to address tumor heterogeneity–PANGEA. Paper presented at: ASCO Annual Meeting Proceedings. Chicago, 2014.

63. Catenacci DV, Ang A, Liao WL, et al. MET tyrosine kinase receptor expression and amplification as prognostic biomarkers of survival in gastroesophageal adenocarcinoma. Cancer 2016.

64. Hack SP, Bruey JM, Koeppen H. HGF/MET-directed therapeutics in gastroesophageal cancer: a review of clinical and biomarker development. Oncotarget 2014;5(10):2866–80.

65. Metzger ML, Behrens HM, Boger C, et al. MET in gastric cancer–discarding a 10% cutoff rule. Histopathology 2016;68(2):241–53.

66. Nakajima M, Sawada H, Yamada Y, et al. The prognostic significance of amplification and overexpression of c-met and c-erb B-2 in human gastric carcinomas. Cancer 1999;85(9):1894–902.

67. Lee HE, Kim MA, Lee HS, et al. MET in gastric carcinomas: comparison between protein expression and gene copy number and impact on clinical outcome. Br J Cancer 2012;107(2):325–33.

68. Graziano F, Galluccio N, Lorenzini P, et al. Genetic activation of the MET pathway and prognosis of patients with high-risk, radically resected gastric cancer. J Clin Oncol 2011;29(36):4789–95.

69. Catenacci DV, Cervantes G, Yala S, et al. RON (MST1R) is a novel prognostic marker and therapeutic target for gastroesophageal adenocarcinoma. Cancer Biol Ther 2011;12(1):9–46.

70. Yu S, Yu Y, Zhao N, et al. C-Met as a prognostic marker in gastric cancer: a systematic review and meta-analysis. PLoS One 2013;8(11):e79137.

71. Iveson T, Donehower RC, Davidenko I, et al. Rilotumumab in combination with epirubicin, cisplatin, and capecitabine as first-line treatment for gastric or oesophagogastric junction adenocarcinoma: an open-label, dose de-escalation phase 1b study and a double-blind, randomised phase 2 study. Lancet Oncol 2014;15(9):1007–18.

72. Jo M, Stolz DB, Esplen JE, et al. Cross-talk between epidermal growth factor receptor and c-Met signal pathways in transformed cells. J Biol Chem 2000; 275(12):8806–11.

73. Yamaguchi H, Chang SS, Hsu JL, et al. Signaling cross-talk in the resistance to HER family receptor targeted therapy. Oncogene 2014;33(9):1073–81.

74. Catenacci DV, Liao WL, Thyparambil S, et al. Absolute quantitation of Met using mass spectrometry for clinical application: assay precision, stability, and correlation with MET gene amplification in FFPE tumor tissue. PLoS One 2014;9(7):e100586.

75. Jardim DL, Tang C, Gagliato Dde M, et al. Analysis of 1,115 patients tested for MET amplification and therapy response in the MD Anderson Phase I Clinic. Clin Cancer Res 2014;20(24):6336–45.

76. Smolen GA, Sordella R, Muir B, et al. Amplification of MET may identify a subset of cancers with extreme sensitivity to the selective tyrosine kinase inhibitor PHA-665752. Proc Natl Acad Sci U S A 2006;103(7):2316–21.

77. Catenacci DV, Henderson L, Xiao SY, et al. Durable complete response of metastatic gastric cancer with anti-Met therapy followed by resistance at recurrence. Cancer Discov 2011;1(7):573–9.

78. Toiyama Y, Yasuda H, Saigusa S, et al. Co-expression of hepatocyte growth factor and c-Met predicts peritoneal dissemination established by autocrine hepatocyte growth factor/c-Met signaling in gastric cancer. Int J Cancer 2012;130(12):2912–21.

79. Zhao J, Zhang X, Xin Y. Up-regulated expression of Ezrin and c-Met proteins are related to the metastasis and prognosis of gastric carcinomas. Histol Histopathol 2011;26(9):1111–20.

80. Shah MA, Cho JY, Tan IB, et al. A randomized phase II study of FOLFOX with or without the MET inhibitor onartuzumab in advanced adenocarcinoma of the stomach and gastroesophageal junction. Oncologist 2016;21(9):1085–90.

81. Cunningham D. Phase III, randomized, double-blind, multicenter, placebo (P)-controlled trial of rilotumumab (R) plus epirubicin, cisplatin and capecitabine (ECX) as first-line therapy in patients (pts) with advanced MET-positive (pos) gastric or gastroesophageal junction (G/GEJ) cancer: RILOMET-1 study. J Clin Oncol 2015;33(Suppl).

82. Shah MA, Bang YJ, Lordick F, et al. Effect of Fluorouracil, Leucovorin, and Oxaliplatin With or Without Onartuzumab in HER2-Negative, MET-Positive Gastroesophageal Adenocarcinoma: The METGastric Randomized Clinical Trial. JAMA Oncol 2016.

83. Shah MA, Wainberg ZA, Catenacci DV, et al. Phase II study evaluating 2 dosing schedules of oral foretinib (GSK1363089), cMET/VEGFR2 inhibitor, in patients with metastatic gastric cancer. PLoS One 2013;8(3):e54014.

84. Kwak EL, LoRusso P, Hamid O, et al. Clinical activity of AMG 337, an oral MET kinase inhibitor, in adult patients (pts) with MET-amplified gastroesophageal junction (GEJ), gastric (G), or esophageal (E) cancer. Paper presented at: ASCO Annual Meeting Proceedings. Chicago, 2015.

85. Kang YK, LoRusso P, Salgia R, et al. Phase I study of ABT-700, an anti-c-Met antibody, in patients (pts) with advanced gastric or esophageal cancer (GEC). Paper presented at: ASCO Annual Meeting Proceedings. Chicago, 2015.

86. Kwak EL, Ahronian LG, Siravegna G, et al. Molecular heterogeneity and receptor coamplification drive resistance to targeted therapy in MET-amplified esophagogastric cancer. Cancer Discov 2015;5(12):1271–81.

87. Mullard A. NCI-MATCH trial pushes cancer umbrella trial paradigm. Nat Rev Drug Discov 2015;14(8):513–5.

88. Su X, Zhan P, Gavine PR, et al. FGFR2 amplification has prognostic significance in gastric cancer: results from a large international multicentre study. Br J Cancer 2014;110(4):967–75.

89. Matsumoto K, Arao T, Hamaguchi T, et al. FGFR2 gene amplification and clinicopathological features in gastric cancer. Br J Cancer 2012;106(4):727–32.

90. Bang YJ, Van Cutsem E, Mansoor W, et al. A randomized, open-label phase II study of AZD4547 (AZD) versus paclitaxel (P) in previously treated patients with advanced gastric cancer (AGC) with fibroblast growth factor receptor 2 (FGFR2) polysomy or gene amplification (amp): SHINE study. Paper presented at: ASCO Annual Meeting Proceedings. Chicago, 2015.

91. Smyth EC, Turner NC, Pearson A, et al. Phase II study of AZD4547 in FGFR amplified tumours: gastroesophageal cancer (GC) cohort pharmacodynamic and biomarker results. Paper presented at: ASCO Annual Meeting Proceedings. Chicago, 2016.

92. Lee J, Bendell JC, Rha SY, et al. Antitumor activity and safety of FPA144, an ADCC-enhanced, FGFR2b isoform-selective monoclonal antibody, in patients with FGFR2b+ gastric cancer and advanced solid tumors. Chicago: ASCO Meeting Abstracts 2016;34(15 Suppl):2502.

93. Doi T, Muro K, Boku N, et al. Multicenter phase II study of everolimus in patients with previously treated metastatic gastric cancer. J Clin Oncol 2010;28(11):1904–10.

94. Ohtsu A, Ajani JA, Bai YX, et al. Everolimus for previously treated advanced gastric cancer: results of the randomized, double-blind, phase III GRANITE-1 study. J Clin Oncol 2013;31(31):3935–43.

95. Mueller A, Bachmann E, Linnig M, et al. Selective PI3K inhibition by BKM120 and BEZ235 alone or in combination with chemotherapy in wild-type and mutated human gastrointestinal cancer cell lines. Cancer Chemother Pharmacol 2012;69(6):1601–15.

96. Serra V, Markman B, Scaltriti M, et al. NVP-BEZ235, a dual PI3K/mTOR inhibitor, prevents PI3K signaling and inhibits the growth of cancer cells with activating PI3K mutations. Cancer Res 2008;68(19):8022–30.

97. Yao F, Kausalya JP, Sia YY, et al. Recurrent fusion genes in gastric cancer: CLDN18-ARHGAP26 induces loss of epithelial integrity. Cell Rep 2015;12(2):272–85.

98. Schuler MH, Zvirbule Z, Lordick F, et al. Safety, tolerability, and efficacy of the first-in-class antibody IMAB362 targeting claudin 18.2 in patients with metastatic gastroesophageal adenocarcinomas. Paper presented at: ASCO Annual Meeting Proceedings. Chicago, 2013.

99. Sahin U, Koslowski M, Dhaene K, et al. Claudin-18 splice variant 2 is a pan-cancer target suitable for therapeutic antibody development. Clin Cancer Res 2008;14(23):7624–34.

100. Al-Batran S-E, Schuler MH, Zvirbule Z, et al. FAST: An international, multicenter, randomized, phase II trial of epirubicin, oxaliplatin, and capecitabine (EOX) with or without IMAB362, a first-in-class anti-CLDN18. 2 antibody, as first-line therapy in patients with advanced CLDN18.2+ gastric and gastroesophageal junction (GEJ) adenocarcinoma. Paper presented at: ASCO Annual Meeting Proceedings. Chicago, 2016.

101. Derks S, Liao X, Chiaravalli AM, et al. Abundant PD-L1 expression in Epstein-Barr virus-infected gastric cancers. Oncotarget 2016;7(22):32925–32.

102. Ma C, Patel K, Singhi AD, et al. Programmed death-ligand 1 expression is common in gastric cancer associated with Epstein-Barr virus or microsatellite instability. Am J Surg Pathol 2016;40(11):1496–506.

103. Muro K, Chung HC, Shankaran V, et al. Pembrolizumab for patients with PD-L1-positive advanced gastric cancer (KEYNOTE-012): a multicentre, open-label, phase 1b trial. Lancet Oncol 2016;17(6):717–26.

104. Le DT, Bendell JC, Calvo E, et al. Safety and activity of nivolumab monotherapy in advanced and metastatic (A/M) gastric or gastroesophageal junction cancer (GC/GEC): results from the CheckMate-032 study. Paper presented at: Proc Am Soc Clin Oncol. San Francisco, January 21, 2016.

105. Chung HC, Arkenau HT, Wyrwicz L, et al. Avelumab (MSB0010718C; anti-PD-L1) in patients with advanced gastric or gastroesophageal junction cancer from JAVELIN solid tumor phase Ib trial: Analysis of safety and clinical activity. Paper presented at: ASCO Annual Meeting Proceedings. Chicago, 2016.

106. Maron SB, LJ, Hovey R, et al. Molecular characterization of T-cell-inflamed gastric carcinoma. WIN Symposium, June 28, 2016, Paris.

107. Bockorny B, Pectasides E. The emerging role of immunotherapy in gastric and esophageal adenocarcinoma. Future Oncol 2016;12(15):1833–46.

108. Melero I, Hervas-Stubbs S, Glennie M, et al. Immunostimulatory monoclonal antibodies for cancer therapy. Nat Rev Cancer 2007;7(2):95–106.

109. Ralph C, Elkord E, Burt DJ, et al. Modulation of lymphocyte regulation for cancer therapy: a phase II trial of tremelimumab in advanced gastric and esophageal adenocarcinoma. Clin Cancer Res 2010;16(5):1662–72.

110. Moehler MH, Cho JY, Kim YH, et al. A randomized, open-label, two-arm phase II trial comparing the efficacy of sequential ipilimumab (ipi) versus best supportive care (BSC) following first-line (1L) chemotherapy in patients with unresectable, locally advanced/metastatic (A/M) gastric or gastro-esophageal junction (G/GEJ) cancer. ASCO Meeting Abstracts 2016;34(15 Suppl):4011. Available at: http://meetinglibrary.asco.org/content/166431-176.

111. Catenacci DV. Expansion platform type II: testing a treatment strategy. Lancet Oncol 2015;16(13):1276–8.

Current Progress in Human Epidermal Growth Factor Receptor 2 Targeted Therapies in Esophagogastric Cancer

Yelena Y. Janjigian, MD[a], Maria Ignez Braghiroli, MD[b],*

KEYWORDS

- Esophagogastric cancer • HER2 • Targeted therapy • Trastuzumab • Pertuzumab
- TDM-1 • Lapatinib

KEY POINTS

- Approximately 20% of EGC have ERBB2 (HER2) gene amplification or oncoprotein over-expression and HER2-directed therapy improves the outcome in metastatic disease.
- Immunohistochemistry analysis for EGC has different parameters than for breast cancer and requires a trained pathologist for evaluation.
- Trastuzumab is the standard treatment in combination with chemotherapy for HER2-positive advanced EGC.
- Studies investigating the use of HER2-directed therapy in early stages of disease are ongoing.
- HER2-directed imaging and patient-derived xenografts might be a useful tool to guide patient treatment and research.

INTRODUCTION

Gastric cancer is the third leading cause of cancer-related deaths worldwide.[1] Most patients are diagnosed with advanced disease and have a median overall survival (OS) of less than 1 year when treated with available cytotoxic chemotherapy.[2] HER2 is a validated therapeutic target in metastatic esophagogastric cancer (EGC). The HER2 proto-oncogene is located on chromosome 17q21 and encodes the 185-kDa transmembrane tyrosine kinase receptor HER2 (also known as HER2/neu, ERBB2, p185). Similarly to breast cancer, the prognosis of patients with HER2 amplified EGC improved when anti-HER2 therapy was added to conventional chemotherapy.[3] Overall, the HER2-positivity rate is around 20% for EGC, with variances according

[a] Gastrointestinal Oncology Service, Memorial Sloan Kettering Cancer Center, Weill Cornell Medical College, 300 East 66th Street, Room 1033, New York, NY 10065, USA; [b] Gastrointestinal Oncology Service, Memorial Sloan Kettering Cancer Center, 300 East 66th Street, Room 1033, New York, NY 10065, USA
* Corresponding author.
E-mail address: ignezbraghiroli@gmail.com

Surg Oncol Clin N Am 26 (2017) 313–324
http://dx.doi.org/10.1016/j.soc.2016.10.005
surgonc.theclinics.com

to tumor histologic subtype and location.[4] The rates of HER2 positivity are the highest in esophagogastric junction and stomach cardia tumors, which is up to 30%.[3] In the mid and distal stomach, it is approximately 15% to 20%, and less than 5% of diffuse or signet ring cell type tumors are positive for HER2 amplification.[5,6]

DIAGNOSIS

Based on the benefit seen from HER2-directed therapy for advanced EGC, testing is currently recommended to all patients on diagnosis. Accurate assessment of HER2 status is essential to determine which patients will benefit from therapy. The test for HER2 in breast cancer is performed using immunohistochemistry (IHC), which shows the HER2 protein expression, and/or fluorescence in situ hybridization (FISH) or chromogenic in situ hybridization, which detects gene amplification.

For EGC, IHC evaluation uses parameters distinct from breast cancer. It is suggested that application of breast cancer scoring to gastric cancer may produce up to 50% false-negative rates on IHC.[7] In comparison with breast cancer, EGC has a higher incidence of tumor heterogeneity. Pathologists should be aware that more focal staining is common in EGC. Expression is mainly restricted to intestinal-type gland-forming cells, and there is incomplete, often basolateral or only lateral membranous IHC staining distribution, appearing as discontinuous HER2 membrane reactivity.[8] A positive IHC in the gastric cancer–specific scoring includes a strong but incomplete membrane staining in greater than or equal to 10% of the cells or greater than or equal to five clustered cells.[9] These criteria showed a high level of concordance between the IHC and FISH testing.

The current recommendation for HER2 evaluation in EGC is that IHC should be the first test performed, using validated assays. Results of IHC 3+, or a FISH ratio of the average HER2 gene copy number to chromosome 17 centromere (HER2/CEP17) greater than or equal to 2.0, are considered positive. Samples with equivocal IHC scores of 2+ should be retested by FISH or other in situ methods. IHC 0 to 1+ is considered HER2 negative.[10]

LOCALLY ADVANCED DISEASE

Currently, there are no definitive data supporting the use of anti-HER2 agents in the adjuvant or neoadjuvant treatment of patients with EGC (Table 1). Based on the encouraging results published with anti-HER2 therapies for localized breast cancer and together with the findings in advanced esophagogastric tumors, anti-HER2 therapies are now under investigation for earlier disease stages.

In 2013, a Spanish, multicenter, phase II study called NEOHX was initially presented and the final results were updated in 2015 (NCT01130337). This study evaluated the efficacy and toxicity profile for perioperative XELOX-T (capecitabine, oxaliplatin, and trastuzumab) followed by 12 cycles of adjuvant trastuzumab in monotherapy for patients with HER2-positive locally advanced but resectable stomach or esophagogastric-junction adenocarcinoma. The primary end point was disease-free survival (DFS) at 18 months and secondary end points included pathologic complete response rate (pCR), R0 resection rate, overall response rate, toxicity of preoperative treatment, and biomarker expression. A total of 63 patients were included. Before surgery, five patients stopped treatment because of toxicity. The overall response rate was 39%. Surgery was performed in 31 patients and 28 (78%) had an R0 procedure. Three patients had pCR (8.3%). After surgical resection, postoperative XELOX-T was administered to 24 patients, 22 of whom underwent trastuzumab monotherapy. With a median follow-up of 24.1 months, the 18-month DFS was 71% (95% confidence

Table 1
Completed clinical studies using anti-HER2 therapies in advanced EGC

Study	Phase	Treatment Line	N	Treatment	Response Rate (%)	Overall Survival (mo)	P
TOGA[3]	III	1	594	Cis + 5-FU	35	11.1	P = ·0046
				Cis + 5-FU + Trastuzumab	47	13.8	
LOGIC[18]	III	1	545	XELOX	39	10.5	P = .3492
				XELOX + Lapatinib	53	12.2	
TyTAN[19]	III	≥2	261	Paclitaxel	9	8.9	P = .1044
				Paclitaxel + Lapatinib	27	11.0	
GATSBY[21]	II/III	≥2	415	Taxane	19.6	8.6	P = .86
				TDM-1	20.6	7.9	
NEOHX[11]	II	Perioperative	63	XELOX-T	39	NR	—
AIO-STO-0310[12]	II	Perioperative	57	FLOT-T	56.2	NR	—

interval [CI], 53%–83%), the 24-month DFS was 60%, and median DFS and OS had not been reached.[11]

The AIO-STO-0310, a German study reported in 2014, was a multicenter phase-II trial testing perioperative chemotherapy with 5-FU, leucovorin, docetaxel, and oxaliplatin (FLOT) in combination with trastuzumab for patients with HER2-positive, locally advanced, resectable adenocarcinoma of the gastroesophageal junction or stomach (NCT01472029). The primary end point was the rate of centrally tested pCR. Fifty-seven patients were included and 69% of them were able to complete all treatment proposed in the study. Twelve patients (21.1%) had a pCR. The R0 resection rate was 93%. There were no unexpected treatment safety findings as described by the investigators.[12]

Among the ongoing trials there is a European study (INNOVATION-TRIAL) and the Radiation Therapy Oncology Group (RTOG) 1010. The first is a phase II study of perioperative treatment of patients with HER2-positive resectable gastric or gastroesophageal junction adenocarcinoma (NCT02205047). Patients are randomized into one of the three arms: (1) standard chemotherapy (cisplatin/capecitabine or cisplatin/5-fluorouracil), (2) standard chemotherapy plus trastuzumab, or (3) standard chemotherapy plus trastuzumab and pertuzumab. Pertuzumab is a humanized monoclonal antibody that binds to extracellular dimerization domain II of HER2, and inhibits heterodimerization of HER2 with other HER family members receptors, especially HER2–HER3, which is the most potent signaling HER heterodimer. The primary end point is the rate of major pathologic response (ie, <10% viable tumor cells present in the pathologic specimen).[13]

The RTOG 1010 is a phase III trial evaluating radiation, paclitaxel, carboplatin with or without trastuzumab in locally advanced HER2 overexpressing esophageal and gastroesophageal junction adenocarcinoma (NCT01196390). The primary end point is DFS. The trial completed accrual and the estimated final data collection for the primary outcome is August 2018.[14]

In the postoperative setting there is a Turkish phase II, single arm, open-label study called TOXAG evaluating the safety and efficacy of the combination oxaliplatin, capecitabine, trastuzumab, and radiation as adjuvant treatment of patients with curatively resected HER2-positive gastric or gastroesophageal junction cancer. Patients will receive concurrent chemotherapy with radiation. Trastuzumab will be continued after radiation for a total of 12 months. The expected completion date is December 2017.[15]

ADVANCED DISEASE
Trastuzumab

Trastuzumab, a monoclonal antibody directed against HER2 receptor, is the first targeted agent approved for the treatment of advanced EGC. The randomized phase III trial that led to the approval of was published in 2010 and is known as the ToGA (Trastuzumab for Gastric Cancer) trial.[3] At that time, previous preclinical models of HER2-overexpressing human gastric cancer xenografts suggested that trastuzumab had some activity when used alone but results were better when it was combined with different chemotherapy drugs. The agents most active were a fluorinated pyrimidine or cisplatin, or both (see Table 1).[16]

In the ToGA study, patients with advanced HER2-positive adenocarcinoma of the stomach or gastroesophagic junction, without previous treatment of metastatic disease, were randomized to receive trastuzumab at an initial dose of 8 mg/kg intravenously followed by 6 mg/kg intravenously every 3 weeks plus capecitabine, or fluorouracil and cisplatin, or chemotherapy alone. The primary end point was OS. In total, 594 patients were included from centers in Asia, Central and South America, and Europe. The trial was closed after the second interim analyses. The median OS in the group treated with trastuzumab was 13.8 months compared with 11.1 months in the control group (hazard ratio [HR], 0.74; 95% CI, 0.60–0.91; P = .0046); progression-free survival was 6.7 versus 5.5 months (HR, 0.71; 95% CI, 0.59–0.85; P = .0002), and overall response rate was 47% versus 35% (P = .0017), respectively.[3] The side effects were comparable between both study groups and grade 3 or 4 toxicities included mainly neutropenia, anemia, nausea, anorexia, and vomiting. Cardiac events, a major concern in patients with breast cancer especially when trastuzumab and anthracyclines are part of the treatment, were rare in this study and cardiac toxicity rate was less than 1% and not different from patients treated with chemotherapy alone.

The FISH test is generally considered positive for HER2 amplification when the HER2/CEP17 ratio is greater than or equal to 2.0, which was one criterion for HER2 positivity on the TOGA trial. A preplaned exploratory analyses showed that the greatest OS benefit with trastuzumab was seen in patients who had tumors with high HER2 protein expression by IHC (HR, 0.65; median OS, 16.0 vs 11.8 months).[5] More recently, a Spanish study analyzed data on 66 patients with HER2 amplification who received anti-HER2 therapy associated with chemotherapy and correlated with clinical outcomes. In this study, the mean HER2/CEP17 ratio of 4.7 (95% CI, 4.0–6.8) was the optimal cutoff value for discriminating between sensitive and refractory patients treated with trastuzumab-based chemotherapy.[17] This criterion, however, has not been validated in clinical practice.

Based on these results, the Food and Drug Administration approved this combination of trastuzumab, cisplatin, and a fluoropyrimidine for the first-line treatment of patients with HER2-positive advanced adenocarcinoma of the esophagogastric junction and the stomach.

Lapatinib

Lapatinib is a small-molecule tyrosine kinase inhibitor that targets HER2 and epidermal growth factor receptor (EGFR). Lapatinib is approved by the US Food and Drug Administration for use in metastatic HER2-positive breast cancer that is refractory to trastuzumab, in combination with capecitabine. The role of lapatinib in the treatment of advanced EGC has been investigated in two phase III studies.

The phase III LOGiC (Lapatinib in Combination With Capecitabine Plus Oxaliplatin in Human Epidermal Growth Factor Receptor 2–Positive Advanced or Metastatic Gastric, Esophageal, or Gastroesophageal Adenocarcinoma) trial studied the use of capecitabine and oxaliplatin with or without lapatinib in the first-line setting for HER2-positive esophagogastric adenocarcinoma with the primary end point of OS.[18] A total of 545 patients were included and the median follow-up was 23 months. Although the final results are negative because there was no statistically significant improvement in OS (12.2 vs 10.5 months; HR, 0.91; 95% CI, 0.73–1.12; $P = .3492$), the response rate was higher in the lapatinib arm (53% vs 39%; $P = .0031$). More patients experienced serious toxicities in the lapatinib arm compared with chemotherapy only, including diarrhea, nausea, vomiting, and fatigue.

In the phase III TyTAN study (Lapatinib Plus Paclitaxel vs Paclitaxel Alone in the Second-Line Treatment of HER2-Amplified Advanced Gastric Cancer in Asian Populations) enrolled patients with HER2-positive EGC after progression on a first-line therapy.[19] The primary end point was OS and they included 261 patients. Median OS was 11.0 months with lapatinib plus paclitaxel versus 8.9 months with paclitaxel alone. This difference was not statistically significant (HR, 0.84; 95% CI, 0.64–1.11; $P = .1044$). Again, there was an increase in the response rate in the lapatinib arm (27% vs 9%).

In breast cancer, HER2 amplification by FISH is a stronger predictor of benefit from lapatinib than HER2 overexpression by IHC. Similarly, in the TyTAN study, those who were treated with lapatinib and whose tumors were strongly HER2 FISH-positive/IHC 3+ had better OS (HR, 0.59; $P = .0176$).[19]

Trastuzumab Emtansine

Trastuzumab emtansine (T-DM1), an antibody-drug conjugate consisting of the trastuzumab linked to the cytotoxic agent emtansine,[20] was explored in the second-line treatment of HER2-positive EGC after trastuzumab progression in the GATSBY trial that was presented in 2016.

The GATSBY trial was initially designed as a three-arm randomized, phase II/III global study of T-DM1 versus a taxane drug in patients with HER2-positive unresectable EGC who had received first-line treatment including a fluoropyrimidine plus platinum agent with or without a HER2-targeted therapy. At first, patients were randomized to T-DM1 3.6 mg/kg every 3 weeks, T-DM1 2.4 mg/kg weekly, or the physician's choice of paclitaxel or docetaxel. After an independent data monitoring committee selected T-DM1 weekly for further study the patients were then randomized to either T-DM1 weekly or a taxane. The primary end point was OS. A total of 415 patients were randomized. The results showed a median OS of 8.6 months for the group treated with a taxane and 7.9 months for the group treated with T-DM1. Objective response rates were 19.6% and 20.6% in the groups treated with a taxane and T-DM1 respectively. Based on these results, T-DM1 showed no benefit in the second-line treatment when compared with a taxane[21] and therefore no standard exists for HER2-directed therapy after trastuzumab progression.

Pertuzumab

Pertuzumab in an antibody that binds to the extracellular domain of HER2 at a different epitope than trastuzumab leading to a more complete blockade of HER2-mediated signal transduction when used in combination with trastuzumab.[22] The JACOB trial explored first-line pertuzumab with trastuzumab and chemotherapy in patients with

HER2-positive metastatic gastric or gastroesophageal junction cancer, and results are expected in 2016 (NCT01774786).[23]

FUNCTIONAL IMAGING

Patients diagnosed with EGC should be tested for HER2 amplification with IHC or FISH and considered for treatment with HER2-directed therapy if the results are positive. HER2 expression can vary over the course of therapy and over the course of the disease.[24,25] Also, HER2 expression may be discordant between the primary tumor and the metastatic lesions.[26] However, repeating multiple biopsies along disease course and therapy may not be feasible or even safe for most patients. A noninvasive method that could access HER2 expression in individual lesions would be an interesting tool in identifying patients who benefit from HER2-targeted therapy.

Specific uptake of molecular biomarkers can be achieved using radiolabeled targeting agents, such as antibodies directed against tumor-associated antigens like HER2 or other cellular receptors. This might be useful to differentiate between HER2-positive and -negative tumors and also to investigate intratumoral and intertumoral heterogeneity in a less invasive approach. An additional benefit would be the possibility to monitor treatment results based on the level of tumor-associated antigen expression.[27]

Specifically for HER2-positive tumors, active investigation has been devoted to radiolabeled trastuzumab. It has been previously combined with 111In, 64Cu, and 89Zr, for in vivo single-photon emission computed tomography and PET imaging of HER2-positive xenograft models of ovarian and breast cancer.[28–31] Because of an extended half-life of 78 hours and its stable ligand disassociation in human serum, 89Zr seems to be an ideal radionuclide for its use.[32] Initial testing in murine models with 89Zr-trastuzumab showed that the accumulation of the tracer was HER2 specific.[33] The first in-human experience was published in 2010 and included 14 patients with metastatic breast cancer. Overall, the uptake of 89Zr-trastuzumab in the tumor lesions in the liver, lung, and bone was high. Moreover, unknown brain metastases were detected. In this study, HER2-overexpressing lesions could be distinguished from non-HER2-expressing lesions. There was no infusion reactions appreciated.[32]

A study using afatinib, a highly selective, irreversible inhibitor of the HER2 family of tyrosine kinase receptors EGFR, HER2, and HER4, in human HER2-positive gastric xenograft models the utility of ^{89}Zr-trastuzumab PET.[27] The ^{89}Zr-trastuzumab PET was demonstrated to be highly specific for HER2-positive gastric tumors, whereas ^{18}F-fluorodeoxyglucose and ^{18}F-fluorothymidine PET were unable to differentiate HER2-positive from HER2-negative tumors. In the NCI-N87 HER2-positive xenografts there was a high degree of accumulation of ^{89}Zr-trastuzumab. To monitor the changes in ^{89}Zr-trastuzumab PET uptake related to therapy, NCI-N87 xenograft–bearing mice were treated with either vehicle or afatinib daily for 21 consecutive days and monitored by PET imaging. Although ^{18}F-fluorodeoxyglucose uptake did not change significantly over time, the ^{89}Zr-trastuzumab tumor uptake decreased, especially over the first 14 days of treatment, reflecting a reduction in tumor weight and decrease in total HER2 as measured by immunoblot and IHC. A pilot study of ^{89}Zr-trastuzumab PET in patients with HER2-positve esophagogastric adenocarcinoma is ongoing (NCT02023996).

GENOMICS OF ESOPHAGOGASTRIC CANCER

As molecular profiling with next-generation sequencing became more widely available, several gene mutations and pathway alterations were linked to different tumors and their pathogenesis, with possible implication for treatment. The data allow a more comprehensive understanding of the acquired genetic, genomic, and epigenetic alterations in cancer cells that could potentially be translated into clinical and therapeutic advances.

The Cancer Genome Atlas reported an analysis of whole-genome sequencing of gastric adenocarcinomas, along with evaluation of DNA copy number, gene expression, and methylation profiling, showed four molecularly distinct tumor subtypes[34]:

1. High Epstein-Barr virus burden (9% of samples) with PIK3CA mutations, PD-L1/2 amplification.
2. Microsatellite instability high tumors (22% of samples) with frequent mutation rates and promoter hypermethylation. The remaining two groups were distinguished by the presence or absence of extensive somatic copy-number aberrations.
3. Chromosomally unstable chromosomal instable (50% of samples) tumors with frequent oncogenic amplifications.
4. Chromosomally stable/diffuse type (20% of samples) tumors with novel mutations of RHOA. Within the 215 nonhypermutated tumors, significantly mutated genes were identified including TP53, ARID1A, KRAS, PIK3CA, RNF43, APC, CTNNB1, SMAD4 and SMAD2, RASA1, and ERBB2.

At Memorial Sloan Kettering Cancer Center, next-generation sequencing is performed using the IMPACT assay (Integrated Mutation Profiling of Actionable Cancer Targets) capable of identifying point mutations, small insertion/deletion events (indels), and large gene-level and intragenic copy number aberrations in 410 cancer-associated genes. Analysis of gastric adenocarcinoma samples revealed an overall increase in alterations in receptor tyrosine kinases and KRAS, PI3-kinase pathway genes, and SMAD4. In the 28 patients with pretrastuzumab and posttrastuzumab exposure testing, there was loss of HER2 amplification in four patients; new amplifications of MET, EGFR, and insulin-like growth factor 1 receptor; mutations in ERBB4, KRAS, PIK3CA, and MTOR; and loss of function of PTEN. The KRAS and PIK3CA mutations are known activating mutations; the ERBB4 and MTOR mutations had unknown significance.[35]

PATIENT-DRIVEN XENOGRAFTS

In general, malignant tumors used to be treated based on their primary location only, and histologic subtypes did not distinguish clinical outcomes. More recently molecular findings are used as important guides for therapy. Still, there are heterogeneous tumor characteristics and clinic outcomes, which is a reflex of the complex mechanisms driving each tumor individually.

Patient-derived xenografts (PDXs) are models developed by transplanting human tumors into immunocompromized mice and have been suggested as a more reflective preclinical cancer model.[36]

Recently, PDX models emerged as a promising translational platform that more accurately predicts human malignancy behavior and may improve the development of effective therapeutics.[37] The tumors are implanted either heterotopically or orthotopically. In the heterotopic PDX model the tumors are implanted into the subcutaneous tissue of the mouse. Orthotopic models involve direct implantation of the tumor into a specific mouse organ.[38] Limitations include the actual process, which is still labor intensive and expensive; the variable rates of engraftment; the inconsistent latency period of the graft; and, more importantly, that models are approximations of the real situation, but not the real situation itself.[39,40]

PDX models in EGC are being studied by our group at Memorial Sloan Kettering. Both heterotopic and orthotopic models using nonobese diabetic/severe combined immunodeficient mouse have been developed. The established PDXs include HER2-positive trastuzumab refractory models, MET-positive models, and signet ring gastric models from patients with germ line CDH1 mutation. The tumor engraftment rates are 46% for orthotopic tumors and 26% for heterotopic implants.[41] These models could be a promising tool to access differences in tumor biology and to guide treatment and trial development. Given the increasing importance of immunity in cancer treatment, the development of PDX models in hosts with humanized immune systems is an emerging approach that requires further study.[42]

MECHANISMS OF RESISTANCE

HER2 is part of a family of transmembrane receptor tyrosine kinases, which includes HER1 (also known as EGFR), HER3, and HER4. When a ligand binds to the receptor, there is either dimerization between two molecules of the same receptor or between two different receptors. When activated, the triggered cascade of signal transduction includes the activation of the Ras-Raf-MAPK signaling pathway and the PI3K-AKT-mTOR signaling pathway, resulting in effects on various cellular processes, including proliferation, apoptosis, adhesion, migration, and differentiation.[43]

The most accepted mechanism by which trastuzumab acts is the inhibition of the MAPK and PI3K/Akt pathways, leading to cell cycle arrest, suppression of cell growth, and proliferation.[44] Patients who are treated with trastuzumab as first-line treatment of advanced EGC experience treatment failure after a median of approximately 6.7 months based on the ToGA results. There are no standard of care HER2-directed options for trastuzumab resistance. The mechanisms by which the tumors stop responding to trastuzumab are under investigation and seem to be related to structural changes in the receptor, alterations in other tyrosine kinases receptors, or alterations in intracellular signaling pathways.[44]

In regard to the HER2 receptor, a truncated isoform called p95HER2 has constitutive kinase activity and no outer cell domain to permit trastuzumab binding. This could be caused by proteolysis or a consequence of mRNA translocation via an alternative route. Reports describe an incidence in up to 30% of HER2-positive tumors[45] and although it is a mechanism of trastuzumab resistance, preclinical data suggest that tumors could still respond to treatment with Lapatinib.[46] The experience at Memorial Sloan Kettering showed that based on biopsy after disease progression on trastuzumab, 34% of the patients had lost HER2 positivity when analyzed by IHC and FISH.[35,47]

The overexpression of HER3 receptors is another mechanism that could result in dimerization and downstream activation. Trastuzumab does not bind to this receptor and HER3 signaling may be a means to overcome the trastuzumab-mediated inhibition of HER2.[48] The phosphorylated EGFR and EGFR/HER2 heterodimers are also not inhibited by trastuzumab and have been shown in cell cultures and xenografts to be a form of treatment resistance.[49] In EGC, EGFR is frequently overexpressed and MKN7 gastric cancer cells, which are insensitive to trastuzumab, when treated with an EGFR tyrosine kinase inhibitor, the sensitivity to trastuzumab is again restored.[49]

One of the most investigated mechanisms involved in trastuzumab resistance is the loss of activity of PTEN.[50] Patients with PTEN-deficient breast cancers have poorer response to trastuzumab compared with those with normal PTEN.[50] In vitro studies on gastric cancer cells with induced resistance to trastuzumab showed that PTEN expression was significantly decreased at the genetic and protein expression level and the phosphorylation of the AKT protein was upregulated.[51,52] These alterations may be one of the most the most prevalent trastuzumab resistance pathways.

The insulin-like growth factor 1 receptor induces the pathways including Ras-Raf-MAPK and PI3K-AKT. In vitro studies have shown that insulin-like growth factor 1 receptor has upregulation of phosphorylation in gastric cancer cell lines that were resistant to trastuzumab, possibly indicating that these signaling pathways might be involved in a resistance mechanism.[52,53]

Also, activating mutations or amplification in PI3K could result in enhanced activity of Akt, which potentially reduces the effectiveness of trastuzumab therapy.[54] The previously mentioned data suggest the need for repeat biopsy, in part to assess potential loss of HER2 expression, to decide on whether or not to continue anti-HER2-based therapy on disease progression.

SUMMARY

HER2-positive EGC is a population under special investigation because of the new medications being developed as treatment options. Most of the knowledge so far was derived from the findings in breast cancer but it is known that EGC has its own peculiarities. Mechanisms of drug resistance and molecular imaging techniques studied might help clinicians understand better the behavior of the tumors and how to better manage patients, and these are areas of active investigation.

REFERENCES

1. Ferlay J, Soerjomataram I, Dikshit R, et al. Cancer incidence and mortality worldwide: sources, methods and major patterns in GLOBOCAN 2012. Int J Cancer 2014;136(5):E359–86.
2. Wagner AD, Unverzagt S, Grothe W, et al. Chemotherapy for advanced gastric cancer. Cochrane Database Syst Rev 2010;(3):CD004064.
3. Bang YJ, Van Cutsem E, Feyereislova A, et al. Trastuzumab in combination with chemotherapy versus chemotherapy alone for treatment of HER2-positive advanced gastric or gastro-oesophageal junction cancer (ToGA): a phase 3, open-label, randomised controlled trial. Lancet 2010;376(9742):687–97.
4. Van Cutsem E, Bang YJ, Feng-Yi F, et al. HER2 screening data from ToGA: targeting HER2 in gastric and gastroesophageal junction cancer. Gastric Cancer 2014; 18(3):476–84.
5. Bang Y, Chung H, Xu J, et al. Pathological features of advanced gastric cancer (GC): relationship to human epidermal growth factor receptor 2 (HER2) positivity in the global screening programme of the ToGA trial. J Clin Oncol 2009;27(15 suppl) [abstract: 4556].
6. Tanner M, Hollmen M, Junttila TT, et al. Amplification of HER-2 in gastric carcinoma: association with Topoisomerase IIalpha gene amplification, intestinal type, poor prognosis and sensitivity to trastuzumab. Ann Oncol 2005;16(2):273–8.
7. Ruschoff J, Dietel M, Baretton G, et al. HER2 diagnostics in gastric cancer-guideline validation and development of standardized immunohistochemical testing. Virchows Arch 2010;457(3):299–307.
8. Ruschoff J, Hanna W, Bilous M, et al. HER2 testing in gastric cancer: a practical approach. Mod Pathol 2012;25(5):637–50.
9. Hofmann M, Stoss O, Shi D, et al. Assessment of a HER2 scoring system for gastric cancer: results from a validation study. Histopathology 2008;52(7): 797–805.

10. Yano T, Doi T, Ohtsu A, et al. Comparison of HER2 gene amplification assessed by fluorescence in situ hybridization and HER2 protein expression assessed by immunohistochemistry in gastric cancer. Oncol Rep 2006;15(1):65–71.

11. Rivera F, Jiménez-Fonseca P, Alfonso P, et al. NEOHX study: perioperative treatment with trastuzumab in combination with capecitabine and oxaliplatin (XELOX-T) in patients with HER-2 resectable stomach or esophagogastric junction (EGJ) adenocarcinoma—18 m DFS analysis. J Clin Oncol 2015;33(suppl 3) [abstract: 107].

12. Hofheinz R, Hegewisch-Becker S, Thuss-Patience PC, et al. HER-FLOT: trastuzumab in combination with FLOT as perioperative treatment for patients with HER2-positive locally advanced esophagogastric adenocarcinoma: a phase II trial of the AIO Gastric Cancer Study Group. J Clin Oncol 2014;32(suppl 5) [abstract: 4073].

13. (NCI) NCI. INNOVATION-TRIAL: radiation therapy, paclitaxel, and carboplatin with or without trastuzumab in treating patients with esophageal cancer (RTOG 1010 Trial); NCT02205047]. Available at: https://clinicaltrials.gov/ct2/show/NCT02205047?term=NCT02205047&rank=1. Accessed March10, 2016.

14. (NCI) NCI. RTOG 1010: Radiation therapy, paclitaxel, and carboplatin with or without trastuzumab in treating patients with esophageal cancer. Available at: https://clinicaltrials.gov/ct2/show/NCT01196390?term=NCT01196390&rank=1. Accessed March 10, 2016.

15. Roche H-L. A Study of the combination of oxaliplatin, capecitabine and herceptin (trastuzumab) and chemoradiotherapy in the adjuvant setting in operated patients with HER2+ gastric or gastro-esophageal junction cancer (TOXAG study). Available at: https://clinicaltrials.gov/ct2/show/NCT01748773?term=NCT01748773&rank=1. Accessed March 10, 2016.

16. Fujimoto-Ouchi K, Sekiguchi F, Yasuno H, et al. Antitumor activity of trastuzumab in combination with chemotherapy in human gastric cancer xenograft models. Cancer Chemother Pharmacol 2007;59(6):795–805.

17. Gomez-Martin C, Plaza JC, Pazo-Cid R, et al. Level of HER2 gene amplification predicts response and overall survival in HER2-positive advanced gastric cancer treated with trastuzumab. J Clin Oncol 2013;31(35):4445–52.

18. Hecht JR, Bang YJ, Qin SK, et al. Lapatinib in combination with capecitabine plus oxaliplatin in human epidermal growth factor receptor 2-positive advanced or metastatic gastric, esophageal, or gastroesophageal adenocarcinoma: TRIO-013/LOGiC-a randomized phase III trial. J Clin Oncol 2016;34(5):443–51.

19. Satoh T, Xu RH, Chung HC, et al. Lapatinib plus paclitaxel versus paclitaxel alone in the second-line treatment of HER2-amplified advanced gastric cancer in Asian populations: TyTAN–a randomized, phase III study. J Clin Oncol 2014;32(19):2039–49.

20. Barok M, Joensuu H, Isola J. Trastuzumab emtansine: mechanisms of action and drug resistance. Breast Cancer Res 2014;16(2):209.

21. Kang Y, Shah MA, Ohtsu A, et al. A randomized, open-label, multicenter, adaptive phase 2/3 study of trastuzumab emtansine (T-DM1) versus a taxane (TAX) in patients (pts) with previously treated HER2-positive locally advanced or metastatic gastric/gastroesophageal junction adenocarcinoma (LA/MGC/GEJC). J Clin Oncol 2016;34(suppl 4S) [abstract: 5].

22. Harbeck N, Beckmann MW, Rody A, et al. HER2 Dimerization inhibitor pertuzumab - mode of action and clinical data in breast cancer. Breast Care (Basel) 2014;8(1):49–55.

23. Tabernero J, Hoff PM, Shen L, et al. Pertuzumab (P) with trastuzumab (T) and chemotherapy (CTX) in patients (pts) with HER2-positive metastatic gastric or

gastroesophageal junction (GEJ) cancer: an international phase III study (JACOB). J Clin Oncol 2013;31(suppl) [abstract: TPS4150].

24. Rasbridge SA, Gillett CE, Seymour AM, et al. The effects of chemotherapy on morphology, cellular proliferation, apoptosis and oncoprotein expression in primary breast carcinoma. Br J Cancer 1994;70(2):335–41.

25. van de Ven S, Smit VT, Dekker TJ, et al. Discordances in ER, PR and HER2 receptors after neoadjuvant chemotherapy in breast cancer. Cancer Treat Rev 2010; 37(6):422–30.

26. Peng Z, Zou J, Zhang X, et al. HER2 discordance between paired primary gastric cancer and metastasis: a meta-analysis. Chin J Cancer Res 2015;27(2):163–71.

27. Janjigian YY, Viola-Villegas N, Holland JP, et al. Monitoring afatinib treatment in HER2-positive gastric cancer with 18F-FDG and 89Zr-trastuzumab PET. J Nucl Med 2013;54(6):936–43.

28. Capala J, Bouchelouche K. Molecular imaging of HER2-positive breast cancer: a step toward an individualized "image and treat" strategy. Curr Opin Oncol 2010; 22(6):559–66.

29. Milenic DE, Wong KJ, Baidoo KE, et al. Targeting HER2: a report on the in vitro and in vivo pre-clinical data supporting trastuzumab as a radioimmunoconjugate for clinical trials. MAbs 2010;2(5):550–64.

30. Mortimer JE, Bading JR, Colcher DM, et al. Functional imaging of human epidermal growth factor receptor 2-positive metastatic breast cancer using (64)Cu-DOTA-trastuzumab PET. J Nucl Med 2013;55(1):23–9.

31. Niu G, Li Z, Cao Q, et al. Monitoring therapeutic response of human ovarian cancer to 17-DMAG by noninvasive PET imaging with (64)Cu-DOTA-trastuzumab. Eur J Nucl Med Mol Imaging 2009;36(9):1510–9.

32. Dijkers EC, Oude Munnink TH, Kosterink JG, et al. Biodistribution of 89Zr-trastuzumab and PET imaging of HER2-positive lesions in patients with metastatic breast cancer. Clin Pharmacol Ther 2010;87(5):586–92.

33. Dijkers EC, Kosterink JG, Rademaker AP, et al. Development and characterization of clinical-grade 89Zr-trastuzumab for HER2/neu immunoPET imaging. J Nucl Med 2009;50(6):974–81.

34. Cancer Genome Atlas Research Network. Comprehensive molecular characterization of gastric adenocarcinoma. Nature 2014;513(7517):202–9.

35. Janjigian YY, Sanchez-Vega F, Tuvy Y, et al. Emergence of RTK/RAS/PI3K pathway alterations in trastuzumab-refractory HER2-positive esophagogastric (EG) tumors. J Clin Oncol 2016;34(suppl) [abstract: 11608].

36. Fichtner I, Slisow W, Gill J, et al. Anticancer drug response and expression of molecular markers in early-passage xenotransplanted colon carcinomas. Eur J Cancer 2004;40(2):298–307.

37. Choi YY, Lee JE, Kim H, et al. Establishment and characterisation of patient-derived xenografts as paraclinical models for gastric cancer. Sci Rep 2016;6:22172.

38. Siolas D, Hannon GJ. Patient-derived tumor xenografts: transforming clinical samples into mouse models. Cancer Res 2013;73(17):5315–9.

39. Aparicio S, Hidalgo M, Kung AL. Examining the utility of patient-derived xenograft mouse models. Nat Rev Cancer 2015;15(5):311–6.

40. Dangles-Marie V, Pocard M, Richon S, et al. Establishment of human colon cancer cell lines from fresh tumors versus xenografts: comparison of success rate and cell line features. Cancer Res 2007;67(1):398–407.

41. Janjigian YY, Vakiani E, Imtiaz T, et al. Patient-derived xenografts as models for the identification of predictive biomarkers in esophagogastric cancer. J Clin Oncol 2014;32(5s) [abstract 4059].

42. Kalscheuer H, Danzl N, Onoe T, et al. A model for personalized in vivo analysis of human immune responsiveness. Sci Transl Med 2012;4(125):125ra30.

43. Tai W, Mahato R, Cheng K. The role of HER2 in cancer therapy and targeted drug delivery. J Control Release 2010;146(3):264–75.

44. Vu T, Claret FX. Trastuzumab: updated mechanisms of action and resistance in breast cancer. Front Oncol 2012;2:62.

45. Tural D, Akar E, Mutlu H, et al. P95 HER2 fragments and breast cancer outcome. Expert Rev Anticancer Ther 2014;14(9):1089–96.

46. Scaltriti M, Rojo F, Ocana A, et al. Expression of p95HER2, a truncated form of the HER2 receptor, and response to anti-HER2 therapies in breast cancer. J Natl Cancer Inst 2007;99(8):628–38.

47. Lordick F, Janjigian YY. Clinical impact of tumour biology in the management of gastroesophageal cancer. Nat Rev Clin Oncol 2016;13(6):348–60.

48. Ma J, Lyu H, Huang J, et al. Targeting of erbB3 receptor to overcome resistance in cancer treatment. Mol Cancer 2014;13:105.

49. Ritter CA, Perez-Torres M, Rinehart C, et al. Human breast cancer cells selected for resistance to trastuzumab in vivo overexpress epidermal growth factor receptor and ErbB ligands and remain dependent on the ErbB receptor network. Clin Cancer Res 2007;13(16):4909–19.

50. Nagata Y, Lan KH, Zhou X, et al. PTEN activation contributes to tumor inhibition by trastuzumab, and loss of PTEN predicts trastuzumab resistance in patients. Cancer Cell 2004;6(2):117–27.

51. Wang JY, Huang TJ, Chen FM, et al. Mutation analysis of the putative tumor suppressor gene PTEN/MMAC1 in advanced gastric carcinomas. Virchows Arch 2003;442(5):437–43.

52. Zuo Q, Liu J, Zhang J, et al. Development of trastuzumab-resistant human gastric carcinoma cell lines and mechanisms of drug resistance. Sci Rep 2015;5:11634.

53. Zuo Q, Liu J, Zhang J, et al. Regulation of trastuzumab resistance in gastric cancer by the PTEN gene, downstream AKT, and bypass IGF-IR signaling pathway. J Clin Oncol 2014;32(suppl) [abstract: e22079].

54. Matsuoka T, Yashiro M. The role of PI3K/Akt/mTOR signaling in gastric carcinoma. Cancers (Basel) 2014;6(3):1441–63.

Nutritional Support in Esophagogastric Cancers

Elliott Birnstein, MD, Mark Schattner, MD*

KEYWORDS

- Malnutrition • Cachexia • Esophageal cancer • Gastric cancer • Enteral feeding
- Parenteral feeding • Immunonutrition

KEY POINTS

- Malnutrition is a common complication of esophageal and gastric cancers.
- Nutritional support is an important aspect of the multidisciplinary care that patients with these cancers require.
- For patients who undergo surgery, nutritional optimization before surgery has been shown to improve outcomes.
- Whenever possible, enteral nutritional support is preferred to parenteral nutrition.
- Nutritional support, either enteral or parental, carries the risk of complications and these should be weighed against the possible benefits when determining the appropriate management course.

INTRODUCTION

Malnutrition is a common complication of esophageal and gastric cancers and it is associated with poorer outcomes.[1] It can occur through multiple mechanisms, including increased metabolic demands, insufficient nutrient intake, or nutrient loss.[2] More specifically, these patients often have poor nutritional intake because of dysphagia, cancer cachexia, surgical resections and their complications, unresectable disease, strictures, chemotherapy, and radiotherapy effects.[3] For these reasons, nutritional support is a critical aspect of the multidisciplinary treatment required by these patients. For clinicians, malnutrition can be defined as an abnormal body composition with functional impairment of organs, caused by an acute or chronic imbalance between energy and protein availability and body requirements.[4] Cancer cachexia is an important aspect of these patients' malnutrition. It has come to carry multiple definitions, but recently Bozzetti and Mariani[5] defined it as a complex

Disclosure: The authors have nothing to disclose.
Division of Gastroenterology and Nutrition Service, Department of Medicine, Memorial Sloan Kettering Cancer Center, 1275 York Avenue, New York, NY 10065, USA
* Corresponding author.
E-mail address: schattnm@mskcc.org

Surg Oncol Clin N Am 26 (2017) 325–333
http://dx.doi.org/10.1016/j.soc.2016.10.003
1055-3207/17/© 2016 Elsevier Inc. All rights reserved.

surgonc.theclinics.com

syndrome characterized by a severe, chronic, unintentional, and progressive weight loss, which is poorly responsive to the conventional nutritional support, and may be associated with anorexia, asthenia, and early satiation. Hence the management of malnutrition and cancer cachexia in these patients is best accomplished via a multidisciplinary approach that includes clinical nutritionists, dieticians, gastroenterologists, medical oncologists, and surgeons.

In general, these patients can be classified into 2 groups: operable and nonoperable. The nonoperable patients can be further subdivided into those who will undergo chemotherapy and/or radiation and those who will receive palliative measures only. Each group of patients faces its own set of obstacles to maintaining adequate nutrition and each group requires a specific approach to nutritional support. For those patients who undergo surgery, there is a significant associated morbidity.[6,7] Undergoing surgery in a malnourished state increases the risk of morbidity. In these cases, nutritional support is an essential aspect of the patient's preoperative and postoperative management. For patients who do not undergo surgery but instead receive chemotherapy and/or radiation, nutritional support is also critical. These therapies can be very toxic to the gastrointestinal (GI) tract and negatively affect the patient's nutritional status. Early nutritional support should be provided when necessary.

Patients who undergo terminal or hospice-based care can present difficult ethical dilemmas regarding their nutrition. Patients and their families may see withdrawal or withholding of nutritional support as hastening death; however, studies have routinely shown that nutritional support in these patients provides no benefit (Box 1).

EPIDEMIOLOGY

In the United States in 2016, esophageal cancer has an estimated incidence of 14,550 new cases and 13,770 deaths are expected. In 2012, there were an estimated 455,800 new cases and 400,200 deaths occurred worldwide. In the United States in 2016, it is also estimated that there will be 22,280 cases of gastric cancer diagnosed and 11,430 deaths are expected.[8] According to the World Health Organization, there were

---

Box 1
Key definitions

Malnutrition

Abnormal body composition with functional impairment of organs, caused by an acute or chronic imbalance between energy and protein availability and body requirements.

Cancer cachexia

A complex syndrome characterized by a severe, chronic, unintentional, and progressive weight loss, which is poorly responsive to the conventional nutritional support and may be associated with anorexia, asthenia, and early satiation.

Enteral nutrition

Providing caloric needs via the GI tract by way of introducing formula either with an nasogastric tube or through percutaneous tubes such as percutaneous endoscopic gastrostomy or percutaneous endoscopic jejunostomy.

Parenteral nutrition

Providing caloric needs via an intravenous solution, which typically contains dextrose, amino acids, lipids, electrolytes, vitamins, and minerals.

952,000 new cases of gastric cancer worldwide and 723,000 deaths attributed to the disease in 2012.

Both of these diseases, because of the organs affected and the treatments they often require, are associated with a significant risk of malnutrition. In patients with esophageal and gastric cancers, malnutrition is reported in 60% to 85% of cases.[9]

MALNUTRITION AS A PROGNOSTIC FACTOR

Malnutrition has been shown to be an independent prognostic factor in patients with esophageal and gastric cancers. In patients with nonoperable esophageal and gastric cancers, Nozoe and colleagues[10] observed that the Prognostic Nutritional Index (PNI) was independently associated with long-term survival. The PNI is a simple tool, because it only requires the patient's albumin level and lymphocyte count to be calculated. Andreyev and colleagues[11] also showed that malnutrition was independently associated with poorer outcomes while undergoing chemotherapy. Malnutrition has also been shown to be an independent prognostic factor in patients who undergo surgical therapy.[12]

NUTRITIONAL SUPPORT IN OPERATIVE PATIENTS

Patients with esophageal and gastric cancers who undergo surgical therapy face considerable obstacles to maintaining nutrition. Malnutrition in these patients can occur because of the patients' inability to consume calories because of mechanical limitations caused by the tumors, such as dysphagia, odynophagia, and early satiety. It may be caused by tumor cachexia, as described earlier. In addition, malnutrition can be caused the effects of the surgeries, including early satiety, nausea, vomiting, pain, anastomotic leaks, and infections. For these patients, attention should be paid to nutritional support in the preoperative and postoperative settings, not only to prevent the long-term nutritional impact of the diagnosis but also to reduce perioperative morbidity and mortality. In a prospective study, Heneghan and colleagues[13] found that malabsorption and malnutrition were prevalent in patients undergoing curative resections of both gastric and esophageal cancers. A study of 205 patients who had undergone esophagectomy showed that 55% of these patients had lost more than 10% of their initial body weight at 1 year after surgery. At 5 years after surgery, 1-year weight loss was one of 3 factors, along with clinical stage and incomplete surgical resection, noted to negatively predict 5-year disease survival.[14]

For these patients, a comprehensive plan of nutrition support should be in place well before the surgery is performed. Mariette and colleagues[2] proposed that, for patients who cannot consume 75% of their goal calories (typically 25–30 kcal/kg/d), oral supplementation of calories should be performed. The investigators proposed that this can be accomplished through nutritional recommendations or dietetic advice as follows:

- Organize a timetable dividing the daily intake into 5 or 6 small meals, eaten in a pleasant environment and with enough time to eat.
- Because smaller volumes are tolerated best, food with high nutritional content should be presented in small quantities.
- Consider the patient's preference in relation to the presentation and preparation of the meals. Dietary recommendations to control symptoms frequently associated with esophageal cancer and gastric cancer include the following.
- In cases of anorexia: meals and drinks should be nutritionally enriched; give small volumes; take advantage of moments when the patient feels like eating.

- In cases of dysphagia: modify the consistency of food and give smaller quantities to ease swallowing and prevent fatigue (which could intensify dysphagia and increase the risk of aspiration); ensure that the patient is in the correct sitting position to ease the progression of the food bolus; avoid food accumulating in the mouth. For dysphagia to liquids, texture should be modified to a gelatinous or creamy consistency; for dysphagia to solids, prepare food with a softer texture.
- In cases of mucositis: eat slowly and take foods at room temperature; maintain optimum oral hygiene; give soft and smooth foods, chopped or mixed with liquids or sauces; avoid irritants, such as skins or spicy, acidic, or fried foods. This advice is intended to prevent the pain of mucositis, alleviate the oral dryness caused by a decrease and modification of saliva production, and improve the flavor of the food.

For patients who cannot consume greater than 50% of their nutritional requirements, enteral feeding is recommended. The route of administration of the enteral feedings depends on many factors, including the length of time the patient is expected to remain on enteral nutrition, the location of the tumor, and provider preference. For patients who require enteral nutrition for a limited period of time (<2–3 weeks), a nasogastric (NG) or nasojejunal tube is recommended. For patients who are likely to require enteral nutrition for an extended period of time, a percutaneous endoscopic gastrostomy (PEG) or percutaneous endoscopic jejunostomy (PEJ) is preferred.[2]

The patients who are not able to meet their nutritional requirements through oral feeding and are not candidates for enteral feeding may benefit from parenteral nutrition (Fig. 1).

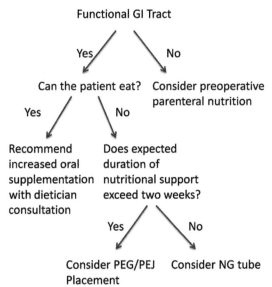

Fig. 1. Proposed nutritional support in a malnourished patient who is to undergo surgical therapy. (1) Determine whether the patient has a functional GI tract or not. (2) If the patient has a functional GI tract and can eat, the patient should attempt to attain the necessary calories via oral intake, with advice by a dietician. (3) If the patient has a functional GI tract but cannot eat, then enteral feeding should be considered. The decision on whether to use an NG tube or place a PEG should be based on the length of time the patient is expected to be receiving the enteral nutrition. If the patient does not have a functional GI tract, then parenteral nutrition should be considered.

NUTRITIONAL SUPPORT IN PATIENTS UNDERGOING CHEMOTHERAPY AND/OR RADIATION THERAPY

Patients with inoperable esophageal and gastric cancers who receive chemotherapy with or without radiation present with their own barriers to adequate nutrition. These patients can have significant toxicity from both the traditional chemotherapies used and radiation. In these patients, enteral nutrition has been shown to prevent weight loss during therapy.[4] Enteral nutritional support can be provided either via NG tube if the duration is expected to be less than 2 weeks or via a PEG/PEJ if the duration is expected to be greater than 2 weeks.

Regarding parenteral nutrition, patients who are malnourished and undergoing chemotherapy may gain some benefit from the use of parenteral nutrition when enteral nutrition is not feasible. Similarly, patients who develop GI toxicity related to their chemotherapy or radiation may tolerate short-term parenteral nutrition better than enteral feeding.[4]

IMMUNONUTRITION

Those patients with esophageal and gastric cancers who undergo surgery often undergo a decline in immune status and, consequently, increase in postoperative mortality and morbidity caused by infection.[2] Immunonutrient formulas are composed of higher omega-3 to omega-6 fatty acid ratios, arginine, nucleic acids, glutamine, and antioxidants compared with standard formulation, providing, in theory, a more antiinflammatory profile. Recent data show that perioperative immunonutrition can reduce infectious complications and length of stay before undergoing intervention in the setting of GI cancers.[15]

COMPLICATIONS OF NUTRITIONAL SUPPORT

Traditional nutritional support modalities such as enteral feeding with PEG or PEJ tubes and total parenteral nutrition (TPN) have risks and complications.

An overall complication rate of up to 70% for patients undergoing PEG placement has been reported; however, most of these complications are deemed to be minor.[16] These complications typically include peristomal leakage, minor bleeding, pain at the PEG or PEJ site, minor skin infections, and tube clogging. However, in about 1% to 2% of cases, patients have more serious complications, such as severe infection, visceral injury, tube dislodgement, buried bumper syndrome, and tumor seeding.[17]

For patients who receive parenteral nutrition, there is an increased risk of blood stream infections compared with patients who have central lines and are not on TPN.[18] Although less commonly used, parenteral nutrition also carries a risk of metabolic complications such as refeeding syndrome, hyperglycemia, Wernicke encephalopathy, and hepatic dysfunction. Even if these patients do not have any of these significant complications, parental feeding has a great effect on overall quality of life. It requires being connected to an intravenous line for a significant portion of the day, and frequent blood draws and doctor visits (Table 1).

PHARMACOTHERAPY

Pharmacotherapy can be an adjunctive therapeutic option in patients with gastric and esophageal cancers. The different classes of medications that have been used include antiemetics, progestational agents, cannabinoids, anabolic agents, and hormonal agents such as anamorelin (ghrelin receptor agonist).

Table 1
Complications of enteral and parental nutrition

Parental Nutrition	Enteral Nutrition
Bacteremia/fungemia	Peristomal leakage
Refeeding syndrome	Pain at tube site
Hyperglycemia	Bleeding
Wernicke encephalopathy	Infection
Hepatic dysfunction	Buried bumper syndrome
	Site metastases

Patients with esophageal and gastric cancers are at very high risk for nausea at any time during their treatment course. Antiemetic and prokinetic agents such as ondansetron and metoclopramide may be used as adjunctive therapies in patients in whom nausea is a primary barrier to oral nutrition.[19]

Progestagens such as megestrol acetate and medroxyprogesterone acetate are approved for the treatment of cancer-related anorexia and cancer cachexia syndrome. These drugs were originally used to treat hormone-sensitive tumors, but weight gain and appetite stimulation were noted to be major effects of the medications. Although their mechanism of action in unclear, these medications have been shown to stimulate weight gain and appetite in patients with cancer cachexia.[20]

The endocannabinoid system is a widespread intercellular signaling mechanism that plays a critical role in body homeostasis. This system is involved in food intake and energy expenditure, and coordinates energy balance. For this reason, cannabinoids have been used in patients with cancer cachexia. Dronabinol has been shown to be effective in stimulating appetite and treating nausea. This class of medication has a significant side effect profile and caution must be used, especially in the elderly and in cannabinoid-naive patients, because of the sedative and hallucinogenic properties of the drugs.[21,22]

Hormonal therapies, more specifically those involved in hunger and satiety, are a growing area of research in the treatment of cancer cachexia such as that seen in patients with gastric and esophageal cancers. Activation of the ghrelin receptor has been shown to increase food intake and body weight.[23] Anamorelin, an oral ghrelin receptor agonist, has been shown to increase lean body mass compared with placebo in patients with cancer cachexia.[24]

PALLIATION AND END-OF-LIFE CONSIDERATIONS

For patients with advanced esophageal cancers in whom dysphagia caused by tumor burden is a significant symptom, esophageal stenting may be a palliative measure. This palliative measure could apply to both patients who continue to undergo therapy and for patients who are to continue on hospice care.[25]

For those patients who continue on hospice care, difficult ethical issues regarding nutrition may arise. For patients with incurable cancers, studies have shown that home enteral nutrition is associated with a significant decrease in overall quality of life.[26] Home parenteral nutrition is also controversial. The current European Society for Clinical Nutrition and Metabolism guidelines recommend that parenteral nutrition should only be considered in patients whose survival is expected to exceed 2 to 3 months.[27]

SUMMARY

The treatment of patients with esophageal and gastric cancers is a complicated endeavor. Among many obstacles, these patients present with barriers to adequate nutritional status. It is critical to first identify these patients and then initiate them on a nutritional support regimen in accordance with their proposed treatment plans. Significant malnutrition in patients who undergo therapy for esophageal and gastric cancers is clearly associated with increased morbidity and mortality, reduced treatment efficacy, and increased hospital stay.

For those patients who are to undergo surgery, nutritional support may be required in the preoperative, perioperative, and/or postoperative setting. This support may be accomplished via increased oral intake with specialized diets and dietician counseling or it may require a more aggressive intervention such as a PEG or PEJ or, if the GI tract is not viable, parenteral nutrition.

Patients who receive chemotherapy and/or radiation tend to have a certain set of causes of malnutrition mainly related to the toxic effects of the chemotherapies and radiation that can include nausea, vomiting, diarrhea, abdominal pain, odynophagia, and so forth. Enteral and parenteral nutritional support can be used to keep these patients on their treatment regimens despite significantly reduced oral intake. Immunonutrition consists of a combination of arginine, glutamine, polyunsaturated omega-3 fatty acids, nucleotides, and antioxidant micronutrients. Preoperative and perioperative immunonutrition, which can be administered parenterally, enterally, or orally, has been shown to decrease rates of postoperative infection complications and length of hospital stay. It has not been shown to affect postoperative mortality.[28–34]

Although nutritional support is generally safe, there are associated risks. The main risks associated with enteral nutrition involve the placement of, and complications related to, PEGs and PEJs. The complications are mostly minor, but can be catastrophic in rare cases. Parenteral nutrition presents its own set of complications, ranging from hyperglycemia to bacteremia and fungemia with sepsis. For these reasons, it is important to only use parenteral and enteral nutrition in those settings in which the benefits clearly outweigh the risks.

A setting in which the boundary between those benefits and risks may be less clear is in the area of hospice and palliative care. Patients who have incurable disease and are no longer candidates for further treatment should not be offered nutritional support because it is likely to only cause decreased quality of life and provide no benefit in terms of mortality reduction.

REFERENCES

1. Van Cutsem E, Arends J. The causes and consequences of cancer-associated malnutrition. Eur J Oncol Nurs 2005;9(Suppl 2):S51–63.
2. Mariette C, De Botton ML, Piessen G. Surgery in esophageal and gastric cancer patients: what is the role for nutrition support in your daily practice? Ann Surg Oncol 2012;19(7):2128–34.
3. Miller KR, Bozeman MC. Nutrition therapy issues in esophageal cancer. Curr Gastroenterol Rep 2012;14(4):356–66.
4. Bozzetti F. Nutritional support in patients with oesophageal cancer. Support Care Cancer 2009;18(S2):41–50.
5. Bozzetti F, Mariani L. Defining and classifying cancer cachexia: a proposal by the SCRINIO Working Group. JPEN J Parenter Enteral Nutr 2009;33(4):361–7.
6. Wright CD, Kucharczuk JC, O'Brien SM, et al. Predictors of major morbidity and mortality after esophagectomy for esophageal cancer: a Society of Thoracic

Surgeons general thoracic surgery database risk adjustment model. J Thorac Cardiovasc Surg 2009;137(3):587–96.

7. Papenfuss WA, Kukar M, Oxenberg J, et al. Morbidity and mortality associated with gastrectomy for gastric cancer. Ann Surg Oncol 2014;21(9):3008–14.

8. Siegel RL, Miller KD, Jemal A. Cancer statistics, 2016. CA Cancer J Clin 2016; 66(1):7–30.

9. Dewys WD, Begg C, Lavin PT, et al. Prognostic effect of weight loss prior to chemotherapy in cancer patients. Eastern Cooperative Oncology Group. Am J Med 1980;69(4):491–7.

10. Nozoe T, Kimura Y, Ishida M, et al. Correlation of pre-operative nutritional condition with post-operative complications in surgical treatment for oesophageal carcinoma. Eur J Surg Oncol 2002;28(4):396–400.

11. Andreyev HJ, Norman AR, Oates J, et al. Why do patients with weight loss have a worse outcome when undergoing chemotherapy for gastrointestinal malignancies? Eur J Cancer 1998;34(4):503–9.

12. Kelsen DP, Ginsberg R, Pajak TF, et al. Chemotherapy followed by surgery compared with surgery alone for localized esophageal cancer. N Engl J Med 1998;339(27):1979–84.

13. Heneghan HM, Zaborowski A, Fanning M, et al. Prospective study of malabsorption and malnutrition after esophageal and gastric cancer surgery. Ann Surg 2015;262(5):803–8.

14. D'Journo XB, Ouattara M, Loundou A, et al. Prognostic impact of weight loss in 1-year survivors after transthoracic esophagectomy for cancer. Dis Esophagus 2011;25(6):527–34.

15. Daly JM, Weintraub FN, Shou J, et al. Enteral nutrition during multimodality therapy in upper gastrointestinal cancer patients. Ann Surg 1995;221(4):327–38.

16. Taylor CA, Larson DE, Ballard DJ, et al. Predictors of outcome after percutaneous endoscopic gastrostomy: a community-based study. Mayo Clin Proc 1992; 67(11):1042–9.

17. Schrag SP, Sharma R, Jaik NP, et al. Complications related to percutaneous endoscopic gastrostomy (peg) tubes. a comprehensive clinical review. J Gastrointestin Liver Dis 2007;16(4):407–18.

18. Kritchevsky SB, Braun BI, Kusek L, et al. The impact of hospital practice on central venous catheter associated bloodstream infection rates at the patient and unit level: a multicenter study. Am J Med Qual 2008;23(1):24–38.

19. Wood GJ, Shega JW, Lynch B, et al. Management of intractable nausea and vomiting in patients at the end of life. JAMA 2007;298(10):1196–207.

20. Ruizb Garcia V, López-Briz E, Carbonell Sanchis R, et al. Megestrol acetate for treatment of anorexia-cachexia syndrome. Cochrane Database Syst Rev 2013. http://dx.doi.org/10.1002/14651858.cd004310.pub3.

21. Gonzalez-Rosales F, Walsh D. Intractable nausea and vomiting due to gastrointestinal mucosal metastases relieved by tetrahydrocannabinol (Dronabinol). J Pain Symptom Manage 1997;14(5):311–4.

22. Hall W, Christie M, Currow D. Cannabinoids and cancer: causation, remediation, and palliation. Lancet Oncol 2005;6(1):35–42.

23. Garcia JM, Polvino WJ. Effect on body weight and safety of RC-1291, a novel, orally available ghrelin mimetic and growth hormone secretagogue: results of a phase I, randomized, placebo-controlled, multiple-dose study in healthy volunteers. Oncologist 2007;12(5):594–600.

24. Garcia JM, Boccia RV, Graham CD, et al. Anamorelin for patients with cancer cachexia: an integrated analysis of two phase 2, randomised, placebo-controlled, double-blind trials. Lancet Oncol 2015;16(1):108–16.
25. Bower M, Jones W, Vessels B, et al. Role of esophageal stents in the nutrition support of patients with esophageal malignancy. Nutr Clin Pract 2010;25(3):244–9.
26. Rogers SN, Thomson R, O'Toole P, et al. Patients experience with long-term percutaneous endoscopic gastrostomy feeding following primary surgery for oral and oropharyngeal cancer. Oral Oncol 2007;43(5):499–507.
27. Bozzetti F, Arends J, Lundholm K, et al. ESPEN guidelines on parenteral nutrition: non-surgical oncology. Clin Nutr 2009;28(4):445–54.
28. Heys SD, Walker LG, Smith I, et al. Enteral nutritional supplementation with key nutrients in patients with critical illness and cancer. Ann Surg 1999;229(4):467–77.
29. Schattner M. Enteral nutritional support of the patient with cancer. J Clin Gastroenterol 2003;36(4):297–302.
30. Kim JM, Park JH, Jeong SH, et al. Relationship between low body mass index and morbidity after gastrectomy for gastric cancer. Ann Surg Treat Res 2016; 90(4):207.
31. Choi WJ, Kim J. Nutritional care of gastric cancer patients with clinical outcomes and complications: a review. Clin Nutr Res 2016;5(2):65.
32. Bozzetti F. Nutritional support of the oncology patient. Crit Rev Oncol Hematol 2013;87(2):172–200.
33. Song GM, Tian X, Liang H, et al. Role of enteral immunonutrition in patients undergoing surgery for gastric cancer. Medicine (Baltimore) 2015;94(31). http://dx.doi.org/10.1097/md.0000000000001311.
34. Fukuda Y, Yamamoto K, Hirao M, et al. Prevalence of malnutrition among gastric cancer patients undergoing gastrectomy and optimal preoperative nutritional support for preventing surgical site infections. Ann Surg Oncol 2015;22(S3):778–85.

Issues in the Management of Esophagogastric Cancer in Geriatric Patients

Elizabeth Won, MD

KEYWORDS

- Geriatric oncology • Elderly • Esophagogastric cancer • Geriatric assessment

KEY POINTS

- Functional, not chronologic age, should be used to determine appropriate treatment strategies for older patients with esophagogastric cancer.
- Geriatric assessment tools may be helpful to identify patient vulnerabilities and to provide an opportunity to implement interventions and support during the management course.
- Definitive chemoradiation can be tolerated as an alternative to surgery in older patients who are not surgical candidates and may provide fair rates of complete response.

INTRODUCTION

Approximately 60% of all cancers and 70% of cancer mortality occurs in individuals aged 65 years or older, defining cancer as a disease of older adults.[1] For esophagogastric (EG) cancers, the median age of diagnosis is 67 years and nearly 30% of patients are 75 years or older.[2] However, despite the demographic shifts, older patients with EG cancers are less likely to be recommended for surgery and less likely to receive chemotherapy compared with younger patients, irrespective of tumor stage.[3] Recent trials in neoadjuvant therapy have clearly shown decreases in recurrence and improvements in overall survival; however, combined modality treatments with chemotherapy and radiation are often not recommended for most elderly patients with localized esophageal cancer.

Clearly, patient-related factors, such as comorbidities, functional status, and limited social support, affect the ability to deliver and tolerate treatment and thus have a direct effect on the survival of older adults. However, there are data that elderly patients have a lower likelihood of being offered treatment based on age alone.[4] This finding is not surprising given the underrepresentation of elderly patients in clinical trials and the limited information to guide oncologists on the management of this population. This

Disclosure Statement: The author has nothing to disclose.
Gastrointestinal Medical Oncology, Memorial Sloan Kettering Cancer Center, 500 Westchester Avenue, West Harrison, NY 10604, USA
E-mail address: wone@mskcc.org

review evaluates the current knowledge and the remaining challenges in optimally managing elderly patients with esophagogastric cancer.

ASSESSMENT OF THE GERIATRIC PATIENT WITH ESOPHAGOGASTRIC CANCER

Advanced age alone should not preclude patients from receiving standard anticancer therapy. We should acknowledge that older patients have unique issues that require careful consideration, including age and life expectancy, functional status, risk of treatment-related morbidity, competing comorbidities, and desire to receive therapy. However, functional, not chronologic, age should guide treatment decisions. Fit older patients may derive the same benefit from aggressive treatments as younger patients. Age-specific modifications of some treatment paradigms, however, may be appropriate, as therapy tolerance and risk of toxicities vary according to patient age and burden of comorbidities.

Conventional performance status measures, such as the Karnofsky Performance Status (KPS) or the Eastern Cooperative Oncology Group (ECOG) performance status are used to predict treatment toxicity and survival in oncology,[5–7] regardless of a patient's age. However, these tools were validated in younger patients and do not address the diversity of health issues of the geriatric cancer population.

Comprehensive geriatric assessment (CGA) has the potential to identify those at risk for treatment complications and functional disability, and to provide an opportunity to implement interventions and support before, during, and after treatment. Geriatricians perform a multidisciplinary assessment that measures independent clinical predictors of morbidity and mortality in older adults[8] (Table 1). This assessment has only recently been evaluated in the oncology setting. One such cancer-specific CGA tool has been developed by Hurria and colleagues.[9] This tool is designed to be mainly self-administered by the patient and feasible in the setting of an outpatient oncology clinic.[10] The Council on Aging Research Group used this tool in a multicenter prospective study to develop a predictive model for chemotherapy toxicity in patients 65 years or older.[11,12] The model identified age 72 years or older, tumor type (gastrointestinal or

Table 1	
Components of a comprehensive geriatric assessment	
Domain	**Description**
Functional capacity	Evaluation of the ability to complete basic activities of daily living (ADLs) and instrumental ADLs (activities required to maintain independence in the community)
Fall risk	Fall history, assessment of balance/gait
Cognition	Evaluation of orientation, memory, concentration
Mood	Screening for depressive symptoms, anxiety
Nutritional status	Evaluation of unintentional weight loss, body mass index, food intake, and eating habits
Social support and financial concerns	Assessment of social/family support and social activity, quality of life, and how physical/emotional/financial problems interfere with well-being
Comorbidity	Number, type, and severity of comorbidities; polypharmacy; vision/hearing difficulties
Goals of care	Patient preferences regarding health, medical treatments, and advanced care planning (health care proxy, discussion of resuscitation wishes)

genitourinary cancers), polychemotherapy, anemia, creatinine clearance, and geriatric assessment variables (hearing, number of falls, and functional status) as risk factors for toxicity. The CGA tool consisting of 11 questions, including 5 geriatric assessment questions and 6 questions captured in routine daily practice, was recently externally validated and shows it is possible to predict chemotherapy toxicity in adults (Table 2). A high score, 10 to 19 points, was associated with high risk (70.2%, $P<.001$) of developing grade 3 to 5 toxicity in the validation cohort. Interestingly, physician-rated KPS was not predictive of chemotherapy toxicity in either the developmental or validation cohorts.

There are ongoing multicenter studies evaluating the efficacy of this tool in predicting toxicity among patients with specific tumor types and treatment regimens. CGAs are being implemented and studied in the preoperative setting to predict and stratify older patients at risk for surgical complications and mortality. Further work needs to be done to implement such tools and could potentially affect the choice of treatment regimens. However, these types of models only just start to improve our understanding of how to best assess and risk-stratify our geriatric patients, and to help determine appropriate treatment plans that go beyond just numeric patient age.

Table 2
Prediction model and scoring algorithm for chemotherapy toxicity developed by cancer in aging research group

Variable	Value/Response	Score
Age of patient	≥72 y	2
	<72 y	0
Cancer type	GI or GU cancer	2
	Other cancer types	0
Planned chemotherapy dose	Standard dose	2
	Dose reduced upfront	0
Planned no. of chemotherapy drugs	Polychemotherapy	2
	Monochemotherapy	0
Hemoglobin	<11 g/dL (men), <10 g/dL (women)	3
	≥11 g/dL (men), ≥10 g/dL (women)	0
Creatinine clearance (Jeliffe, ideal weight)	<34 mL/min	3
	≥34 mL/min	0
How is your hearing (with a hearing aid, if needed)?	Fair, poor, or totally deaf	2
	Excellent or good	0
No. of falls in the past 6 mo	≥1	3
	None	0
Can you take your own medicine?	With some help/unable	1
	Without help	0
Does your health limit you in walking 1 block?	Somewhat limited/limited a lot	2
	Not limited at all	0
During the past 4 wk, how much of the time has your physical health or emotional problems interfered with your social activities (eg, visiting with friends, relatives)?	Limited some of the time, most of the time, or all of the time	1
	Limited none of the time or a little of the time	0

Abbreviations: GI, gastrointestinal; GU, genitourinary.
Data from Hurria A, Mohile S, Gajra A, et al. Validation of a prediction tool for chemotherapy toxicity in older adults with cancer. J Clin Oncol 2016;34(20):2366–71.

SURGERY FOR ESOPHAGEAL CANCER

The only predominant curative approach for esophagogastric cancer is surgical resection. Esophagectomy is a complex, invasive procedure with potentially high rates of morbidity and mortality. This risk of the increased postsurgical morbidity in older patients has been debated in the literature and appears to be closely related to hospital volume, surgical expertise, and patient selection.[13,14] Single-institution reports have demonstrated that esophagectomy can be performed safely in patients 80 years and older[15-21]; however, most of the data suggest that older patients are at increased risk for pulmonary and cardiovascular complications. Nationally, mortality risk has been shown to significantly increase proportionally with age: 8.8% of patients aged 65 to 69 years, 13.4% of patients aged 70 to 79, and 19.9% of patients aged 80 years or older.[22]

Tan and colleagues[23] examined the Nationwide Inpatient Sample database for the presence of geriatric events after surgery in patients older than 65. These events included dehydration, delirium, falls, fractures, failure to thrive, and pressure ulcers, which are not commonly reported in the surgical literature. A quarter of all patients undergoing stomach cancer surgery experience a geriatric event, with even higher rates seen in those 75 years and older (data were not provided for esophageal cancer surgery). These geriatric events were associated with prolonged hospitalization (odds ratio [OR] 5.97; 95% confidence interval [CI] 5.16–5.80), higher cost (OR, 4.97; 95% CI 4.58–5.39), lower likelihood of discharge to home (OR 0.27; 95% CI 0.26–0.29), and higher likelihood of death during the index hospitalization (OR 3.22; 95% CI 2.94–3.53) compared with patients who did not experience such events. This is consistent with the surgical literature reporting higher postoperative complications and longer hospitalizations in older patients.[15-21]

As part of the consideration in determining the optimal approach in elderly patients, the relative benefit of surgery needs to be considered in the context of the high proportion of patients developing metastatic disease within the first 2 years of diagnosis, even with initial presentation of localized disease. Surgery remains the mainstay of early-stage T1 and node-negative esophagogastric cancer. However, the risk of metastatic disease development escalates to reach 60% or higher in patients with T2 or higher T-stage disease, and node positivity at surgery portends a risk in excess of 70% to 80% to develop metastatic disease.[24,25]

Therefore, the role of esophagectomy in an elderly patient needs to be considered carefully in a select group of robust individuals based on assessment of their physiologic and functional status. These patients may be best served by referral to a high-volume center with appropriate expertise. Preoperative CGA to identify and prevent potential complications specific to older patients, such as early mobilization, avoidance of polypharmacy, and early recognition of postoperative delirium may reduce both cardiopulmonary and geriatric-specific complications and optimize treatment outcomes.[26-29] Postoperative management of elderly surgical patients needs to be specialized to avoid geriatric events, including delirium, malnutrition, pressure ulcers, falls, infection, functional decline, and polypharmacy. With adequate and collaborative perioperative care between the surgical and geriatric teams, the risk of morbidity and mortality for older patients may be mitigated.

NEOADJUVANT CHEMORADIATION

For locally advanced esophagogastric cancers (T3 or node-positive disease), preoperative chemoradiation (CRT) has become an accepted standard treatment. The Chemoradiotherapy for Esophageal Cancer followed by Surgery Study (CROSS) randomized 368 patients with esophageal and gastroesophageal junction cancers to surgery alone or weekly carboplatin and paclitaxel for 5 weeks with concurrent radiotherapy followed by surgery. The CRT arm showed a significant improvement in median survival of 49 months versus 24 months compared with surgery alone.[30] The long-term follow-up data show 14% improvements in 5-year survival in the CRT group compared with surgery alone, as well as significantly lower rates of locoregional and distant progression.[31] Toxicity data show that the treatment can be well tolerated with low rates of grade 3 or 4 toxicity in the CRT arm. However, the median age of the patients in the CROSS trial was 60 years (range 36–79 years), with more than 80% of patients having a World Health Organization performance status score of 0. There is no subset analysis provided for age, making it difficult to generalize the findings to a geriatric patient population.

There are few small, mostly retrospective, studies focused on older patients who have received preoperative chemoradiation followed by esophagectomy. Fogh and colleagues[32] reported no significant difference in mortality in patients older than 70 years compared with younger patients (7% vs 5%) but reported higher rates of cardiac arrhythmias and pulmonary complications requiring intubation in the older patients undergoing surgery. Similar data were reported by Ruol and colleagues,[33] who showed no difference in mortality rates in patients older than 70 years compared to those younger than 70 years old receiving neoadjuvant chemoradiation with 5-fluorouracil (5-FU)/cisplatin with 45 to 50 Gy of radiation followed by esophagectomy. The study was limited by the small number of older patients (n = 31). This study showed similar median survival rates in the older and younger patients (23.1 vs 23.7 months) with similar partial complete response (pCR) rates (26% vs 23%). Older patients had significantly higher rates of cardiovascular complications, with 22% of patients experiencing a myocardial infarction, severe arrhythmia, pulmonary edema, or pulmonary embolism compared with 5% of younger patients ($P = .003$).

These studies suggest that a select group of older patients who are good surgical candidates appear to tolerate neoadjuvant treatment with no significant increase in mortality compared with younger patients, but higher rates of cardiopulmonary complications are seen. The limitations of these data are the retrospective nature of the studies and they do not include data on quality of life and functional recovery after treatment.

Definitive Chemoradiation as an Alternative to Surgery

There are many more elderly patients who are not good candidates for esophagectomy on the basis of frailty, medical comorbidities, advanced age, or patient preference. Definitive chemoradiation is an alternative for such patients who can potentially achieve long-term disease control. It is an accepted practice for squamous cell histology.[34] The data are limited but there are studies suggesting that chemoradiotherapy is not only feasible in elderly patients with esophageal cancer, but also those with good functional status can obtain comparable benefit seen in younger patients (Table 3). For elderly, frail patients, this approach of definitive chemoradiation can provide fair rates of clinical complete response of approximately 50% to 60% with median 2-year survival rates of 30% to 40%.

It clearly needs to be acknowledged that the pathologic complete response rates for adenocarcinoma histology are much lower than those for squamous histology (23% vs 49%) with chemoradiation, as reported on CROSS. However, this needs to be placed in the context of esophagogastric cancers being aggressive malignancies with high rates (70%–80%) of developing distant metastases for patients with lymph node–positive disease at the time of surgery.[24,25] This approach of definitive chemoradiation provides a potentially curative and tolerable treatment plan for most elderly patients for whom surgical resection would not be indicated. Providers need to have an open discussion with

Table 3
Chemoradiation studies in elderly patients with esophagogastric cancers

Authors	Type of Study	Regimen	Definition of Elderly, Age in Years	Patient Characteristics	Conclusions
Tougeron et al,[35] 2008	Retrospective review	5-FU/cisplatin or cisplatin/irinotecan with 50–55 Gy	≥70 y	n = 109 Mean age 74 y Range 70–88 WHO PS 1–2: 78%	• CCR in 58% with 2-y survival of 36% • Median OS 15.2 ± 2.8 mo • Grade 3 or higher toxicity in 24%, 1 death from febrile neutropenia • 30% required chemotherapy dose reduction; 41% chemotherapy delays >1 wk; 16% treatment discontinuation
Anderson et al,[36] 2007	Retrospective review	5-FU/mitomycin with 50.4 Gy	≥65 y	n = 25, all were deemed not to be surgical candidates Median age 77 Range 66–88 Median KPS 80 (70–90)	• CCR rate 68% with 2-y survival of 64% • Median OS 35 mo • 36% (9 pts) required admission for toxicity management; 36% developed grade 3 or 4 hematological toxicity
Takeuchi et al,[37] 2007	Retrospective review comparing outcomes of CRT between elderly and nonelderly patients	5-FU/cisplatin with 60 Gy	≥71 y	Japanese population n = 178 (33 "elderly" pts ≥ 71 y, 145 "nonelderly" pts <70 y)	• CCR rate similar in elderly group 63.6% vs 63.4% nonelderly • Inferior median survival in elderly group 14.7 vs 35.1 mo, P = .01 • 94% of elderly pts were able to complete planned radiation therapy; 33% of elderly required chemotherapy dose reduction
Servagi-Vernat et al,[38] 2009	Prospective phase II study	Cisplatin or oxaliplatin with 50 Gy	≥75 y	n = 30 Mean age 85 Range 79–92	• CCR 53% with 3-y survival of 22% • 28 completed treatment • 2 patients died from pneumonitis

Abbreviations: 5-FU, 5-fluorouracil; CCR, complete clinical response; CRT, chemoradiation; KPS, Karnofsky Performance Status; OS, overall survival; pts, patients; PS, performance status; WHO, World Health Organization.

the patient regarding the expectations and limitations of treatment for an aggressive malignancy as well as the potential toxicities and impact on quality of life.

For patients with residual disease after chemoradiation, surgical resection is an option for those who are candidates for esophagectomy. For elderly patients who defer surgery or are not surgical candidates, brachytherapy may provide palliation. Data reported from single institutions show that brachytherapy after prior external beam radiation can be safely administered. One study reported improvement in dysphagia in 28% of patients, with median overall survival of 7 months.[39] In another small cohort of 10 patients, the overall survival after brachytherapy was 55% at 18 months.[40] The most common serious complications include strictures and ulceration/fistula.

Management of advanced/metastatic disease

Systemic chemotherapy More than 50% of patients present with metastatic or unresectable esophageal cancer at diagnosis. In addition, as stated previously, the vast majority of patients with locally advanced disease undergoing chemoradiotherapy with or without surgery will develop recurrent metastatic disease. Improving or maintaining quality of life and symptom relief are paramount goals. Best supportive care is the appropriate treatment option for some patients with compromised functional status. Chemotherapy, which is palliative, should be individualized based on a patient's performance status and comorbidities. Chemotherapy can potentially improve or maintain stability of quality of life and relieve dysphagia in 60% to 80% of patients.[41–43] Typical clinical and radiographic responses last for fewer than 4 months, with a median overall survival time of 8 to 10 months.

Chemotherapy can be given as a single agent or in combination based on the patient's functional status and comorbidities (Fig. 1). Active agents include cisplatin, oxaliplatin, carboplatin, fluorinated pyrimidines, taxanes, ramucirumab, irinotecan, gemcitabine, and mitomycin. Response rates to single chemotherapy agents range from 15% to 30%.[44] Complete responses are rare and usually are not durable remissions. Capecitabine can be used interchangeably with 5-FU, although caution is warranted in patients with renal dysfunction and infusional 5-FU may be better tolerated in patients with dysphagia.[45] Cisplatin and oxaliplatin can be used interchangeably,[46] although oxaliplatin is generally better tolerated. One phase III study indicated improved response rates and survival in patients older than 65 treated with oxaliplatin compared with cisplatin in combination with infusional 5-FU.[47]

Combination chemotherapy can be considered in patients with an intact performance status and preserved physiologic reserve. Combination regimens, usually

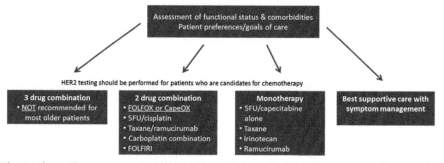

Fig. 1. Chemotherapy recommendations for elderly patients with metastatic/advanced disease. CapeOX, capecitabine, oxaliplatin; FOLFIRI, 5-FU, Leucovorin, Irinotecan; FOLFOX, 5-FU, Leucovorin, Oxaliplatin.

containing a platinum backbone, can result in higher response rates of 30% to 57% in the first-line setting, with occasional patients achieving complete responses of 0% to 11%.[41,42,48–52] Three-drug combinations, which produce higher response rates and slightly increased survival benefit, should be reserved for only the physically fit younger patient given the very high rates of grade 3/4 toxicity reported with these regimens.[52] Al-Batran and colleagues[53] compared FLO (5-FU, leucovorin, infusional 5-FU 2600 mg/m^2 as 24-hour infusion) versus FLO plus docetaxel in patients older than 65 with locally advanced and metastatic disease. The triple combination improved response rates and progression-free survival in a subgroup of patients between 65 and 70, but not in the metastatic group or patients older than 70. There was significant toxicity with the triplet combination (82% had grade 3/4 events) and deterioration of quality of life in this group.[53] Trastuzumab should be added to the chemotherapy regimen in patients who have HER2-positive esophagogastric tumors based on the Trastuzumab for Gastric Cancer (TOGA) trial data showing improved survival.[54] The rates of cardiac failure were less than 1% in the study.

The use of a combination drug regimen for metastatic cancer needs to be considered very carefully in robust older patients with a quick response to adverse reactions. Given the overall goal of palliation and the significant toxicity associated with triplet regimens, it is difficult to recommend this treatment approach for the average elderly patient with advanced esophageal cancer.

Palliation and supportive measures Patients with poor functional status, a KPS $\leq$60, or an ECOG performance score $\geq$3 should probably be offered best supportive care alone. Palliative interventions provide symptomatic relief and may result in prolongation of life, and improvement in quality of life and well-being for the patient and caregivers.

Dysphagia is the most common symptom in patients with esophageal cancer and a cause of significant source of discomfort. Older patients with esophageal cancer are likely to be at the highest risk of malnutrition due to increased medical comorbidities compounded by normal physiologic changes of decreased muscle mass and geriatric issues of altered cognition, mobility, mood, and social support/access to nutrition. Poor nutrition has been identified as a predictive risk factor for death in elderly patients undergoing chemotherapy for cancer.[55] Malnutrition also has been associated with reduced response to treatment and survival in patients with esophageal cancer, as well as detrimentally affecting quality of life and increasing health care costs.[56–58] Despite this, there are few guidelines regarding nutritional and dysphagia management to guide oncologists. At Memorial Sloan Kettering, a pilot study of a nutritional algorithm to optimize the nutritional status of older patients with locally advanced esophageal cancers undergoing chemoradiation is being conducted.[59]

Palliative treatment options for dysphagia include chemotherapy, which can relieve dysphagia; however, with short time to progression or for those patients who are not candidates for chemotherapy, additional management of dysphagia is often required. Options include endoscopic dilatation, placement of a temporary or permanent self-expending metal stent, or palliative radiation. The use of a feeding tube for hydration and nutrition can be considered. The management method needs to be individualized to the patient's overall wishes and medical condition.

SUMMARY

Older adults respond differently to cancer treatments than younger people. This is in part due to physiologic changes associated with aging as well as increased incidence of comorbidities in older adults. Chronologic age should not be the determinant for the selection of patients for treatment of esophagogastric cancer, as there is wide heterogeneity in the health of older adults. Functional age provides a more accurate portrayal of a patient's overall health status and potential tolerance of treatment. Fit older adults may derive the same benefit from aggressive treatments as younger patients. Modifications of some treatment paradigms may be appropriate in older patients because therapy tolerance and risk of toxicity vary according to a patient's functional status and comorbidities. The underrepresentation of older adults in clinical trials means clinicians have limited evidence on how to treat this rapidly growing patient population. Clearly, more research focused on older adults is necessary; and clinical trials should make concerted efforts to include older adults in the study design and recruitment to ensure all patients receive high-quality evidence-based care.

REFERENCES

1. Siegel RL, Miller KD, Jemal A. Cancer statistics, 2015. CA Cancer J Clin 2015;65: 5–29.
2. Howlader N, Noone AM, Krapcho M, et al, editors. SEER cancer statistics review, 1975-2009 (vintage 2009 populations). Bethesda (MD): National Cancer Institute; 2012. Available at: http://seer.cancer.gov/csr/1975_2009_pops09/. Based on November 2011 SEER data submission, posted to the SEER web site.
3. Steyerberg EW, Neville B, Weeks JC, et al. Referral patterns, treatment choices, and outcomes in locoregional esophageal cancer: a population-based analysis of elderly patients. J Clin Oncol 2007;25:2389–96.
4. Bouchardy C, Rapiti E, Blagojevic S, et al. Older female cancer patients: importance, causes, and consequences of undertreatment. J Clin Oncol 2007;25: 1858–69.
5. Bajorin DF, Dodd PM, Mazumdar M, et al. Long-term survival in metastatic transitional-cell carcinoma and prognostic factors predicting outcome of therapy. J Clin Oncol 1999;17:3173–81.
6. Motzer RJ, Bacik J, Schwartz LH, et al. Prognostic factors for survival in previously treated patients with metastatic renal cell carcinoma. J Clin Oncol 2004; 22:454–63.
7. Albain KS, Crowley JJ, LeBlanc M, et al. Survival determinants in extensive-stage nonsmall-cell lung cancer: the Southwest Oncology Group experience. J Clin Oncol 1991;9:1618–26.
8. Extermann M, Hurria A. Comprehensive geriatric assessment for older patients with cancer. J Clin Oncol 2007;25:1824–31.
9. Hurria A, Gupta S, Zauderer M, et al. Developing a cancer-specific geriatric assessment. Cancer 2005;104:1998–2005.
10. Hurria A, Togawa K, Mohile SG, et al. Predicting chemotherapy toxicity in older adults with cancer: a prospective multicenter study. J Clin Oncol 2011;29:3457–65.
11. Hurria A, Mohile S, Gajra A, et al. Validation of a prediction tool for chemotherapy toxicity in older adults with cancer. J Clin Oncol 2016;34(20):2366–71.
12. Birkmeyer JD, Siewers AE, Finlayson EV, et al. Hospital volume and surgical mortality in the United States. N Engl J Med 2002;346:1128–37.
13. Swisher SG, DeFord L, Merriman KW, et al. Effect of operative volume on morbidity, mortality, and hospital use after esophagectomy for cancer. J Thorac Cardiovasc Surg 2000;119:1126–34.
14. Kuo EY, Chang Y, Wright CD. Impact of hospital volume on clinical and economic outcomes of esophagectomy. Ann Thorac Surg 2001;72:1118–24.

15. Adam DJ, Craig SR, Sang CTM, et al. Esophagectomy for carcinoma in the octogenarian. Ann Thorac Surg 1996;61:190–4.
16. Bonavina L, Incarbone R, Saino G, et al. Clinical outcome and survival after esophagectomy for carcinoma in elderly patients. Dis Esophagus 2003;16:90–3.
17. Rice DC, Correa AM, Vaporciyan A, et al. Preoperative chemoradiotherapy prior to esophagectomy in elderly patients is not associated with increased morbidity. Ann Thorac Surg 2005;79:391–7.
18. Moskovitz AH, Rizk NP, Venkatraman E, et al. Mortality increases for octogenarians undergoing esophagogastrectomy for esophageal cancer. Ann Thorac Surg 2006;82:2031–6.
19. Morita M, Egashira A, Yoskida R, et al. Esophagectomy in patients 80 years of age and older with carcinoma of the thoracic esophagus. J Gastroenterol 2008;43:345–51.
20. Pultrum BB, Bosch DJ, Nijsten MEN, et al. Extended esophagectomy in elderly patients with esophageal cancer: minor effect of age alone in determining the postoperative course and survival. Ann Surg Oncol 2010;17:1572–80.
21. Cijs TM, Verhoef C, Steyerberg EW, et al. Outcome of esophagectomy for cancer in elderly patients. Ann Thorac Surg 2010;90:900–7.
22. Finlayson E, Fan Z, Birkmeyer JD. Outcomes in octogenarians undergoing high-risk cancer. J Am Coll Surg 2007;205:729–34.
23. Tan H-J, Saliba D, Kwan L, et al. Burden of geriatric events among older adults undergoing major cancer surgery. J Clin Oncol 2016. http://dx.doi.org/10.1200/JCO.2015.63.4592.
24. Abate E, DeMeester SR, Zehetner J, et al. Recurrence after esophagectomy for adenocarcinoma: defining optimal follow-up intervals and testing. J Am Coll Surg 2010;210:428–35.
25. Gu Y, Swisher SG, Ajani JA, et al. The number of lymph nodes with metastasis predicts survival in patients with esophageal and esophagogastric junction adenocarcinoma who receive preoperative chemoradiotherapy. Cancer 2006; 106:1017–25.
26. Korc-Gordzicki B, Downey RJ, Sharokni A, et al. Surgical considerations in older adults with cancer. J Clin Oncol 2014;32:2647–53.
27. PACE Participants, Audisio RA, Pope D, Ramesh HS, et al. Shall we operate? Preoperative assessment in elderly cancer patients (PACE) can help—a SIOG surgical task force prospective study. Crit Rev Oncol Hematol 2008;65:156–63.
28. Fukuse T, Satoda N, Hijiya K, et al. Importance of a comprehensive geriatric assessment in prediction of complications following thoracic surgery in elderly patients. Chest 2005;127:886–91.
29. Inouye SK, Bogardus ST, Charpentier PA, et al. A multicomponent intervention to prevent delirium in hospitalized older patients. N Engl J Med 1999;340:669–76.
30. Van Hagen P, Hulshof MC, van Lanschot JJ, et al. Preoperative chemoradiotherapy for esophageal or junctional cancer. N Engl J Med 2012;366:2074–84.
31. Shapiro J, van Lanschot JJB, Hulshof MCCM, et al. Neoadjuvant chemoradiotherapy plus surgery versus surgery alone for oesophageal or junctional cancer (CROSS): long-term results of a randomised controlled trial. Lancet Oncol 2015;16:1090–8.
32. Fogh SE, Yu A, Kubicek GJ, et al. Do elderly patients experience increased perioperative or postoperative morbidity or mortality when given neoadjuvant chemoradiotherapy before esophagectomy? Int J Radiat Oncol Biol Phys 2011;80: 1372–6.

33. Ruol A, Portale G, Castoro C. Effects of neoadjuvant therapy on perioperative morbidity in elderly patients undergoing esophagectomy for esophageal cancer. Ann Surg Oncol 2007;14:3243–50.
34. Stahl M, Stuschke M, Lehmann N, et al. Chemoradiotherapy with and without surgery in patients with locally advanced squamous cell carcinoma of the esophagus. J Clin Oncol 2005;23:2310–7.
35. Tougeron D, DiFiore F, Thureau S, et al. Safety and outcome of definitive chemoradiotherapy in elderly patients with oesophageal cancer. Br J Cancer 2008;99: 1586–92.
36. Anderson SE, Minsky BD, Bains M, et al. Combined modality chemoradiotherapy in elderly oesophageal cancer patients. Br J Cancer 2007;96:1823–7.
37. Takeuchi S, Ohtsu A, Doi T, et al. A retrospective study of definitive chemoradiotherapy for elderly patients with esophageal cancer. Am J Clin Oncol 2007;30: 607–11.
38. Servagi-Vernat S, Bosset M, Crehange G. Feasibility of chemoradiotherapy for oesophageal cancer in elderly patients aged ≥75 years: a prospective, single-arm phase II study. Drugs Aging 2009;26:255–62.
39. Sharma V, Mahantshetty U, Dinshaw KA, et al. Palliation of advanced/recurrent esophageal carcinoma with high-dose-rate brachytherapy. Int J Radiat Oncol Biol Phys 2002;52:310–5.
40. Folkert M, Cohen GN, Wu AJ, et al. Endoluminal high-dose-rate brachytherapy for early stage and recurrent esophageal cancer in medically inoperable patients. Brachytherapy 2013;12:463–70.
41. Bleiberg H, Conroy T, Paillot B, et al. Randomized phase II study of cisplatin and 5-fluorouracil 5-FU (5-FU) versus cisplatin alone in advanced squamous cell oesophageal cancer. Eur J Cancer 1997;33:1216–20.
42. Conroy T, Etienne P-L, Adenis A, et al. Vinorelbine and cisplatin in metastatic squamous cell carcinoma of the oesophagus: response, toxicity, quality of life, and survival. Ann Oncol 2002;13:721–9.
43. Ajani JA, Moiseyenko VM, Tjulandin S, et al. Quality of life with docetaxel plus cisplatin and fluorouracil compared with cisplatin and fluorouracil from a phase III trial for advanced gastric or gastroesophageal adenocarcinoma: the V-325 study group. J Clin Oncol 2007;25:3210–6.
44. Shah M, Schwartz G. Treatment of metastatic esophagus and gastric cancer. Semin Oncol 2004;31:574–87.
45. Cunningham D, Rao S, Starling N, et al. Capecitabine and oxaliplatin for advanced esophageal cancer. N Engl J Med 2008;358:36–46.
46. Cunningham D, Rao S, Starling N, et al, for the NCRI Upper GI Study Group. Randomised multicentre Phase III study comparing capecitabine with fluorouracil and oxaliplatin with cisplatin in patients with advanced oesophagogastric (OG) cancer: the REAL 2 trial. J Clin Oncol 2006;24(18 suppl) [abstract: LBA4017].
47. Al-Batran S, Hartmann J, Probst S, et al. Phase III trial in patients with advanced adenocarcinoma of the stomach receiving first-line chemotherapy with fluorouracil, leucovorin and oxaliplatin or cisplatin: a study of the Arbeitsgemeinschaft Internistische Onkologie. J Clin Oncol 2008;28:1435–42.
48. Webb A, Cunningham D, Scarffe H, et al. Randomized trial comparing epirubicin, cisplatin, and fluorouracil versus fluorouracil, doxorubicin, and methotrexate in advanced oesophagogastric (OG) cancer. J Clin Oncol 1997;15:261–7.
49. Ilson DH, Forastiere A, Arquette M, et al. A phase II trial of paclitaxel and cisplatin in patients with advanced carcinoma of the esophagus. Cancer J 2000;6:316–23.

50. Ilson D, Saltz L, Enzinger P, et al. A phase II trial of weekly irinotecan plus cisplatin in advanced esophageal cancer. J Clin Oncol 1999;17:3270–5.

51. Ilson DH, Ajani JA, Bhalla K, et al. Phase II trial of paclitaxel, fluorouracil, and cisplatin in patients with advanced carcinoma of the esophagus. J Clin Oncol 1998;16:1826–34.

52. Van Cutsem E, Moiseyenko VM, Tjulandin S, et al. Phase III study of docetaxel and cisplatin plus fluorouracil compared with cisplatin and fluorouracil as first-line therapy for advanced gastric cancer: a report of the V325 Study Group. J Clin Oncol 2006;24:4991–7.

53. Al-Batran SE, Pauligk C, Homann N, et al. The feasibility of triple-drug chemotherapy combination in older adult patients with oesophagogastric cancer: a randomised trial of the Arbeitsgemeinschaft Internistische Onkologie (FLOT65+). Eur J Cancer 2013;49:835–42.

54. Bang YJ, Van Cutsem E, Feyereislova A, et al. Trastuzumab in combination with chemotherapy versus chemotherapy alone for treatment of HER2-positive advanced gastric or gastro-oesophageal junction cancer (ToGA): a phase 3, open-label, randomised controlled trial. Lancet 2010;376:687–97.

55. Soueyran P, Fonck M, Blanc-Bisson C, et al. Predictors of early death risk in older patients treated with first-line chemotherapy for cancer. J Clin Oncol 2012;30:1829–34.

56. Bollschweiler E, Herbold T, Plum P, et al. Prognostic relevance of nutritional status in patients with advanced esophageal cancer. Expert Rev Anticancer Ther 2013;13(3):275–8.

57. Gupta D, Vashi PG, Lammersfeld CA, et al. Role of nutritional status in predicting the length of stay in cancer: a systematic review of the epidemiological literature. Ann Nutr Metab 2011;59(2–4):96–106.

58. Conti S, West JP, Fitzpatrick HF. Mortality and morbidity after esophagogastrectomy for cancer of the esophagus and cardia. Am Surg 1997;43:92–6.

59. Won E, Ilson DH. A nutritional management algorithm in older patients with locally advanced esophageal cancer. Bethesda (MD): National Library of Medicine (US); 2000. ClinicalTrials.gov [Internet]. Available at: http://clinicaltrials.gov/show/NCT02027948. Accessed June 24, 2014.

Printed and bound by CPI Group (UK) Ltd, Croydon, CR0 4YY

07/10/2024

01040506-0015